D0138522

10.75A9

BEHAVIORAL METHODS FOR CHRONIC PAIN AND ILLNESS

BEHAVIORAL METHODS FOR CHRONIC PAIN AND ILLNESS

WILBERT E. FORDYCE, Ph.D.

Professor of Psychology, Department of
Rehabilitation Medicine and Pain Clinic, University
Hospital, University of Washington School of Medicine,
Seattle, Washington

with 31 *illustrations*

THE C. V. MOSBY COMPANY

Saint Louis   1976

Printed in the United States of America

Distributed in Great Britain by Henry Kimpton, London

Library of Congress Cataloging in Publication Data

Fordyce, Wilbert Evans, 1923-
   Behavioral methods for chronic pain and illness.

   Bibliography: p.
   Includes index.
   1. Pain. 2. Behavior modification.
3. Chronically ill—Care and treatment. I. Title.
[DNLM: 1. Behavior therapy. 2. Pain—Therapy.
3. Chronic diseases—Therapy. WL700 F713b]
RB127.F67   616'.047   75-31782
ISBN 0-8016-1621-2

VH/VH/VH 9 8 7 6 5 4 3 2 1

To
Lundy

Preface

This book results in part from two different sets of observations or developments. One stems from the obvious shortcomings of traditional health care approaches for resolving adequately many problems of chronic pain. After traditional methods and perspectives have had their day, a significant number of people will still continue to display pain problems that bedevil them, their physicians, and insuring and compensation agencies. The second is the emergence of behavioral methods and concepts as important evaluation and treatment tools for a variety of human problems. The term *behavior modification* is the most frequently used label. This book brings together behavioral concepts and methods to combat one of the major continuing problems in health care: chronic pain.

The approach used in this book is to reanalyze chronic clinical pain from a behavioral perspective and to describe both evaluative and treatment methods that are indicated by this analysis.

This book has been written with two kinds of readers in mind. One is the health care professional: physician, nurse, physical therapist, or occupational therapist. The other is the behavioral scientist or other human services professional with developing interests in the use of behavioral technology to help people with chronic illness problems. This latter group may include psychologists, psychiatrists, social workers, or perhaps members of yet other professions.

Newly graduating students in these various professions are increasingly likely to have received at least some exposure to the concepts and methods of behavioral technology. In some instances the training will have been extensive. For them, this book may serve to relate their behavioral training to a new context and a new set of problems. Practitioners in the field from these various professions are much less likely to have had training in or to have had more than superficial exposure to behavioral concepts and methods. For them, this book has a dual objective. One is to describe another way of looking at chronic pain. The second is to equip them with enough relevant behavioral technology that they can begin to add new dimensions to their evaluation and treatment procedures.

The concepts and procedures on which this book is based represent the work of many people. The tactical steps for applying operant-based methods to the management of chronic pain evolved from the conjoint efforts of many. It would be impractical to list the names of all of those who have made significant contributions to the process. We must be content with acknowledging that the development and application of the procedures represent a team operation. Certain individuals have made special kinds of contributions for which specific mention can be made. The names that follow report some of those contributors. Many others also could have been named, were space limitations not a factor.

A major part of the initial impetus for the operant program came from Justus F. Lehmann, Chairman of the Department of Rehabilitation Medicine, University of Washington. His encouragement and support were indispensable to development and growth of the program. His conceptual and procedural contributions were and continue to be equally important. Roy S. Fowler, Jr., Associate Professor of Psychology, in the same department, played a key role from the outset, as did several other psychologists, including Patricia Sand, Roberta Trieschmann, and Lynn Caldwell. Physician support and procedural contributions were also vitally important. Among the many who have played a role in program development, mention should be made particularly of Barbara DeLateur, Kendall Holmes, Thaworn Hongladarom, George Kraft, Phil Morrison, Clyde Nicholson, Walter Stolov, and Janet Whitmore. Nursing also played a key role, and special mention should be made of Rosemarian Berni, Michelle Kenney, Hannah Kuhn, Laura Heard, and their many ward service colleagues. In physical therapy, Ann Nourse, Maureen McGee, and their colleagues, and in occupational ther-

apy, Marilyn Wittmeyer and her colleagues were instrumental in providing a suitable treatment environment for testing the methods. Social workers Jane Itzkow, Katherine Chambers, Grace Schertzer, and others, and the Prevocational Unit directed first by Janet Hart and later by Mike Clowers, all have made their contributions.

To all these people and to their colleagues, who are far too numerous to mention, goes a special note of thanks for their help, their ideas, and their support.

The list would be incomplete without mentioning that any number of patients braved what often appeared to them to be the unknown and the unlikely-to-succeed. But they did it, and they let all of this evolve.

Wilbert E. Fordyce

Contents

Introduction, 1

SECTION ONE   Conceptual background

1   Pain as a clinical problem, 11

2   Psychogenic pain, 26

3   The acquisition of operant pain, 41

4   Techniques of behavioral analysis and behavior change, 74

SECTION TWO   Evaluation

5   Treatment goals, 103

6   The behavioral analysis of pain, 120

7   Patient selection, 141

SECTION THREE   Treatment

8   Patient and spouse orientation, 150

9   Managing pain medications, 157

10   Exercise and the increase in activity level, 168

11   Distorted gait—a problem of shaping, 184

12   Attention and social responsiveness, 190

13   Generalization and the maintenance of performance, 211

Bibliography, 222

Appendix   A   Diary analysis form, 225
            B   Daily diary page, 226

BEHAVIORAL METHODS FOR CHRONIC PAIN AND ILLNESS

Introduction

This book concerns chronic clinical pain. It analyzes from a behavioral perspective the complex set of problems involved in chronic pain and considers diagnostic and treatment methods suggested by the behavioral approach.

The question as to what behavioral concepts have to do with pain is to be expected. Pain is ordinarily viewed in neurophysiological terms. It is considered to be a medical problem with so-called organic or physical characteristics. If, in a given case, diagnostic evidence suggests that the reports of pain do not have the expected basis of physical findings, the problem may be shunted into another conceptual pathway where the problem is viewed as nonorganic, that is, psychogenic, psychiatric, or emotionally based. It will be argued in this book that these distinctions have limited utility. Furthermore, whatever their merits, they leave untouched a number of other important issues about pain that involve behavior and factors that guide or change such behavior.

Before proceeding further, since the concept of behavior is being considered, a beginning definition of the term is needed. The concept will receive more detailed treatment in Chapter 4. Briefly, the term *behavior* refers to observable and potentially measurable actions of the organism; in this context, it includes patients, family members, and health care professionals. Behavior is, therefore, movement; it is observable movement. The definition is not intended to imply that there are not other organism activities, such as neural impulses, glandular secretions, mental images, or covert arithmetical calculations. The definition means that it is only the observable,

countable behaviors that will be dealt with here. This constraint provides a number of important logistic and pragmatic advantages to both the professional and the patient.

The expression or display of pain is itself behavior. A moan or grimace or verbalized complaint is behavior. As such, it is vulnerable to influence by factors that influence all behaviors. This matter is the major—although not the sole—focus of this book. There are many other behaviors or actions of the person with a pain problem that are associated with the pain. They may influence its course or the interpersonal and social consequences of the pain problem. There is, for example, the effect of activity or inactivity stemming from the pain on the pain itself and on other body processes. Is there excessive disuse producing unnecessary atrophy? Would more action or movement create distraction and thereby decrease pain? Would systematic stimulation better activate inhibitory mechanisms that might dampen the pain experience? Is pain being produced or aggravated by other body processes such as muscle tension or deficient peripheral circulation? Each of these phenomena often can be influenced by behavior change methods.

In addition to the more immediate pain and pain-related behavior relationships, there are many complex social and interpersonal effects relating to a pain problem. The chronic pain patient, for example, often develops a dogged and persistent set of strategies for seeking additional help from the health care system. The pain patient who develops multiple sources of analgesics or narcotics is one prime example. The whole set of behaviors making up

1

health care use, excessive or otherwise, provides further examples.

There are yet more interconnections between behavioral concepts and what happens to people with problems of chronic pain. Restricted activity leads to unemployment and to altered social and recreational patterns. It may also lead to activation of wage replacement systems. This brings in the complex issue of compensation and its effects on illness. There is the question of how effectively a patient who is moderately impaired by a pain problem finds vocational or avocational outlets by which to maintain productivity. If he or she does not, the pain problem or its side effects often will worsen. Finally, a pain problem or the effects of the treatments used to deal with it may leave the person unemployable or in major ways restricted in social or avocational activities. What actions or behaviors can the person engage in that would make life more enjoyable?

Pain happens to people. People have behavior. The two, pain and behavior, are inextricably related.

The ideas, the methods, and the results on which this book is based reflect the efforts of a number of people working together since 1966. Results were positive, providing immediate impetus to proceed with further trials.

John Kenneth Galbraith (1958) once commented, "Events and the ideas used to explain them often have a way of pursuing an independent course." Such a comment undoubtedly can be applied to the methods described here. There is, as yet, limited empirical data from which to assess closely the effectiveness of individual segments of the behavioral approach to chronic pain. There is sufficient evidence to indicate that the methods, in their collective effect, are capable of producing significant positive results with many patients. Sometimes the results are dramatic (Fordyce and associates, 1973). In every case thus far treated, the patient had previously undergone multiple treatment programs for his or her pain problems without finding a solution. Each of those patients who displayed and maintained progress when treated by behavioral methods did so after failure to be helped by other approaches.

Chronic pain viewed in behavioral terms leads one to recognize that many chronic pain patients, to use a phrase gained from a colleague, Dr. Roy S. Fowler, Jr., suffer more than they need to. Pain patients pay a terrible price. It is not only that they suffer pain. Their ways of living are disrupted and perhaps virtually shattered. There may be enormous economic losses. But perhaps most of all, life is passing them by. As the years pass and treatment programs repeatedly fail to yield durable results, the sufferers must sit on the sidelines and watch their only chance at life slip past.

The burden is often made heavier by the very sources of help to which the patient turns. As will be shown in detail later in this book, the actions families take to help are often not only ineffective but actually serve to make things worse. The health care system also may add to the problem rather than help it. Multiple surgeries that fail to solve the pain problem and that produce additional functional impairments are a case in point. There are more subtle but often just as burdensome actions by the health care system. Methods of handling pain medications, activity, and rest, for example, sometimes worsen the problem or at least maintain it beyond what otherwise would have been a point of positive resolution.

The health care system, as well as family and friends, sometimes adds to the burden in another way. If the source of pain cannot be seen and the problem has not responded well to treatment based on the system's understanding of what the pain problem is, it is all too often the case that the patient's pain comes to be labelled as imaginary, psychogenic, or all in the head. Now the patient is trapped. The pain and its associated functional impairments persist. The only source of help, the health care system, has failed to solve the problem. More than that, the system may have begun to question the authenticity of the problem. Family members or work associates may pick up the chorus and allude one way or another to doubts about the reality of the pain. Where is the patient to turn?

Experience with operant conditioning–based approaches to selected problems of chronic pain suggests that the difficulties just described often stem from insufficient awareness of the importance of learning or conditioning on the course of chronic pain.

The major concern here is pain, the chronic pain encountered in clinical settings. But chronic pain may also be seen as a ubiquitous member of a larger set of problems: chronic illness. The relationships between chronic pain and chronic illness, taken generally, become even more evident when viewed in behavioral terms.

More than is often recognized, illness is made up largely of behavior. It is a patient doing or not doing something or changing the way of doing something. Behavioral patterns and problems associated with acute or short-term illness are only temporary. The illness events might then be said to be under control of the pathogenic factor, and what follows is treatment aimed at removing that factor. So long as treatment is successful, the process is straightforward. The task facing the patient and his or her family is also simple: follow the treatment plan to minimize the interruption in life-style from the illness.

Adding the dimension of chronicity changes the picture radically. Chronicity ensures the need for behavior change by both patient and family. The health care system will therefore need skills for changing behavior, just as it needs skills for diagnosis and treatment. If essential patient and family behavior changes do not occur, treatment effectiveness will be diminished and sometimes eradicated altogether.

Chronicity of illness adds another dimension. The patient comes time and again to interact with the physician or other therapist. These interactions, in addition to whatever other characteristics they may have, are learning trials. Learning will occur. The question arises, however, as to whether the learning inevitably occurring is always to the benefit of the patient.

Careful examination of the situation in regard to almost any chronic illness, when viewed in behavioral terms, indicates that a significant part of what is involved focuses on the need for the patient and perhaps family members to:

1. Decrease, modify, or stop altogether some behaviors or actions they have been doing and which were enjoyed or had some value
2. Start to do some things not necessary before, not desired, and for which the negative consequences of failure to perform are remote and not previously experienced

The newly diagnosed diabetic must alter eating habits and must develop skill at checking blood sugar levels. He or she may also need to begin injecting insulin. These things must be done consistently and forever. The emphysema patient needs to stop smoking. The chronically obese person whose cardiac status is now compromised must stop eating so much. The paraplegic must relinquish life plans involving ambulation and start to go in new directions. He or she must also learn to check for skin breakdowns and to maintain a high level of fluid intake to protect bladder and kidney function. The post–myocardial infarction patient must learn to discriminate between too high and too low levels of exercise and must remain within that band of activity. The left hemiplegic patient must learn how to move about and how to scan to the left, when he or she cannot reliably judge distance, position, movement, and surface variations, all of which threaten to cause falls and hip fractures.

The examples are endless. The point is that chronic illness requires behavior change. Behavior change is not automatic. It most certainly is not automatically brought about simply by informing someone about what and why to change. Behavior change often requires the careful application of behavior change technology.

A secondary intent of this book is to stimulate the analysis of chronic illness in behavioral terms. The problems and the methods described here will have pertinence to many forms of chronic illness for which pain is of little or no significance. The behavior change technology, as an operational tool, bears essentially the same relationship to chronic illness as it does to chronic pain. Stated another way, many patient management problems encountered in relation to chronic illness are likely to profit from the methods outlined in this book.

The objectives of the book can now be stated in behavioral terms. They are, first, to increase the extent to which physicians and other health care professionals analyze chronic illness, particularly chronic pain, in terms of the behavior of the people who have the pain and the people who interact with them. Behavioral analysis will of necessity also consider environmental cues and consequences that influence the pertinent behavior. The second objective is to describe use of these methods in the evaluation and treatment of chronic pain and in the prevention of some chronic pain and associated problems, with the hope they will be used more than at present.

The book is divided into three sections. The first section provides a conceptual context. It reviews the concepts of pain, psychogenic pain, and how learning or conditioning may play a role in the development and character of pain problems. The second section describes behavioral technology and considers how to apply it to treatment planning and patient evaluation. The third section details clinical methods for using behavior change technology in selected problems of chronic pain.

Since the ideas and the methods presented in this book represent somewhat of a departure from traditional perspectives in regard to chronic pain, some consideration should be given to the evolution of what might be called modern behaviorism.

Any choice of a starting point is arbitrary and ignores preceding developments. The earliest applications of behavioral concepts to illness began mainly in the context of mental illness and mental retardation.

This is understandable, for, by the very nature of the problems encountered in those settings, there was bound to be an initial concern about what the patient or client did, his behavior. In the final analysis it was not that the people called mentally ill *were* mentally ill, but that they *behaved* in strange ways. It was what they did that got them into a kind of trouble: the trouble associated with being identified as having problems about which some kind of remedial or custodial action was necessary or with feeling distress severe enough to interfere with daily living and performance.

In the case of mental retardates, the emergence of behavior methods and supporting concepts had probably an even easier and more direct evolution. Clearly, the mental retardate could be seen as one who had deficient performance. The conern was with what he could not *do*. Moreover, working with mental retardates often did not have the same appeal as working with those identified as mentally ill or emotionally disturbed. There was less professional attention to the retardates and correspondingly less competition of ideas or establishment dogma. It was simply easier to find opportunities to try behavioral methods in programs for the mentally retarded.

Whatever the case, by the late 1950s and early in the 1960s, the professional literature began to be spotted with reports of behaviorally based work on various kinds of human problems. The work was based mainly on foundations laid by B. F. Skinner (1953) in relation to concepts of operant conditioning. Two early and often-cited publications certainly should be mentioned: Ayllon and Michael (1960) and Ullmann and Krasner (1965). Innumerable other significant pioneering efforts could be mentioned. It is not the intent, however, that this become a historical treatise. What is of some importance in providing a contextual perspective is to note that two kinds of changes were emerging from these and other early works. One was that a tool or technology was being developed. It began to be more possible and logistically and ethically more practical to help people change; to solve or to ameliorate problems that previously had not lent themselves to cost-effective, or even simply effective, solutions. This is not to suggest that all problems of mental illness or emotional disturbance and of mental retardation were solved or significantly helped by behavioral methods. Nor does it imply that other methods were incapable of helping. But it can be asserted with confidence that a host of problems, some of which were not previously readily helped by existing methods, were and are being helped with these behavioral methods to the marked advantage of the patient or client and the funding sources, personal or organizational, for such services.

The second change was in how problems were characterized or identified. The sometimes startling results when behavioral methods were applied to problem behavior raised difficulties for some theorists and conceptualizers. The prevailing wisdom asserted that the actions of an emotionally disturbed (perhaps a ritualistic handwasher or a compulsive eater) person were controlled by underlying neurotic mechanisms evolved as a defense against some symbolic threat relating to earlier experiences, *and* that solution to the problem required somehow working through or retroactively reliving the earlier trauma. In contrast, behavior changers sometimes concerned themselves solely with helping the patient to establish a different behavior in place of handwashing or excessive eating. A positive result often followed and persisted, accompanied by more effective performance in other spheres. When only the symptom (for example, handwashing) and not the alleged cause was treated, the patient did not revert to his symptom behavior, nor did he display anxiety or other symptoms in its place. To the contrary, he often began to do better in many parameters of behavior.

It was an awkward task to explain this kind of outcome in prevailing conceptual modes. The least that could be drawn from, for example, the numerous case illustrations reported in Ullmann and Krasner (1965), to mention but one of many possible references, was that traditional conceptual models underlying professional methods should be reexamined. And, indeed, they were.

Behavioral technology and behaviorally based conceptual models, as now seems inevitable, began to be tested in yet other parameters besides those of mental illness and mental retardation. Chief among these other areas of application, pertinent to this book, are illness and health care. Perhaps the tool was the chicken and the problems to which it was to be applied or tested were the eggs. At any rate, the behavioral perspective, and the tools for change that relate to it, are now being used in many aspects of what heretofore has been considered physical illness.

The use of biofeedback technology as a means of trying to reverse or modify body processes that have been functioning to the disadvantage of the patient is but one set of examples. This work has been directed toward such targets as blood pressure, heart rate, brain wave activity, skin temperature, peripheral blood flow, and muscle tension. The procedures take direct aim at the process or phenomenon. To paraphrase, one way to help a person to relax painfully tense muscles (such as in tension headaches) is to teach him or her how to do that. Notably lacking in this approach is the assumption that one must always first understand and eliminate the alleged underlying causes for the tension.

The work with selected problems of chronic pain, which serves as the underpinning to this book, is another case in point. Essentially, as will be described in detail, the added element is to examine closely what the patient does—and does not do—and then to apply behavior change technology to help make desired and relevant changes in these behaviors. This kind of approach necessitates a frame of reference and a technology for doing something about the problem. This book will be concerned with the conceptual framework and the technology.

If the events of the past decade or so are understood at all correctly, it seems apparent that the next few years will see many reexaminations of illness-related problems and the applications of methods derived from behavioral science to the health care system.

It is essential to recognize that awareness of the importance of learning or conditioning in chronic illness leads to major changes in how these phenomena are perceived. This seems particularly to be the case in regard to chronic pain. The evidence is all around us that traditional methods, although scoring many successes and helping untold thousands of patients, also result in many patients failing to find relief and solutions to their problems. The rapidly expanding number of pain clinics now appearing on the scene is one kind of evidence of the not infrequent failures of traditional treatment to resolve pain problems.

This book will examine chronic pain, as one form of chronic illness, from a different conceptual perspective. When illness becomes chronic, one of the inevitable consequences is the opportunity for learning or conditioning to occur. That is, it becomes possible for sequences of illness-related behaviors and their consequences to occur repeatedly. That is how learning occurs. It will be shown that many of the key elements making up a problem of chronic pain are organism responses that are subject to conditioning or learning effects. It follows that chronic pain, as is true of other chronic illness states, needs to be examined in terms of the learning or conditioning that is occurring, has occurred, or might occur. In short, in addition to its numerous other characteristics, chronic illness is learning opportunity. Not all of the learning is to the patient's advantage, nor does it contribute to the reduction of the illness.

The time dimension of chronicity, with its attendant learning opportunities, leads one to recognize that chronic pain is usually both the presence of something and the absence of something. Pain is commonly the presence of some ongoing body damage factor producing, among its effects, distress or the subjective experience of pain. There is something wrong, or there may be. At the same time, the fact of chronicity is likely to mean that the patient's way of life will have been altered in some degree through the course of the illness. He or she is not only sick (in pain) but also has gaps in well behavior. There are things he cannot do or has not done for perhaps many months, even years. There are absences of well behaviors. The protracted reduction in or abstinence from well behaviors also creates sequences of behavior-environmental consequences, which, when repeated, may become learned or conditioned. These gaps in well behavior (that is, things the patient does not do or has not been doing because of the pain problem) almost always involve others around the patient. Elaborate networks of learned behavior patterns involving patient and family emerge, are rehearsed, and are selectively and effectively conditioned. Modification or resolution of the pain or illness problem does not inevitably result in concomitant change of the learned behavior patterns associated with gaps in well behavior. To put it another way, chronic pain provides opportunity for the network of pain behaviors to be influenced by learning and conditioning. Chronicity also makes it possible for corresponding gaps in effective or well behavior performance to develop, to be conditioned, and to persist, even after the pain problem has been resolved. It follows that treatment of chronic pain must look at both the presence of pain problems and the absence of well behavior. Both sets of problems play crucial roles in treatment outcome.

One final preparatory comment seems in order. It is intended to help make the shift in perspective presented in this book an easier one. What does it mean to loosen one's hold on the traditional concepts of motivation and personality, of adjustment and defense mechanisms to which we have all been so long exposed and committed? It is easy for the issue to become an intellectualized conceptual battle of interest only to a few. It is perhaps even easier for it to become a tug-of-war between dogmas or to seem that crusaders are attacking the bastions. This book is not intended as a doctrinaire treatise. It is aimed instead at a particularly vexing problem in health care. But the approach sets out from a different view of the way humans function. The differences between this behaviorally based view and the conventional wisdom from which it varies in some degree can be related to the concept of sensitivity. This matter will receive more formal treatment later in the book. Let me take a few lines to deal with it more informally and in a more introductory way now.

Each of us has a continuity. We are certain persons with certain names and fairly consistent physical and functional characteristics. Each of us tends in considerable degree to see these consistencies or continuities almost as constants. In regard to physical appearance and attributes, we are nearly always surprised at the amount of change when we see a snapshot taken as recently as 6 months or a year before. The consistencies of appearance and the like are not as consistent as we think. The same is true of our actions. We may think of ourselves as having certain styles of behavior or, if we use the technical term, certain traits or personality characteristics. We tend to see ourselves as displaying a consistent way of behaving to others. Indeed, there are consistencies. But change and variability are also ever present, more than we recognize, because we tend to be aware mainly of the consistencies.

The discrepancy between what we see as consistency in our actions and what instead is a greater degree of variability and ongoing change can be thought of in terms of sensitivity. We are more sensitive as functioning beings to our immediate environments than we often recognize. What we do, how we act, what we say, how we move, what decisions we make have a significant ongoing interaction with what is going on around us—and with what we anticipate will soon be going on. To put the point another way, our behavior tends to be more influenced by the immediate and the immediately anticipated environment than we often recognize. We make more use of cues and environmental feedback in our ongoing behavior than we think we do. We tend to overestimate the importance of our personalities and to underestimate the skill and sensitivity with which we perceive and use cues and guidelines from our surroundings.

Personalized examples are risky affairs because they do not necessarily apply to the next person, but one will be ventured to illustrate the point. I recently had my first experience at driving in England and did so for a few weeks and several hundred miles. The conventional wisdom often voiced in this context is that driving on the right-hand side is a well-established habit and is therefore difficult to break. Habit, in this context, can be likened to a well-established trait or behavioral disposition; it is part of the driver's personality, so to speak. The truth of the matter is that about the only real hazard to the change of driving on the left is in the first few seconds of each driving period. It takes a moment or so to remember to watch for the cues. Thereafter, if one relaxes, it rapidly becomes apparent that there is an abundance of continuously presented environmental cues that guide driving. In England, these cues are to keep to the left. The cues are not simply signs saying, "Keep to the left," although a few of those are encountered. There are a host of other and continuously present cues that guide. Roadside advertising signs are placed differently. Each car on the road is a reminder. Road directional and curve indicator signs are placed differently. Instead of driving behavior being dominated by habit or personality, this experience suggests that it is a flexible process, sensitive to environmental cues and anticipated consequences.

As we learn to watch our own behavior, we can become aware of how sensitive we are. This is not a doctrinaire position or a bit of dogma. It is simply an observation. This book, just as is true of much of the work presently being done with behavioral methods, is simply being responsive to the flexibility and sensitivity of the human organism.

The importance of the environment and

our interactions with it on behavior will be referred to repeatedly in this book. It means, of course, that the diagnostic or evaluation process, as well as treatment, must take into account and deal with the patient's environment. To focus solely on the patient is to ignore a major set of highly influential factors.

There are many implications to the preceding point. One is that once a pain problem has become chronic, it also has become a family affair. Inevitably, patient-family interactions will be playing significant roles in the maintenance of pain behavior or the failure to reinforce or support well behavior or both. It follows that diagnosis and treatment almost certainly need to involve the family as well as the patient. We *are* sensitive to our environments. Our pain behaviors, as well as other behaviors, will reflect this.

The primary focus of this book is on the use of behavioral methods in the evaluation and management of certain types of chronic clinical pain. It is not intended to be an exhaustive analysis, or even an extensive set of the many facets of the subject of pain. There will be a not inconsiderable review and discussion of the broad context of pain to provide as many touch points as possible between the ideas and methods described here and what is known about pain. But it is well to remember that although this book presents some different perspectives and tactical treatment procedures regarding aspects of clinical pain, it does not purport to redefine pain nor to challenge theories about the nature of pain.

There are additional limits of coverage that should be set forth in these introductory comments. In the first place, this book focuses only on parts of the subject of pain, the parts that appear to have the greatest relevance to behavioral concepts and methods. Many pressing and important pain problems are not mentioned or referred to, much less dealt with. This is not a book about how to diagnose and treat pain. It is a book about how to add behavioral concepts and behavioral methods to one's diagnostic and treatment armamentarium. To do so will augment the professional's capability for dealing with some but not all pain problems.

There are further constraints to the information and methods that should be identified at the outset. I am a psychologist. I am not a physician or a pharmacologist or a physical therapist, to name but a few. The approach in this book, as it bears on specific diagnostic or treatment issues, is to describe behavioral aspects of what are broader processes. For example, consider the use of exercise in relation to various forms of back pain. This book does not specify when to use exercise nor which exercises to use for a given kind of pain problem. The reader will need to look elsewhere to sources competent to address themselves to such matters. What this book does is to describe how to program exercises in such a fashion as to better organize and control learning or conditioning factors. The exercises selected on the basis of competencies other than those of this book can then be delivered in a manner to maximize performance and to minimize functional impairment associated with the pain. A similar illustration pertains to the use of pain medications. I have limited knowledge about the pharmacological properties of analgesics, narcotics, and the like. There will be no suggestions here as to which medications to prescribe or to avoid. There will be attention to the manner of delivery of the medications selected. Prolonged medication regimens provide situations fraught with potential for learning, addiction, habituation, or whatever term one chooses. There are delivery strategies that draw on learning principles and that can have significant influence on the course of the pain and the medication problems.

Finally, at a philosophical level, the reader will not find here a comprehensive definition of pain—either what it is or what it is not. This is basically a methods book. It will leave to others the task of deciding precisely what the semantic and logical boundaries are to the concept.

SECTION ONE
Conceptual background

Section One is concerned with the theoretical, conceptual, and technical background to the evaluation and management of chronic pain by behavioral methods. Chapter 1 presents a review of basic concepts relating to pain and of studies that help to characterize pain. Chapter 2 is concerned with an analysis of the concept of psychogenic pain and a redefinition in behavioral terms. The next step in the sequence is to examine in behavioral terms how problems of chronic pain may come under the influence of learning or conditioning. Chapter 3 reviews and discusses the more common ways in which learning factors may appear in problems of chronic pain and may, in some cases, maintain the pain problems after the initiating body defect has been resolved. One more background element in the evaluation and management of chronic pain by operant conditioning methods is essential: the methods of behavior change or conditioning. Those are presented briefly in Chapter 4.

1 Pain as a clinical problem

The subject of pain has been likened by Mortimer (1968) to the fable of the blind men and the elephant. Each of the blind men "saw" and understood the elephant only as that particular part of the subject with which he came in contact. Similarly, pain may be viewed differently by the neurophysiologist concerned with study of nociceptive stimuli or neural transmission; the experimental psychologist concerned with psychophysical methods in the measurement of sensory thresholds; the physician or dentist faced with a patient who reports severe, nagging, unending pain; and the patient who both hurts and sees his way of life disrupted by what may seem to be a threatening and potentially unresolvable illness. Each of these perspectives may include, at least implicitly, a definition of pain. To the definer, that is what pain is; but the definitions are likely to vary considerably.

Clark and Hunt (1971, p. 374) provide an invaluable entry into the subject by noting, "Most discussions of pain begin with a definition, which quickly reveals its inadequacy, followed by a quasi-philosophical discussion of the mind-body problem, with the author finally opting for dualism, psychophysical parallelism or some kind of monism in which pain experience is epiphenomenal to the 'real' events taking place in the tissues and nervous system." Since this book does not aspire to a definitive statement about the total complex of pain, perhaps some of the problems Clark and Hunt note can be avoided by simply asserting that pain is not an entity or thing; it is a label that observers, including the pain sufferer, have attached to relevant phenomena they have observed or experienced. Both the phenomena and the concepts used to describe or explain them may vary, according to the particular circumstances of the observer. It can surely be agreed that the term pain involves a complex set of events or phenomena. As a consequence, efforts at precise definition carry the assurance that elements or terms important to some observers probably will be omitted.

There will not be presented here a final, precision statement about pain that has a broad range of applications. From the brief review of the subject of pain that follows, a limited number of facets of the subject will be the concern of this book.

A story is told about days at Harvard of the late comedian, Robert Benchley. According to the story he was taking a course in economics. He chose to spend much of the weekend preceding the final examination in nearby taverns. He reported for the examination in something less than a state of high readiness. The examination was to write on the effects of recent legislation on the fishing industry of the Grand Banks. Benchley achieved an "A" by writing to the question from the point of view of the fish.

Pain, most particularly chronic pain, needs also to be viewed from the "point of view of the fish"—in this case, the patient. Most scientific studies of pain have focused on neurophysiological events. This is not to imply that the patient has been neglected nor that there has been limited work on what methods serve to relieve pain and solve pain problems. There is a tendency to accord to the neurophysiological events a greater sense of importance. They seem to be more real. The subjective experience of pain and the related functional impairments (pain "from the point of view of the fish") are sometimes viewed as unfortunate by-products. Moreover, these by-products are further influenced or distorted by psychic factors to the end that some of what patients may report as pain is not really pain at all but something else. Some or all of their pain is not real; it is called psychic, a term that ordinarily connotes that the pain is thought to be imagined or unreal.

The issue of so-called psychogenic pain will be dealt with in Chapter 2. The point for now is to recognize something of what pain is not. Pain is not simply a neurophysiological event. To hold that it is, is to fail to come to grips with what happens to patients.

It is equally true that pain is not simply what a patient says it is. There are at least two reasons why this statement is true. One is that the patient's knowledge and perceptions will limit his ability to discriminate well enough what is going on. Patient reports about pain will be subject to influence and distortion by a host of factors deriving from ongoing cortical activities, from the immediate stimulus situation, and from prior experience. Each of these factors will be analyzed in some detail in this first section. There is a most important second reason why the patient's pain is not necessarily what he or she says it is, which relates to the first reason but which should be viewed from a different perspective.

For the problem to be identified, the person must in some fashion communicate to the surrounding environment that he or she is experiencing pain. The report of pain, particularly chronic pain, may be verbal or by some other form of audible or visible action: some behavior. What the patient *says* the pain is (the verbal report) is not to be considered the final, definitive answer of what it is, even for him or her. That is of course true because of inherent patient limitations to observe the total system or to have the knowledge properly to interpret the data gained from experiencing current bodily states. But it is also true because there is no inherent reason why what patients say and what they do will correlate highly or be the same. This is a discussion of chronic pain, but the same point could be made about virtually any other human activity. The point is that verbal statements

about pain are one kind of behavior, and the *other* visible and audible methods by which the problem is communicated to the environment are another. For the moment they will be distinguished as verbal and nonverbal pain behaviors. The latter group includes nonlanguage sounds (such as moans and gasps), body posturing and gesturing (limping, rubbing a painful area, grimacing), and displaying functional limitations or impairment (reclining excessively to rest or staying home from work because it hurts too much.) Each of these sets of behaviors meets different contingencies or consequences in the environment. As a result, verbal and nonverbal behaviors are not only somewhat free to vary from each other; they in fact do vary from each other far more than we often are ready to accept.

The discrepancy between what people say and what they do is not simply a question of honesty or candor. Verbal and nonverbal behaviors each meet consequences. These consequences are often not the same. Since consequences influence behavior, it follows that verbal and nonverbal behaviors—even when focused around a single conceptual theme or topic—can be expected to vary from each other. The variation is an inevitable result of learning or conditioning. When verbal behaviors receive one set of consequences and nonverbal behaviors receive another, they will begin to diverge. When differential learning or conditioning has had more time in which to assert itself, the opportunities for greater discrepancy obviously increase. That is certainly the case in chronic pain. The problem has been active a long time. There has been opportunity for learning or conditioning. The verbal and the nonverbal behaviors may well have been receiving different consequences. If so, they will have tended to go their separate ways—certainly not totally unrelated, but no longer synonymous and perhaps downright discrepant.

An illustration in another context may make the point clearer. An easy example concerns smoking. Verbal behavior about smoking meets one set of consequences, puffing on cigarettes another. When the Surgeon General's report was released several years ago, social consequences of smoking began to change. Instead of being fashionable to smoke, it began to be unfashionable. Moreover, the information about lung cancer and other smoking-related health problems received increasing visibility. Many people quit smoking. But many did not quit and of those who did, many did so only after a number of false starts. Some people who tried to quit and failed, or who succeeded only after several false starts, and some who made no serious attempt at all, will have been observed to display markedly discrepant verbal and nonverbal smoking related behavior. They talked about quitting. They voiced determination, even vows, to quit. These verbal behaviors tended initially to receive positive encouragement and reinforcement from people around them. But the social consequences were not likely to have been delivered systematically. They did not occur consistently or with the right timeliness, nor did they always have much impact or emotional horsepower. They were not effective consequences by which to change smoking behavior. At the same time, the smoking activity itself continued to receive the reinforcement of the body need factor associated with addiction. This reinforcement was systematic, consistent, ever present, and usually rather powerful. Other reinforcing consequences to smoking behavior also will have played a part. Discrepancies between smoking talk and smoking action began to emerge. The smoker often began to understate how much he or she was smoking or overstate the length of the intervals between cigarettes. To do so was to continue to receive the social approval attendant to seeming-to-quit behavior. What the smoker said and what he or she did began increasingly to diverge. Eventually, in the case of smoking the discrepancy became so visible as to elicit negative reactions from others. These negative reactions usually led the smoker who had not yet succeeded in quitting to voice reasons why quitting was unimportant. The rationalizations against quitting serve the purpose of minimizing negative or aversive responses from others when smoking behavior persists.

Applied to chronic pain, the verbal/nonverbal discrepancy points to differences often observed between what a pain patient may say and what he or she may do. The patient may, for example, provide an exquisitely detailed description of the quality, intensity, and circumstances of the pain. Some long-time pain patients provide the examiner with a typed statement containing both a description of the pain and the history of medical interventions that have occurred to attempt to resolve the problem. These accounts may include such statements as, "I cannot sit in a moving car for more than 20 minutes before the pain becomes severe," or "I cannot walk more than a city block before I must sit down to rest and to ease my pain." That same patient may report, when asked, that analgesics are taken only when needed and as rarely as possible, perhaps once or twice a day or "a few times a week." If directly observed, the same patient may be noted periodically to sit fishing in a gently rocking boat for hours on end. He or she may walk several blocks to attend a movie or sporting event and sit through either with few or no interruptions. The patient may also be taking analgesics far in excess of what has been reported, using multiple prescription sources to maintain a high level of intake.

Such discrepancies may be viewed as reflecting dishonesty or some form of malingering. That choice is an unfortunate one. It fails to recognize that the verbal and the nonverbal behaviors have long been receiving different consequences. They should be expected to vary as a natural result of learning or conditioning. To consider such behavior as dishonest or as malingering is but to call the patient a dirty name. The patient is already suffering enough without the health care system viewing their encounters as fraught with the dishonesty of malingering.

The verbal/nonverbal discrepancy plays another important role in the analysis of chronic pain, one which is perhaps even more important. As will be considered in more depth in the discussion of psychogenic pain in Chapter 2, the evaluation of pain is dependent in large part on information imparted by the patient in the form of verbal reports. The examiner should recognize the extent to which these verbal reports are sets of behaviors that have for at least the life of the pain problem, to say nothing of earlier pain episodes, been receiving systematic consequences. These consequences may shape, direct, or modify pain reports somewhat independently of the underlying neurophysiological events that first occasioned their expression. To fail to recognize this is to lay oneself open to misinterpretation of key diagnostic data. Patients should be listened to most carefully, but their actions deserve attention equal to their words. One should remain mindful of the perfectly logical and reasonable possibility that the words and the actions may vary, perhaps markedly, 'as a natural consequence of the manner in which the patient's environment has been responding to the pain problem. Particularly in regard to chronic pain, it is of the utmost importance to study what the patient does as well as what he or she says. They are two sets of data. They tend to correlate positively, but there is no assurance that the correlation is high.

To sum up the point, one of the things pain is *not* is simply what the patient says it is. The scope and definition of a clinical pain problem is to be found in what the patient does as well as what he or she says. Patient behavior is a critically important element.

From the perspective of the neurophysiologist, pain is likely initially to be viewed as some form of activity in a sensory system. This approach is usually concerned with sensory receptor and transmission mechanisms and the stimulus characteristics adequate to activate them. Historically, the neurophysiological study of pain led to two major theories as to the nature of pain as a body system or process. Von Frey proposed in 1894 (Melzack and Wall, 1965) a specificity theory that held that there are specific pain receptors, which, when stimulated, result in the sensation of pain. Moreover, stimulation of these receptors (free nerve endings) resulted only in the sensation of pain. The specificity theory thus holds that pain has its own central and peripheral mechanisms, as do other body senses.

In the same year, 1894, Goldschneider, drawing on earlier work as well, proposed (Melzack and Wall, 1965) a contrasting and allegedly mutually exclusive pattern theory of pain. Pattern theory proposes that it is not the adequate stimulation of specific receptors but the transmission of nerve impulse patterns coded at the periphery that yields the sensation of pain. Rather than a more or less discrete and specific receptor and transmission system, there is the coded, intense stimulation of nonspecific receptors. As pattern theory has evolved, it has come to propose both the coding/patterning function at the periphery and the modulation of resulting impulse patterns during transmission by central nervous system inputs, as in emotional state, prior experience, alertness, and the like.

For many years the specificity theory held major sway, with most medical texts considering pain mainly in those terms. Excellent reviews of both conceptualizations of pain can be found in, for example, Clark and Hunt (1971), Melzack and Wall (1965) and, more briefly, Melzack (1968). Specificity theory correctly recognizes that some receptors indeed have responsivity only to specific kinds and amounts of stimulus energy. It would be a mistake to discard specificity theory in its entirety. For example, the specific, unique, and under appropriate stimulation, consistently occuring pain experience originating in the skin, has been described by Bonica. He states:

A quick light stab of a sensitive portion of the skin results in an immediate short, slight flash of pain which disappears, and after a brief interval is followed by a second pain which lasts longer and is more intense. . . . Most of the experimental evidence seems to demonstrate rather decidedly that the double pain response is due to transmission of impulses in two sets of nerve fibers which have well separated velocities of conduction . . . and which are of two types, one mediating impulses which give rise to the sensation of prickling pain, and the other mediating impulses which reach the sensorium slowly and give rise to the sensation of burning pain.*

Thus there are two sets of fibers having stimulus-specific as well as differentiated conducting properties that clearly are involved in pain.

There are a number of lines of approach that indicate that specificity theory is, by itself, insufficient to account for the phenomena of clinical pain. Hill and associates (1952) have shown that subjects experiencing experimentally induced anxiety feel electric shock or burning heat to be more painful. Reduction of the anxiety results in lowered intensity of perceived pain. They have also shown that morphine reduces pain if the anxiety level is high but has no effect if anxiety is low. Thus, with pain stimulus constant, pain response varies according to other factors; this is a challenge to strict specificity theory.

Beecher's (1959) well-known work studying the effects of combat wounds at Anzio demonstrated clearly that psychological factors can and do have a profound influence on the perception of and response to pain. A significant number of soldiers sustaining obvious tissue damage from combat wounds nonetheless reported little or no pain because the wound was perceived as an assurance of their being removed from the life-threat scene of battle. Here, then, is yet another break in the tie between pain stimulus and pain response.

Christopherson (1966) studied relationships between Anglo- and Mexican-American subjects in regard to responses to chronic pain. His findings demonstrated what other

studies and anthropological observations have indicated—there are often to be found discernible differences in magnitude of pain responses to given pain stimuli, as a function of cultural identity.

One more example of challenge to specificity theory should suffice to indicate that we must look beyond such a perspective and consider other factors as well in dealing with pain. When specificity theory emerged, surgeons began using this knowledge in attempts to alleviate clinical pain. From the periphery to such central sites as frontal lobotomy, attempts have been made to disengage connections between the site of peripheral body damage and the central experience of pain. If such procedures had enjoyed consistent success, it would have represented compelling evidence in support of both specificity theory and the key role of peripheral stimulation in the experience of pain. Such success has not been enjoyed. Surgical approaches to a broad spectrum of pain problems have not had sufficiently consistent success to warrant reliance solely on a specificity theory of pain.

Without discarding all elements of specificity theory, it can be seen that the numerous indications of variations in the relationship between peripheral stimulus and pain response require dealing with additional factors.

Pattern theory, perhaps more accurately phrased as a family of pattern theories, is also flawed. In strict construction, it fails to account for the physiological evidence of nerve fiber specialization (Bonica, 1953; Melzack and Wall, 1965). However, that is not to suggest a total rejection of pattern concepts. Livingston (1943) proposed that peripheral stimulation emanating from body damage may set up reverberating circuits in spinal internuncial pools, which, by their summating effects, account for the common observation of modest but rapidly repeated peripheral stimulation (as in pinpricks) leading to intense pain. In that kind of example, the stimulus-response relationship is not one-to-one, but it does make sense.

Another pattern theory proposal by Noordenbos (1959) suggests that central

---

*From Bonica, J. J.: The management of pain, Philadelphia, 1953, Lea & Febiger, pp. 92-93.

summation may be prevented by the action of rapidly conducting fibers inhibiting transmission by slow conducting fibers.

It is from variations of pattern theory that most significant advances in our understanding of the neurophysiology of pain have come. Melzack and Wall (1962) proposed that skin receptors have specialized physiological properties by which they may transmit particular types and ranges of stimuli in the form of patterns of impulses. They further proposed that every somesthetic perception is elicited by a unique pattern of nerve impulses. These propositions were coupled with additional data and observations to formulate a new theory of pain, the gate control theory (Melzack and Wall, 1965). They drew on the work of Wall (1962), which indicated that impulses arriving at the spinal cord stimulate spinal cord fibers, which transmit on to the brain and which also influence the substantia gelatinosa. Mendell and Wall (1964) had further shown that the substantia gelatinosa can both inhibit and facilitate transmission of sensory input from the periphery to central cells. These and other of their observations and observations of other investigators indicate there are efferent fiber systems that run from the brain down to different pathways and that can inhibit or modify afferent input pattern enroute centrally. They also noted that dorsal column and dorsolateral systems of the spinal cord may have a function of stimulating central attention, memory, and prior experience processes, which can then act downward on afferent impulses. In short, their theory proposes that central or cortical mechanisms are capable of influencing transmission of noxious stimuli (that is, modulating or diminishing them, as one possibility) and that the initial transmission of such impulses is capable of stimulating these central mechanisms to take action.

The gate control theory is summarized by Melzack as follows:

The theory proposes that (1) the *substantia gelatinosa* functions as a gate control system that modulates the amount of input transmitted from the peripheral fibers to the dorsal horn transmission (T) cells; (2) the dorsal column and dorsolateral systems of the spinal cord act as a central control trigger, which activates selective brain processes that influence the modulating properties of the gate control system; and (3) the T cells activate neural mechanisms that constitute the action system responsible for both response and perception. . . . The theory proposes that pain phenomena are determined by interactions among these three systems. For example, a marked loss of the large peripheral-nerve fibers, which may occur after traumatic peripheral nerve lesions or in some of the neuropathies, such as postherpetic neuralgia, would decrease the normal presynaptic inhibition of the input by the gate control system. The input arriving over the remaining large and small fibers is transmitted through the unchecked, open gate produced by the small-fiber input. This, together with the opportunity for summation of inputs into the *substantia gelatinosa* from other parts of the body and from the brain, provides the basis for the triggering of pain by a variety of stimuli that are normally not noxious.*

The gate may be closed or partially closed by the interaction between large and small fiber activity reaching the dorsal horn of the cord from the periphery, which is the presumed site of body damage or pain stimulation, and by the influence from central control centers activated by stimulation of the dorsal column and dorsolateral spinal cord systems. These central control centers in turn will be influenced by ongoing organism activity, by prior experience, and by competing stimuli. Keep in mind that effective closing of the gate means the pain is not experienced. Functionally, it is as if there had not been peripheral stimulation or as if it had been of minor intensity.

There is a time dimension to gate control of particular importance here. Mild

---

*From Melzack, R.: Pain. In Sills, D. L., editor: International encyclopedia of the social sciences, vol. 2, New York, 1968, The Macmillan Co., p. 362.

sensory stimulation may activate the large myelinated sensory fibers involved with non-painful tactile stimuli. This activation may then modify the ratio of large to small fiber activity, causing partial closing of the gate and decreased T cell activity. However, large fibers tend to adapt rapidly, and so their input to the gate may soon diminish, thereby re-altering the large/small fiber ratio and permitting pain sensation to pass on to be perceived. Subsequently, additional stimulation of large fibers, for example, through rubbing the skin, could serve to renew closure of the gate.

Noxious stimulation of smaller A fibers, as noted previously, gives rise to rapidly transmitted and quickly experienced prickling pain. The effect is virtually immediate and well correlated with stimulation. The gate has little effect. The slower C fiber impulses, when stimulated, are capable of producing dull, diffuse, burning pain. Because these impulses are slower, a gating effect may occur to reduce or eliminate their impact. For that to happen, there must be activation of the system of nonpainful stimulation receptors, the large A fibers. The influence of the central control centers enters in, as well. Both peripheral and central factors, then, may serve to inhibit transmission of the slow pain impulses and, therefore, of the pain experience.

Time becomes an issue in at least two ways. One is in regard to whether slow- or fast-transmitting fibers are stimulated. Moreover, if it is fast-arising pain, as in cardiac pain, there probably will not be enough time for the gate to close to inhibit pain sensation. This aspect of the time factor, although of considerable neurophysiological importance, is not likely to be of lasting significance in regard to the problems of chronic pain, which endure for months and even years.

A second relevance of time in regard to the gate control theory is that the gating effect is an unstable arrangement, constantly capable of change. Noxious stimulation varies, not only according to which fibers are stimulated but also as to when. Move-

ment or changes in body position, for example, may evoke renewed pain stimulation. Rubbing adjacent skin areas to activate large A fibers and thereby promote gate closure may ease pain or inhibit sensation. But this kind of peripheral stimulation, although exerting influence on the ratio of active fibers and therefore on the gate, is not likely to be continued indefinitely. These are short-term time considerations, which may further limit control of pain by gate closure.

There are also long-term time factors that must be considered. Assuming the continuing presence of peripheral noxious stimulation adequate to evoke the sensation of pain, there are inherent limitations in how much one can do by way of movement, skin rubbing, promotion of distraction, generation of competing stimuli, and so on. One sees this in the increase of the sensation of pain often reported when trying to fall asleep at night. Activation and competing stimuli are at a minimum. The gate may not close well. Viewed from the perspective of the treatment or management of chronic pain, gate control is not a fixed solution. Strategies and tactics derived from gate control theory and relating mainly to activation through nonpainful stimulation have an important role in pain management. This role is mainly in the short-term time sense, although the short-term application may be a continuing and repeated one. The studied use of activation as part of a remediation effort for pain will be returned to later.

The gate control theory represents a major step forward in organizing information about pain. The physiological mechanisms postulated as underlying the theory have not all yet been verified, but the theory itself is a most important contribution.

The major points in the material thus far covered can now be summarized:

1. Pain is not a discrete entity but a complex network of phenomena about which there is a broad range of perspectives. Approaches to the subject must be prepared to identify which facets are being dealt with and to

recognize that others may view the problem differently.

2. There is but a loose linkage between noxious stimulation peripheral to the central nervous system and sensations presumed to emanate from this stimulation, even when viewed in strictly neurophysiological terms. For example, under certain conditions of peripheral noxious stimulation, there is a neurophysiological basis for anticipating the modulation or reduction of experienced pain by forms of activation, that is, stimulation of large A fibers.

3. Previous experience and ongoing cortical activity are ensured a role in even the simple detection of a pain stimulus, to say nothing of how the sensation is perceived and what responses ensue.

To continue the development of the conceptual roots and data basis for the role of behavioral methods in working with chronic pain, the nature of the influence of prior experience and ongoing cortical activity must also be examined.

Gate control theory concerns factors influencing the *sensation* of pain. The theory provides a rationale for a role of central factors (competing stimuli, prior experience, and so on) and of activation or counterstimulation, in whether a currently active noxious stimulus will be perceived as painful. The theory does not address itself to what people *do,* that is, their responses when they experience pain. Beecher (1959) made the distinction between a sensory (afferent input) and a reactive component. What people do in regard to pain is a complex mixture of both sensory and reactive components. Melzack and Wall have shown how cortical factors can play a role in sensation, but this book must also be concerned with the impact of cortical factors on the reactive component. Neurophysiological issues regarding sensation, transmission, reception, and, in part, perception of pain have thus far been considered. The picture would be incomplete without also considering organism responses to these stimuli and the interactions between the responses and the environment around the responder.

One of the main difficulties in understanding and working with clinical pain is that it happens to people. People are complicated. Each patient brings to the clinical pain experience a learning or conditioning history, which predisposes him or her to bring to bear on stimuli perceived as painful the unique products of that learning history. Beecher made the point when he said:

> Many investigators seem grimly determined to establish—indeed, too often there does not seem to have been any question in their mind—that for a given stimulus there must be a given response; that is, for so much stimulation of nerve endings, so much pain will be experienced, and so on. This fundamental error has led to enormous waste. . . . It is evident in work in our laboratory that there is no simple relationship between stimulus and subjective response. It is also made evident that the reason for this is the interposition of conditioning, of the processing component, of the psychic reaction. It is clear that this component merits and must have extensive consideration. It must be taken into account not only for pain but for all subjective responses.*

There is evidence to suggest that a reasonably broad or normal conditioning history is important to the mere perception of pain. Melzack described responses to pain stimuli in dogs reared under conditions of extreme isolation:

> We were surprised to find that when these dogs grew up they failed to respond normally to a flaming match. Some of them repeatedly poked their noses into the flame and sniffed at it as long as it was present. If they snuffed it out, they reacted similarly to a second flaming match and even to a third. Others did not sniff at the match but made no effort to get away when we touched their noses with the flame repeatedly. These dogs also endured pinpricks with

---

*From Beecher, H. K.: Measurement of subjective responses: quantitative effects of drugs, New York, 1959, Oxford University Press, p. x.

little or no evidence of pain. In contrast, littermates that had been reared in a normal environment recognized potential harm so quickly that we were usually unable to touch them with the flame or pin more than once.°

Thus it appears that receptivity or the readiness to perceive and respond to pain in the expected manner itself requires experience. Sternbach (1963) considered this issue in a different way. He studied records of people born without the ability to feel pain. Typically, such people learned at a far less rapid and effective rate than normal people to avoid hazardous, tissue-threatening stimuli. Burns, severe bruises, and major wounds were often sustained because of the absence of the pain experience as a moderating influence on behavior.

Prior experience, reflected in the cortical elements in receptivity, perception, and, later in the sequence, response, enter in in yet several other ways. Consider the matter of attention. We are capable of focusing our attention or perceptual processes on certain kinds of incoming sensory information, to the exclusion of other inputs. When that happens we are said to be attending selectively. Selective attention may occur as a more or less voluntary matter, as when one concentrates on a single subject, or it may occur as a consequence of the arrival of interest-arousing, attention-demanding stimuli. The hypnotic trance state is generally considered to be another, and extreme, form of attentional focus, one in which the person in the trance state is capable of exercising extraordinary selectivity of attention.

The psychological or cortical process of attention may exert considerable influence on the perception of pain stimuli, as well as on the ensuing responses or pain behaviors. Kanfer and Goldfoot (1966) studied tolerance for the cold pressor test (immersion of arm in icy water), under varying conditions of attention. The experimental groups showing the most tolerance were one that was

distracted by being required to view and describe slides during the experiment and another that produced distraction by watching a clock to time their tolerance. This study confirms with formal data what is already well recognized, that presentation of attention-demanding stimuli can provide an effective distraction effect, thereby diminishing the perception of pain.

Selectivity of attention is itself subject to influence by prior experience or learning effects. People are capable of constituting or reconstituting in symbolic form anticipated or imagined events through fantasy or thinking. Daydreaming is one obvious example. One may exercise selective attention in an active sense by deciding to think about or fantasize some state of affairs. What is thought about will reflect the effects of prior experience. One may think about something that was pleasant when previously thought about or actually experienced. Thinking about it now yields again some of the pleasantness. The pleasantness may be direct, or it may be only that the distraction of thinking about the subject is less unpleasant than what one was experiencing moments before. The fantasy or thinking-about-something-else is in this case a way of escaping or avoiding the pain stimulus. The benefit that it yields may lead to continued repetition, a learning or conditioning effect.

Whether attentional mechanisms are actively employed to seek direct reinforcement through pleasant experience or function as escape or avoidance tactics, they are likely to be influenced further by actions of those around the person. The chronic pain patient often displays a preoccupation with pain and other major or minor somatic signals. Much of his or her thought or attention seems riveted to the subject of the pain. When that occurs, there would appear to be two logical alternative explanations. One is that the pain stimulus is so ever present and compelling as to command the patient's attention to it, to the relative exclusion of other ongoing events. Support for this alternative requires evidence that the body damage factor is active, noxious, compelling, and

---

°From Melzack, R.: The perception of pain, Sci. Am. 204:41-42, Feb., 1961.

incessant. An alternative explanation is that the preoccupation itself leads to positive reinforcement. Thinking about the pain presumably does not avoid the pain experience and so cannot be rewarding in this sense. But thinking about the pain may generate or lead to certain other effects in the immediate environment that are themselves more pleasant or rewarding.

Meldman (1970) examines the whole process of illness and disease in attentional terms. One aspect that he deals with is the interactions between people, which, in attentional terms, he labels as attender-attendee relationships. In mature interpersonal exchanges, each participant is capable of shifting from one of these roles to the other, and frequently does so. The person who is preoccupied with illness, as in chronic pain, however, tends to remain excessively in the attendee role. That is, by his actions, he casts others into the role of attender, of paying attention to him and of acting in ways that support his attention-seeking behaviors. This perspective is an example that illustrates the effects of learning or experience on attentional behavior. In the context of chronic pain, it illustrates how displays of pain behaviors may elicit systematic effects in the environment that reward or sustain the pain behaviors. It is but one of a number of ways to illustrate how cortical or experiential factors can and do play a major role in shaping the ongoing behavior of pain patients. This matter will be considered in much greater detail at several later points in this book when dealing with relationships between the occurrence of pain behaviors, on the one hand, and the responses of family, physicians, and others, on the other.

The effects of attentional factors on pain also enter into the picture in a passive sense. That is, regardless of whether one's attention is focused on pain or on something else, exposure to distracting stimulation may seize attention and thereby reduce the pain experience. Conversely, exposure to reduced distraction may increase the pain experience, as when the lights are out and one is trying to fall asleep.

Set or anticipation is another aspect of attention that is capable of influencing whether and how pain is experienced. The matter of set may enter in in several ways and will receive further consideration later in this chapter in the context of placebo effects and hypnosis. The point should be made here that what one is set to experience, the anticipation of what is to follow, can itself modulate considerably the nature of the ensuing experience. This is illustrated by Nesbitt and Schacter (1966), who studied the effects of instructional set on pain detection and pain thresholds and on tolerance of painful shock. Subjects were led to believe that the study concerned determination of shock levels appropriate for electroconvulsive therapy. Subjects were given a placebo pill. Half were told the pill would produce side effects approximating emotional arousal; the other half that the side effects would be unlike arousal. Pain detection and thresholds proved to be comparable in the two groups. However, the group *expecting* arousal side effects from the placebo showed reliably higher tolerance for suprathreshold electric shocks. The effects of instructional set were so great that subjects even failed to attribute their arousal symptoms to the shock but instead to the anticipated effect of the placebo. These results show that there can be significant influence on both perception and response to clearly painful stimuli as a function of how one labels what is expected.

The studies cited deal with situations that have two important characteristics potentially differentiating them from chronic clinical pain. One is that there is a known stimulus readily identifiable as to type, timing, and intensity. The stimulus is a given in the studies, and it is the responses that are observed. In clinical pain, in contrast, the stimulus may be identified only by inference or speculation. It is far from a given fact. A second difference in these studies concerns the social context in which they occur. Experimental pain subjects were aware that they were engaged in a time-limited research enterprise that might be noxious or painful but that would not pose a threat to the maintenance of their way of life. As a result, only limited aspects of previous life experiences were evoked by the experimental conditions. Which aspects were evoked varied according to the instructional set of the particular study, but it would be a mistake to consider the studies as having characterized the limits of the role of cortical and social factors in pain perception and response.

These reservations are voiced particularly at this point because the subject of the measurement of pain will now be considered. It will receive additional consideration further along. The study of cortical input on pain perception and pain response is necessarily shaped and limited by the response parameters measured. If one could but settle on a set of responses that met the criterion of reproducibility or reliability and that could be systematically correlated with stimulus conditions, the study of pain would be eased no end. But regardless of whether the study is experimental and exercises considerable regulation over the noxious stimulus, or whether it is clinical and must contend with the complex social context and interaction of a hurting patient and a health care professional, the elements of set, attention, experience, and so on will intrude to attenuate the correlation between stimulus and response.

The emergence of signal detection measurement for experimental study of pain has been a most productive step. Green and Swets (1966), in the context of psychophysical measurement of pain, outlined procedures by which one can isolate response bias of the individual from his own stimulus discrimination performance. This work is tangential to our objectives and so will only be touched on. The major point about signal detection theory here is that it illustrates how subject response can carry obfuscating bias, even at the level of psychophysical measurement in experimental situations that provide stimuli of relatively known characteristics. Signal detection theory is demonstrably useful in controlling bias effects. Its utility is in the special case in which the observational setting provides precision stimulus measurement, as well as response measurement. The position taken here is that signal detection methods are not sufficient to deal with the measurement problems of the clinical setting.

One who would measure pain is often attracted to the use of nonverbal mediated responses, such as physiological indicators. They seem as if they would be less subject to measurement distortion. Hilgard (1969) and his colleagues have addressed themselves to relationships between verbal report and physiological indicators of pain, using hypnosis as one of the key experimental variables. Sachs (1970), as part of this work, measured both subjective report and simultaneously observed physiological measures under conditions of hypnotically induced analgesia and, separately, generalized suggestions of relaxation. He found that hypnotic analgesia changed both the verbal pain report and the nonverbal, physiological measure of blood pressure, although it changed the former much more than the latter. In contrast, under general relaxation, the two remained correlated. He thus demonstrated that it is possible to produce both changes in and significant differences between these two sets of pain measures, subjective report and blood pressure, under conditions of hypnosis. Hilgard (1969) has shown that verbal report measures yielded finer stimulus discriminations and were more systematically correlated with stimulus variations than the physiological measures. So, in still another way, it has been shown that a pain measure has not yet been found that functions free of verbal mediation and that bypassing verbal measures in favor of physiological ones does not necessarily lead to more precise measurement. This work is another indication of the importance of cortical factors in observable indications of pain.

A definitive measure of pain is not offered here, although specific measurement methods will be described later on. The point for the moment is that analysis of the role cortical and subcortical factors play in pain perception and response indicates that these factors cannot somehow be circumvented or controlled by settling on nonverbal mediated measures. Nor, in the instance of persisting clinical pain occurring in vivo, under conditions in which there cannot be precise stimulus identification and measurement, can such sophisticated measurement strategies as signal detection theory clear away the response biasing effects of attitudinal, subcortical, cortical, and experiential elements. It would be nice if they could.

Placebo and hypnosis effects have been touched on. They both require a bit more detail. Beecher (1959, p. 169) studied, among others, such unambiguous types of problems as postoperative wound pain. He noted that about 75% of such patients received significant relief from morphine but that 35% also received approximately comparable relief from placebos (for example, saline solution or sugar), suggesting that about half the effect of morphine may be a placebo effect. The Nesbitt and Schacter (1966) study cited earlier in relation to instructional set also illustrated a placebo effect on tolerance for experimentally produced electric shock. Clark and Hunt (1971) discussed the work of Hass and co-workers (1959), who reported that placebo effects produced relief of infections and rashes and changes in such physiological observables as corticosteroid levels. Precisely how placebos have their effect is not clear, and, of course, it may be a family of effects and not simply one. There appear to be two lines of evidence that bear on this and that are of concern here. One derives from work with hypnosis, the other from studies manipulating instructional set and experimental situational variables. The concern at this point is with the broader issue of cortical factors influencing pain response, and so instructional set and hypnosis can be brought into the discussion.

A study by McGlashan and associates (1969) compared groups of subjects of high and low hypnotic susceptibility. Both groups worked under conditions of control, anal-gesic-hypnosis, and placebo. They produced ischemic pain in each subject. The question was, Under which of the three conditions was pain threshold more greatly influenced? The findings were that the hypnotically nonsusceptible subjects showed a rise in pain threshold under hypnotic analgesia but only equal to their rise under placebo. They did not show a rise under the control condition. Hypnotically susceptible subjects showed a marked rise in pain threshold under hypnosis, greater than the rise under placebo. They interpreted their results as suggesting that two factors were operating. One was the instructional set or demand characteristics of the situation in which all subjects were influenced by placebo and by hypnotic-induced analgesia but not by control conditions. The second was that the subjects susceptible to hypnosis were significantly further influenced by trance induction. Thus the relatively simple or discrete element of pain threshold also shows itself to be vulnerable to cortical and subcortical influence.

There have been a number of studies that indicate that mere information that the research concerns pain or that the experimental pain stimuli presented can be anticipated as of high or of low intensity will influence the rate and magnitude of subjects' response and of pain threshold. The effect of subject expectation or the demand characteristics of the situation can be so great that subjects can be brought by instructional set to deliver to others highly painful and even tissue-threatening levels of shock or experimental pain.

Clearly, there is an abundance of evidence to indicate that the current set or expectation of the individual receiving a potentially pain-producing stimulus, or even anticipating that he might receive such a stimulus, can produce pain-related responses or behaviors of compelling magnitude and persuasiveness. The distortion effect is capable of working to increase or to decrease threshold and reported intensity of pain, according to the design of the study. As noted before, the problem with pain is that it happens to people, and people are complicated. It is small wonder that the clinician, confronted with a compelling display of pain by his patient on the one hand and ambiguous or speculative diagnostic data alleging to account for the pain displays on the other, may experience uncertainty and frustration in his efforts to gain secure measurement. The data with which he must deal originate primarily in the form of a verbal report from the patient. During formulation by the patient, the verbal report will have been exposed to an array of potentially influential factors. If there was a noxious stimulus at the periphery, with what fidelity was it perceived? The status of the gate on transmission to the central nervous system is a factor to consider. There is the distinct possibility that the stimulus-perception correlation will have been attenuated significantly. Add the ongoing cortical or mental activity of the patient, including prior experience and perceptions of what is expected or appropriate in the diagnostic interpersonal transaction, and the picture becomes more clouded.

There are a number of lines of evidence illustrating that anxiety and depression can also be expected to play roles in the perception of and response to pain. Merskey and Spear (1967), for example, compared medical and psychiatric populations with medical patient subgroups displaying chronic pain. Their data show that pain patients differed from patient controls reporting no pain in many ways. They were older, more neurotic, had poorer marital and sexual adjustments, tended to have more hostile feelings, and had histories of more painful experiences, to name a few. The sufferer identifies what is experienced as pain when it may, at least in part, be some other form of emotional distress. That is not surprising. In childhood, pain is usually associated with injury or illness and with punishment. The former is a threat to the body and thereby produces anxiety or fear as well as pain. The latter produces a sense of alienation from parental authority and therefore a sense of loss of love. These associations between pain, on the one hand, and anxiety or loss of love (a form of depressive feelings), on the other,

occur repeatedly during childhood. The opportunities for learning are ample. The nature of associative processes are such that when one member of the class of responses or feelings of distress (for example, anxiety, depression, or pain) is elicited by adequate stimulation, other members of the response class may also be experienced.

The person suffering from whichever stimulus and emotional state response is being experienced could find it difficult to discriminate which stimuli are present. In effect, what is felt is depression or anxiety, or whatever the case may be. The precise stimuli eliciting the distress may not be so clear. What is perceived as pain arising from suspected body damage may instead be anxiety relating to some status threat. This kind of misidentification of the precise character of one's distress can become more complete and persistent if the subsequent behavior of the sufferer effectively minimizes distress or leads to other positive effects. Here, then, is yet another element of ongoing cortical activity, in this case emotional state, that complicates efforts to understand why a patient signals he is experiencing pain. The interplay of pain and emotional problems will receive considerably more examination in the next chapter in the course of an analysis of psychogenic pain.

There is one more thread of data that bears on chronic pain: the matter of cultural patterns and cultural training. The repertoire of each of us is capable of being influenced profoundly by those around us. People in the rural South, when they speak, do not sound like residents of New England, or vice versa. The accents, rates of speech, and tonal inflections have been modeled by the immediate environment in which the person was raised. The topic of modeling is dealt with further in Chapter 3.

Let a man raised in New England marry a woman raised in the rural South. Let that new family unit settle in the Bronx to raise children. The voice sounds of these children will likely be discriminable from those heard typically in New England, the South, or the Bronx. Lasting exposure to and shaping by a voice-shaping environment containing elements of each will have their effects. In similar vein, one finds cultural modeling effects on pain expression. The impact of modeling appears not to be strong, producing effects markedly specific to the culture involved, except in certain extreme and culturally isolated situations. Christopherson (1966, p. 2) quotes from a novel by Ruesch describing polar Eskimos as responding to pain with laughter, "even when one's arm is being mangled by a polar bear." This illustration and others have been reported from relatively isolated cultures, describing pain responses markedly contrasting with prevailing Western experience. For the most part, however, studies making cultural comparisons have yielded only modest and sometimes inconsistent differences among subcultures in regard to pain display. The fact that these differences appear to increase as a function of cultural discreteness from our reference norms suggests that the people around us, by their behavior and their responses to our behavior, indeed have a significant effect on our pain displays. The magnitude of the effect, however, as will be considered in some detail later when focusing on social reinforcement, probably depends a great deal on the consistency and intensity of these responses of others. Had the progeny of the New England/South marriage been raised in rural Arkansas where, except for one parent, all those around spoke in similar style, the loading of Arkansas environmental feedback on speech and language would have been more consistent and intense. The accents of the children, although probably carrying elements of New England, almost certainly would be heavily laden with the influence of Arkansas.

There is another way to consider the influence of cultural factors on pain perception and response in addition to impact of cultural modeling. There is the matter of probable experience. The athlete engaged in such explosively violent contact sports as professional football is not likely to display expressions of pain after each collision with a muscular opponent. He will have been involved in the subculture of football for many years. He will have evolved any number of counter-stimulant procedures to help with gate closure. He will, as well, have had years of repeated exposure to the selective responses of those around him to displays of pain and nonpain after vigorous collisions. The social consequences to open displays of debilitating pain will have been nonreinforcing, to say the least. The football subculture supports nonpain displays after impact and actively discourages pain displays. The experienced football player has both set and expectation to influence perception of the noxious stimulus, and he has the social training provided by his subculture regarding pain response. The point is also made in a study reported by Clark and Mehl (1971). Using signal detection theory methods to factor out response bias from stimulus perception, they studied the criterion for pain of older subjects. These subjects consistently required stronger stimulation from radiant heat before reporting pain, although the data indicated there was no reduction in ability to perceive the stimulation as such. They concluded that older people may develop definitions of what constitutes pain that are different from younger subjects. They went on to consider that this difference may reflect such factors as the relationship of the pain stimulus to various currently active body distresses attendant to old age or the different meaning of pain to one who has experienced it numerous times, or both.

This chapter has been concerned with developing a historical and data base perspective on factors influencing the sensation and perception of pain. The evidence clearly indicates that a host of factors can operate to attenuate the correlation between arrival of ordinarily adequate noxious stimuli at effective sensory receptors and the sequence of events that follows, including inferences by observers that the person receiving the noxious stimuli is experiencing pain. The report by a patient or experimental subject of pain that is experienced does not provide a sure basis for inferring there is or is not a currently active noxious stimulus by which to account for some or all of the reported pain.

In the course of the chapter it has been essential to consider cortical factors influencing sensation and perception of pain, as well as the ensuing responses. This subject, however, opens Pandora's box of personality, motivation, and so-called psychogenic pain. Since the concern of the book is chronic clinical pain, Pandora's box must indeed be opened, if only a little. That will follow in the next chapter.

2 Psychogenic pain

The work reviewed in the preceding chapter was based almost solely on studies of experimental pain. Experimental and clinical pain have many important differences. One key difference is that experimental pain works with a pain stimulus of known characteristics. It is the responses to that stimulus that are the center of attention. They are studied in the context of, for example, subject characteristics, instructional set, or the like. Schematically it is a stimulus-response paradigm. Given the pain stimulus and the particular defining interests of the study (old-young, male-female, medication-placebo, special instructional sets), pain responses or behaviors are measured.

The situation is different in the clinical setting. The given or known facts are limited at the outset to the report that pain is being experienced. The diagnostic enterprise then works backward (relative to the situation with experimental pain) to try to identify the stimulus.

When diagnostic efforts fail to reveal a convincing relationship between reported pain and a body damage or noxious stimulus condition, the working diagnosis frequently becomes "psychogenic pain." But the concept of psychogenic pain is complex and often misleading. Issues about it are central to this book, so they will be considered in some detail.

There are other and equally important differences between experimental pain studies and clinical settings concerned with chronicity. The concept of pain tolerance is illustrative. It is one thing to sit in a laboratory, one's hand immersed in icy water or with a dolorometer beating its heat onto the blackened forehead, knowing that the scene is time-limited. It is a different matter to experience persisting pain, if even for but a

few minutes or hours, without being able to determine whether or when that pain will abate. The time dimension to pain tolerance as it relates to chronic pain cannot be dealt with realistically by experimental pain studies.

The contrast between experimental and chronic clinical pain becomes even greater when one considers two additional elements to the time dimension. When a patient's pain problem has persisted, not for seconds or minutes, but for months and years, the process becomes vulnerable to the effects of learning or conditioning. It is premature to deal with that point in any depth here. It is a central part of later chapters. It suffices for the moment to repeat that chronicity ensures learning trials, that is, the opportunity for learning or conditioning to occur. It remains to be determined for each case whether and in what form learning effects will be displayed. It seems clear, however, that the opportunity for learning effects to become significant is an inherent part of chronic pain.

Finally, when pain persists, the effects the pain has on patient performance, or ability to do things, will begin to touch and to interact with the patient's way of life. The experimental pain subject is not likely to leave the laboratory and face a job or an evening of study or a weekend of recreation influenced in any discernible degree by whatever pain was experienced during the course of the pain study. In contrast, the chronic pain patient's job, marital interactions, recreational activities, even aspirations and life plans, may come face-to-face with the pain and whatever debilitating effects it has. Interactions between the patient's expressions of pain and indications of functional impairment associated with it, and the immediate environment, may influence yet further the course of the problem. Pain and its effects may pose a threat to job survival. The associated anxiety and tension may increase pain, or they may decrease pain via distracting and counter-stimulation effects, to cite but two possibilities. The way in which those around the patient respond to his displays of pain will have an influence, as well, a point that will be explored later.

One way to summarize some of the major differences between experimental and clinical pain is to note that experimental pain subjects are usually lifted out of the natural environment, installed in the special environment of the laboratory, and then exposed to the special conditions of the pain study. One of the by-products of that relative detachment from the natural environment is the experimenter's ability to exercise degrees of control over and have knowledge about the interplay of experimental subjects and the pain conditions. The clinician, faced with diagnosing a chronic pain problem, is dealing with a patient embedded in the natural environment. All of the ongoing concerns and events, which will be reflected in cortical activity, can influence the exchanges of information essential to the diagnostic process. These factors can and do blur the picture. When physical findings do not mesh closely with pain displays, some clarifying alternative explanation is sought. The diagnostician often turns to the concept of psychogenic pain in an effort to account for the blurred picture.

The term *psychogenic pain* is often used in two rather different ways, and the user is not always clear as to whether he is using one, the other, or a mixture of the two. The broad use of the term is an attempt to label or identify situations in which there is or appears to be a discrepancy between displays of pain behavior (Fordyce and associates, 1968, 1973; Sternbach and Fordyce, 1975) and observations about the probable cause of that behavior in the form of peripheral nociceptive stimuli. For example, a subject's hand may be placed in icy water. After a period of time the subject

withdraws the hand and thereby signals that he or she is experiencing pain or distress. The observer is aware of the noxious stimulus of icy water, and, judging the timing and magnitude of the pain behavior as appropriate or as adequately correlated with the stimulus, concludes that the pain behavior displayed is not psychogenic. If, however, the water is not icy but tepid, and a given subject suddenly withdraws the hand after a decent period of immersion, the observer concludes that some intracortical and therefore psychic phenomenon accounts for the pain behavior of hand withdrawal. The correlation between noxious stimulus and pain behavior is inferred to be low. The pain behavior is to be accounted for in some other fashion, namely, psychic. It is psychogenic pain. The referent for that use of the term is only the inferred or observed low stimulus-response correlation. The use only labels a discrepancy. It explains nothing.

The second use of psychogenic pain is more specific and goes beyond the first. When a patient is inferred or observed to display pain behaviors that appear not to be consonant with currently active noxious stimulation acting on peripheral receptors, the discrepancy may be considered in terms of some alleged underlying personality or motivational problem. A patient may be seen, for example, as displaying a conversion reaction, or as having a hysteric-type personality. This use of the concept of psychogenic pain adds to the observations about stimulus-response discrepancies (observed or inferred) some attempts to explain the discrepancies in terms of a particular view of human functioning.

When one reviews the clinical records of long-standing clinical pain patients, it is apparent that the term psychogenic pain is often used. Moreover, it is used in both of the ways described above but with the user not always being clear as to which.

As Sternbach and Fordyce (1975) point out, when the term psychogenic is added to comments about pain, the user is embarking on an attempt to explain events and not simply to describe them. Even in the more cautious first use of the term described above, there is the implication that the mind is exercising control over pain behaviors. The pain behaviors are the events. Adding psychogenic brings into the picture cause-and-effect and mind-body dualism concepts. Naming something psychogenic does not *establish* that there is a cause-effect relationship, much less establish that the cause has been adequately explained.

The more ambitious second use of psychogenic, in which the user seeks to place us within the context of a particular conceptualization of behavior or personality functioning, indeed carries a heavy load. Not only is it laden with problems of mind-body dualism and cause-effect, but it also must be concerned with the conceptual and empirical adequacy of its particular descriptive framework of patient functioning. Such an important matter cannot be accepted uncritically.

The whole matter of psychogenic pain is a central issue for this book. The frequent misuse of the term and the unvalidated assumptions that often accompany its use can and too frequently do lead to a failure to understand the nature of a patient's pain problem. As a consequence, treatment may go down blind alleys.

It is when the medical diagnostic process fails to reveal a correlation of convincing magnitude between tissue damage stimulus and pain behavior responses that the psychogenic diagnosis is entertained. Thus, initially, it is a diagnosis by exclusion. The data are that pain behavior is occurring in the relative or total absence of demonstrable body damage or noxious stimulation. The apparent explanation, however, is in terms of some personality function intruding to cause the pain behavior.

To quote Sternbach and Fordyce (1975, p. 122), "the essence of the problem lies in assuming that there are real mental and physical events which can and do interact. In fact, there are simply phenomena which we describe in physical language or mental language; we delude ourselves to believe

that because we can impose both mental and physical concepts on such an abstraction as 'pain,' that, in fact, such a causative sequence exists."

It is well established and was amply documented in Chapter 1 that there are many reasons why the linkage between pain behaviors and antecedent stimuli may be loose, sometimes to the point of obscurity. The current state of the gate—open, closed, or partially closed—as a function of the amount of stimulation of A fibers is but one example. It is apparent that any mix of a number of ongoing cortical states or activities is capable of influencing whether pain is signalled and whether such displays, when they occur, were preceded by stimulation from body damage. Let us now examine the matter of the pain stimulus-pain behavior linkage in the clinical context.

Sternbach (1968, p. 13) has said, "In order to describe pain, it is necessary for the patient to do something . . . in order for us to determine that he is experiencing pain." There must be some form of pain behavior. Diagnostic inferences and treatment judgments lean heavily on interpersonal communications from the patient. He says he hurts. He grimaces or moans. He flinches when put through certain motions or into certain positions. He describes the quality and quantity of the pain he is experiencing. He asks for analgesics. Those forms of social communications are readily subject to many distortions. Lasagna (1960) has stated, "the investigator who would study pain is at the mercy of the patient, upon whose ability and willingness to communicate he is dependent." In similar vein, Kast and Collins (1966) commented, "In judging the intensity of pain by verbal exchange, one must be willing to accept the premise that the descriptive terms applied to degree of pain refer to definite quantities. However, it is not known that these degrees of pain are elicited by the same sensory input in different individuals." It belabors the obvious to conclude that what the patient says about the pain, whatever the diagnostician's impressions about his or her candor and honesty, is to be considered useful but by no means definitive information. Clinically, chronic pain is necessarily viewed initially through the prism of patient pain behaviors.

Chapter 1 considered in theoretical terms some of the factors involving cortical or mental processes that may influence patient descriptions of the experience of pain, even when there may be only modest or no stimulation arising peripherally from body damage. Emotional factors and prior emotional conditioning are important as potentially obfuscating elements in the diagnosis of pain. They require more detailed consideration than the overview of Chapter 1.

Much of the data that bear on this subject are analyses of case material by psychotherapists, usually psychoanalysts, of patients characterized as displaying much psychogenic pain. Case reviews and discussions, and in some instances more formal measurement data, may be found in Engel (1959), Kolb (1954), Szasz (1957), Tinling and Klein (1966), and Janis (1958). Janis's work is in relation to surgical patients. Melzack and Chapman (1973), Sternbach and co-workers (1973), and Sternbach and Fordyce (1975) also provide discussions of these matters.

Taken together, these studies arrive at fairly consistent inferences, which enhance confidence in their findings. They appear also to concur with other work reported, as will be noted.

There is agreement that the report of pain is, for the patient, a real experience, one that he can describe with detail and specificity. Subjectively, he hurts. It is usually not a difficult process to elicit from such patients associations to and recollections of earlier pain experiences, particularly those experienced in childhood.

The pattern that emerges in these childhood associations about pain is to relate them to injury, illness, or punishment. When children experience illness or injury, depending on its severity and on concurrent distress levels of whatever origin, they are likely also to experience some degree of threat to survival or to the restoration of function of an injured body part. By the nature of things, this association between pain relating to illness or injury and anxiety is likely to occur a number of times during maturation. And, of course, some children experience it more frequently than others. There may be more illness or injury, or these may be more severe or more lingering. The more frequent, severe, or lingering illnesses may also have produced more anxiety. An alternative pattern is for a child's anxiety levels to be high or persisting, for whatever reason, and that he or she is exposed to illness or injury. In either case, the learning trials will have been repetitive, intense, or both.

Anxiety, psychodynamically, may be seen as based on a fear of body harm or a fear of loss of love. When either is experienced, as is inevitably the case for at least some limited time intervals during childhood, the affect of anxiety may be accompanied by the affect of depression, that is, a sense of loss. Depression, as a sense of loss, occurs also in later life when there is a loss of body function through trauma or illness or a waning of function through aging. Similarly, depression may follow loss of some source of positive reinforcement from the environment, as when one suddenly loses a job or a marital partner. These emotional states are likely to have had at least some early occurrences in conjunction with pain.

The situation in regard to punishment is more direct than for anxiety but yields the same effect. The punished child probably will experience at least momentary concern that he is rejected by or alienated from his parents, as well as whatever physical discomfort or pain was evoked by the form of punishment used. The sense of alienation from parents may lead to depressive affect and to further momentarily the guilt feelings probably already aroused by the misdeed that led to the punishment. The more frequent or severe the punishment, the more intense and enduring may be the depressive feelings and the pain. When, after punishment, there is reassurance or restoration of nonstressful communication with parents, the depression and the guilt are relieved concomitant with the naturally occurring reduction of pain. This pattern promotes punishment, and perhaps pain, as a cue to be followed by the reduction of guilt. The opportunities for learning or association between the affective distress and pain and between both of these and reduction of guilt are readily available. The more fraught with conflict, punishment, and sense of alienation from the parents has been the childhood, the more learning of these associations can be expected. That finding, as noted in Chapter 1 in reference to the work of Merskey and Spear (1967), has been demonstrated at least in part in formal empirical studies as well as in case analysis data. Chronic pain patients tend to report childhoods more fraught with pain experiences and with conflicts than do non-pain patients. Studies using the Minnesota Multiphasic Personality Inventory (MMPI) by Pilling and associates (1967) report comparable findings. They compared medical and surgical patients having physical complaints who were referred for psychiatric consultation because of the absence of physical findings. Some of them had the complaint of pain as part of the symptom picture, and others did not. The patients reporting pain showed greater elevations on the hypochondriasis and hysteria scales than the patients reporting other body problems but not pain. Measures of psychic distress (anxiety and depression) were elevated in both groups.

Pilowsky (1967) further analyzed hypochondriasis. He identified three major dimensions: "bodily preoccupation," "disease phobia," and "conviction of the presence of disease with nonresponse to reassurance." Such characterizations fit aptly with the clinical picture of chronic pain, where there are minimal organic findings. Sternbach and co-workers (1973) also have reported indications of pervasive depression in many chronic pain patients. Their findings indicated that acute and chronic pain patients, with or without physical findings, showed markedly elevated depression scale scores on the MMPI.

Depression as an emotional state appears to bear special relationships and importance to the effect of reinforcement/nonreinforcement, as well as to chronic pain. It will therefore receive additional consideration in the following chapter after a foundation of reinforcement principles has been presented.

Yet another affect or emotion, anger, should be added to the picture. It is reasonable to expect and is confirmed by these clinical studies that the child who receives punishment may experience anger or hostility toward the source of his distress. The anger cannot prudently be expressed directly, for to do so would elicit further punishment and pain. The anger may be withheld. Clinically, withheld anger is observed often to lead to depressive and guilt feelings or to muscle tension or headaches, often to both. When, in the course of events, communication and rapport are reestablished with the punishing parent, the anger, tension, guilt, and depressive feelings are likely to diminish but not disappear altogether. The finding of greater hostile feelings as yet another characteristic of chronic pain patients was reported by Merskey and Spear (1967).

There is the risk of a snowballing or vicious cycle effect when these kinds of problems arise in childhood. The frequently anxious or depressed child can be expected to be correspondingly less effectively involved in normal relationships. The net result is greater preoccupation with inner events: depression, anxiety, and so on. This, too, promotes relative alienation from the social world and correspondingly greater likelihood of more anxiety and depression. Later in life, these disturbed feelings may lead the person to seek psychiatric assistance. For others, however, and, one would expect, particularly those for whom the anxiety and depression occurred more commonly in juxtaposition to pain, the preoccupation with internal states may focus more on body sensations. The focus of interest on pain and body sensation may also be reinforcing. Depending on parental styles, displays of pain and body distress by the child may elicit more supportive or positive parental response. In other parents, of course, that may not be true. When it is the pattern, it would appear to be the breeding ground for hypochondriasis and the often encountered readiness of chronic pain patients to focus their attention virtually exclusively on pain and body distress. To do so has been and to some degree continues to be reinforcing.

These psychodynamic analyses of patients who display much so-called psychogenic pain should be understood also as analyses of learning opportunities.

Anxiety, depression, guilt, anger or hostility, and pain have been considered. It has been shown how in the natural state of things, they are likely to occur together during maturation. Moreover, it has been shown how they are likely to be reduced or eliminated concomitantly. To some degree, then, they may be elicited together in some combination, and the events that terminate one or more may also serve to terminate or reduce the others. It is small wonder that they often appear to be associated.

In learning terms, these emotions or subjective feeling states can be seen as members of a single response class, the general term for which could be labelled distress. The members of the class share elements of feeling states and common stimuli capable of eliciting them. They also share circumstances in the environment or in interpersonal communication that may alter or reduce the distress. It is therefore to be expected that cues or stimuli that elicit one member of the class can be expected to be capable of eliciting any mix of the other members. In addition, cues, actions, or events that lead to alteration or reduction of one may lead to alteration of another. For example, some cue (that is, some social stimulus or environmental event) that elicits anxiety in a given person might also elicit the sensation of pain. Either anxiety or pain, or both, may be experienced. The person may not discriminate between the two, nor will he necessarily discriminate whether the distress he feels is because of the environmental event eliciting anxiety or whether the distress relates to some anticipated source of pain. If he has a history of pain or a recent series of pain episodes, he may well confuse his distress experiences and feel pain, which he assumes is coming from his recent or long-active source of pain, when anxiety or fear would be a more appropriate response to the stimulus situation. Clark and Hunt (1971, p. 394) describe a vivid example of this phenomenon while studying experimental pain: ". . . the strongest verbal, autonomic, and skeletal response of pain ever emitted by one of the writers occurred when the radiant heat stimulus was misdirected at the wall instead of his arm; instead of the expected pain, there was a bright flash of light. The result was an extreme 'pain' response, after which he was forced to admit that absolutely no pain had been experienced." There had been a mental set to experience pain produced in this case by the fact they were engaged at the moment in observations of pain responses. An equally potent mental set could be expected in a person long besieged by pain. Anxiety occurs when he is anticipating pain, and so it is pain he feels and reports. In the Clark and Hunt example, it was easy subsequently to make the correct discrimination. But in the example of a chronic pain patient, that discrimination might not be so easy because the patient probably will have evolved certain protective actions taken when what he perceives to be pain is experienced, which yield at least some and perhaps much relief. Those protective actions may also reduce anxiety. When he feels the distress, he takes the protective action and thereby feels better. As will be considered in more depth later in the context of avoidance learning, each time this error of stimulus discrimination is followed by an effective action (that is, one which successfully reduces distress), it will be reinforced, and the discrimination error is thereby increasingly likely to recur. Thus there may be an error as to what stimulus is being encountered and perpetuation of the error because the response or action taken was helpful even though it was aimed at the wrong stimulus.

It is important to keep in mind that the process and the products of learning are automatic. If circumstances are favorable, learning will occur. That, in turn, means that cues or stimulus situations initially relating to anxiety or threat but now evoking pain (instead of or in addition to anxiety) will indeed produce a realistic experience of pain. There is nothing imaginary about it, nor is it reasonable to expect that the sufferer will be able reliably to discriminate. The pain he experiences is as real as the saliva of Pavlov's dog was wet.

Psychodynamic findings are comparable when there is a currently active and proportional noxious stimulus relating to body damage (that is, a physical source of pain) as shown by Janis (1958) in relation to surgical patients and by LeShan (1954) in relation to terminal cancer patients. That kind of patient, too, is likely to have a network of associations from earlier experiences that interrelates anxiety, depression, guilt, and anger with pain. When one member of the response class of distress is experienced, other members of the response class are also likely to occur. The power of learning or association is manifest regardless of whether one deals with demonstrable organic pathology. The terminal cancer patient, even while episodically bombarded with stimuli evocative of severe pain, is likely also to have other members of the distress response class elicited. He is also likely on occasion to fail to distinguish which stimulus is coming in and may behave in ways appropriate to pain when, at the moment, it may be cues or stimuli relating to depression or anxiety that are present.

The automatic character of learning and the natural likelihood that these various forms of distress may be associated and elicited by common stimuli does not, however, ensure a causal or functional relationship in any given instance. The demonstration of the presence of anxiety or depression or some such emotional disturbance, when the medical evaluation has failed to reveal an adequate organic stimulus, does not in itself permit the inference of psychogenic pain. It does make such an inference potentially tenable. Our clinical experience suggests a not inconsiderable number of people have anxiety or depression and also have pain for which initial medical diagnostic efforts fail to find the organic factor when it is there to be found. To state the point another way, if indeed one is to use the term psychogenic pain at all, it is not enough to find a stimulus-response discrepancy (that is, pain behavior with little or no identifiable organic stimulus) and to find that the patient has emotional problems. There needs to be, as well, some demonstration that the cues and responses associated with the emotional problems, but allegedly evoking reports of pain, have some systematic relationship to when pain does and does not occur. In short, a diagnosis of psychogenic pain is not to be reached by exclusion. It should be shown that displays of distress bear systematic relationships to environmental cues and consequences and not just that no organic basis can be found.

The immediately preceding review and discussion of the psychodynamics of pain and emotional states is intended to rationalize one important set of reasons why a patient may report that pain is experienced when the clinical evidence is that it is a misperception to infer that the source of distress is body damage. The distress experienced may instead relate to some emotional problem or the like. The emotional problem may have its genesis in the past, but it is cued into action by current events. A second objective of this section has been to open a challenge as to the adequacy and utility of the term psychogenic pain.

There are a number of assumptions underlying the diagnosis of psychogenic pain that need further examination. One of these is the assumption that the patient diagnosed as having psychogenic pain is different in other relevant ways from those patients for whom the tissue damage–pain response correlation is adequate. Further, those dif-

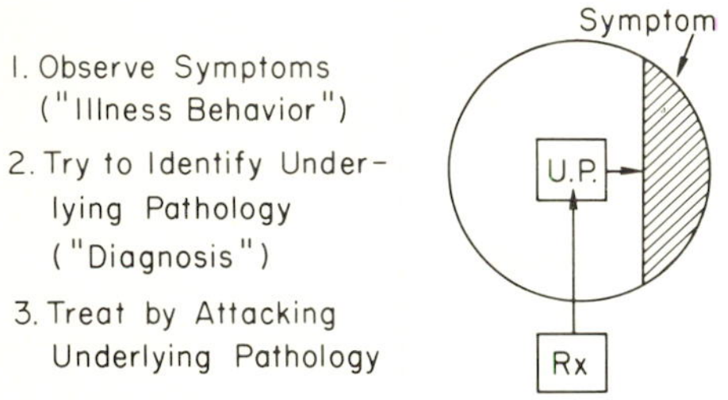

1. Observe Symptoms
   ("Illness Behavior")

2. Try to Identify Under-
   lying Pathology
   ("Diagnosis")

3. Treat by Attacking
   Underlying Pathology

Fig. 1. *Disease model.*

ferences, it is assumed, would bear a causal relationship to the displays of pain behavior. A second assumption is that it is the patient who should be examined and not the social interaction between patient and those around him, including the diagnostician. These assumptions will be examined separately.

The assumption that psychogenic pain, in the relative absence of tissue damage, is caused by and associated with some personality, motivational, or situational problem, appears to derive primarily from the continued use of a disease model perspective on pain (Fig. 1) as described by Fordyce and associates (1968, 1973). The essential characteristic of a disease model is that it assumes that the symptoms or illness events are under control of some form of underlying pathogenic factor. Although such a perspective was not always the predominant view of illness by medicine, it has been central to the diagnostic process for many decades. It has been a useful perspective in regard to the diagnosis and treatment of pain as well as innumerable other problems. It is, however, in the final analysis, a theory or descriptive system and not a statement of facts. The factual basis for such an approach to viewing and understanding chronic pain or any other condition must have an empirical foundation. If it is to be the sole perspective, it should also be required to establish that alternative approaches are not only less plausible but also empirically of clearly lesser merit. If it is the only approach one is going to use, the user had better be sure it is the best one available.

The long and honorable history of the disease model perspective in regard to illness, including chronic pain, need not be recounted. It is proposed, however, that a disease model perspective has two shortcomings in the context of chronic pain. One is that the signs, symptoms, or public displays of pain by patients are, as has been shown, subject to influence by a host of factors besides so-called underlying pathology. Displays of pain or pain behaviors are modulated to almost any conceivable degree by the intervening events of cortical activity and of prior experience or conditioning, of which the cortex is the repository. When pain behavior is displayed, it may mean that there is a peripheral stimulus arising from the body damage, but then again it may mean something different. Therefore, to limit oneself to the search for an antecedent pathogenic pain stimulus is to ignore numerous equally tenable alternatives.

The second problem with the disease model perspective in regard to chronic pain concerns the concept of psychogenic pain. As noted previously, it is usually the case that psychogenesis, as a provisional diagnosis, begins with finding—or seeming to find—an unacceptably low correlation between the quality, quantity, or location of reported pain and evidence of body damage or tissue pathology. When an organic explanation for the pain is found wanting, the alternative of psychogenic enters. But with the almost irresistible pull of a powerful magnet, the user of the term almost always begins to think in terms of personality disturbance, conversion reactions, and so on. Almost without thought, one falls into the path of thinking in mind-body dualism terms. But even more, one begins to think of underlying mental mechanisms, in the form of one or another kind of personality deviation, exerting causative control over displays of pain behaviors. If it is not physical, it must be mental. If it is mental, it must be some form of personality problem.

It is not argued here, as is apparent from the preceding section, that personality problems are not often present and central to many problems of chronic pain. The point for the moment is that it should not automatically be concluded that such problems are the *only* viable alternative to an organic cause. Nor should it be concluded that the demonstration of convincing relationships between personality problems and current displays of pain automatically indicates that treatment must change personality or inferred underlying motivational problems to succeed.

The assumption that displays of problem behavior are under control of underlying personality malfunctions of one sort or another is itself a use of the disease model perspective. It assumes both that the symptom behaviors are related to alleged underlying personality conflicts or problems *and* that, as with, for example, an infectious process, the underlying causative agent must be eliminated or modified before the symptoms will depart from the scene. There are solid grounds for questioning these assumptions.

For at least a decade now, there have been careful, reasoned, and empirically based challenges to the traditional psychodynamic or disease model–based view of human functioning or behavior. It is too much to expect that there be an exhaustive review here of the theoretical and empirical bases for calling into question the adequacy of traditional views of the role of personality factors in behavior. But these issues are so central to the whole matter of chronic pain and particularly of so-called psychogenic pain that they cannot be skirted completely. They will be dealt with as briefly as seems defensible.

Such authors as Albee (1966), Bandura and Walters (1963), and Ullmann and Krasner (1965), to name but a few, have pointed out that the disease model perspective, as described in Fig. 1, which won its spurs in the context of infectious processes, body injury, and the like, has been applied by *analogy* to other behaviors or actions of people, particularly to events or behaviors going under the general rubric of mental illness or emotional disturbance. Psychogenic pain is traditionally viewed as one example.

There are several bases for challenging that model as it relates to behavior generally. One is logical. The model has often proved useful and precise, although not always so, in regard to what might for the moment be called "physical illness." That does not ensure validity in regard to other kinds of problems. The adequacy of the disease model in regard to interpersonal behavior must be established empirically, not by analogy.

A second basis for challenge is empirical. Mischel (1968, p. 147) carried out an extensive review of empirical studies bearing on the subject. He says, in part, "The initial assumptions of trait-state theory were logical, inherently plausible, and also consistent with common sense and intuitive impressions about personality. Their real limitations turned out to be empirical—they simply have not been supported adequately." At another point he comments, "with the possible exception of intelligence, highly generalized behavioral consistencies have not been demonstrated, and the concept of personality traits as broad response dispositions is thus untenable" (Mischel, 1968, p. 146).

There are a number of other reviews of empirical data bearing on this issue (for example, Ullmann and Krasner [1965], Neuringer and Michael [1970]). There are also precision tests of the question in the form of empirical studies, a number of which are reported in Bandura and Walters (1963) and Krasner and Ullmann (1966).

The challenges come in another way as well. As noted previously, the disease model perspective, as it relates to interpersonal behavior, characteristically assumes both that the behaviors of interest are under control of or caused by underlying motivational or personality mechanisms and that change can be affected only by changing those alleged underlying mechanisms. This is, of course, another extension of the analogy drawn from disease; namely, treat the cause and not the symptom. Alternative treatment or behavior change approaches proceed from a different view. Rather than postulating control of behavior by underlying basic personality structures, they approach the behavior change process more directly. Gendlin and Rychlak, in reviewing some of these new approaches, state:

> The therapies written about tend to reject the older conception of maladjustment as a long-term illness needing long-term treatment . . . instead of deep dynamics, the therapies now tend to make the difficulty a mode of interaction . . . or behavior pattern which is to be knocked out, not by years of treatment, but simply by taking up some other mode of interaction. . . .*

It has proved practical in a wide variety of situations to approach interpersonal, social, behavioral, or so-called mental illness problems by the direct modification of behavior, without recourse first to modifying alleged underlying personality mechanisms or motivational patterns. The whole movement of behavior modification, which is now so prevalent, is based on that approach. The efficacy of these methods stands as a persuasive challenge to the adequacy of a disease model perspective in accounting for problem behavior. This is not to say that the concept of basic personality and of underlying motivation is without merit nor that traditional psychotherapies are not of value. The challenge, rather, is that the explanatory value of the traditional perspective warrants only partial acceptance. Moreover, the treatment strategies derived from it are not the only approaches to be considered, nor are their rationalizations as to why they have whatever effect they do have to be considered the only possible explanations. They may be right or partially right, but alternative explanations of their effects may work as well.

In a number of different ways it has been proposed that patients identified by traditional psychodynamic perspectives (or, simply, by a diagnostician concluding from observations of a pain stimulus–pain behavior response discrepancy that the problem must be psychogenic) are not neces-

sarily different from pain patients for whom the antecedent pain stimulus is found in relation to body damage. There are empirical data that support this proposition.

Woodforde and Merskey (1972) compared so-called organic and psychogenic pain patients with neurotic patients on a series of personality measures. There were no differences except that males with organic pain had more phobic and obsessive behavior, as reflected in the personality test scores. All groups, neurotic and pain, had increases in scores on neuroticism and depression.

Fordyce and associates (1975), studied Minnesota Multiphasic Personality Inventory (MMPI) scores of chronic pain patients previously arranged by physician clinical judgments along a continuum from organic to psychogenic and found no differences. Consistent with the Woodforde and Merskey data, these patients, organic and psychogenic, showed consistent elevations on measures of distress (scale 2: depression) and on measures of hypochondriasis and hysteria. Sternbach and co-workers (1974), also using the MMPI and studying low back pain patients, some of whom had physical findings while others did not, found the same results: elevations in hypochondriasis, depression, and hysteria scores, but no differentiation between organic and psychogenic.

Bond (1971) studied women with cervical cancer. Both those who did and those who did not report pain had elevated hypochondriacal scores, although patients with pain had significantly higher scores than those who were relatively pain free.

Each of these studies illustrates that when there is a report of chronic pain, there are likely to be increases in depression or psychic distress, hypochondriasis, hysteria, or other such neurotic measure scores. Further, the indications of increased emotional distress are approximately equally true of patients identified independently of the emotional or personality measures as organic or psychogenic.

These data must be interpreted cau-

---

*From Gendlin, E., and Rychlak, J.: Psychotherapeutic processes, Ann. Rev. Psychol. **21**:156, 1970.

tiously. There are other ways of trying to measure differences in personality or emotional status than those reported in these studies. Yet the burden of proof would appear to lie with those who assert that patients identified as having psychogenic pain are reliably and discriminably different from those whose pain is labelled as organic. The MMPI has a formidable record of reliability by itself and in comparison to other methods of personality measurement. The absence of evidence of reliable differences in personality measurement between organic and psychogenic, as reported in these studies, is not to be discounted lightly.

The major inference drawn here is not that organic and psychogenic pain patients have no differences. Instead, it is proposed that examining alleged underlying personality or motivational patterns is the wrong place to look for the critical differences. It is proposed that the differences are to be found in the systematic interactions between occurrences of pain behavior, on the one hand, and environmental cues and responses, on the other. That brings us to the second assumption about the use of the concept of psychogenic: that it is the patient who should be examined and not the social interaction between patient and those around him—including, of course, the physician who seeks to diagnose and treat.

Earlier in this chapter Mischel (1968, p. 146) was quoted to the effect that ". . . highly generalized behavioral consistencies have not been demonstrated, and the concept of personality traits as broad response dispositions is thus untenable." That is an extreme position, one which appears to overstate the case. But regardless of whether one agrees, it is not germane to the issue here to arrive at a precise judgment on the matter. What is central to the issue is whether immediate or perceived-as-impending environmental cues and events, as distinguished from the idea of personality traits or underlying motivations, exert significant influence on behavior. Our concern is with chronic pain. In that context, one can properly ask whether signals of pain (that is,

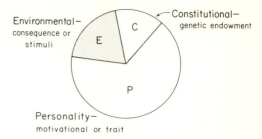

Fig. 2. *Behavior influence factors—motivational model.*

pain behaviors) that occur when physical findings are minimal are to be accounted for by the action of underlying personality or motivational mechanisms or in some other fashion.

The traditional psychodynamic view of the matter might be said to allocate sources of influence in somewhat the fashion shown in Fig. 2. The precise proportions are totally arbitrary; it is a schematic presentation.

Traditional analyses of personality or motivation recognize that genetic or personal endowment factors exercise some constraining influence on our behavior. They also recognize that behavioral sequences are triggered by cues (and also misperceptions) of the immediate environment. In the main, however, the thesis advanced is that it is basic personality structure that guides, shapes, or controls behavior. As noted previously, one common expectation derived from that perspective is that enduring behavior change *requires* change in underlying motivation or personality. It is the alleged underlying mechanisms that have the major role in the control of behavior.

One need not look beyond the context of chronic pain to develop an alternative. Skinner (1953) made the distinction between respondent and operant behavior. Work in more recent years (for example, Miller, 1969) suggests that many responses of the organism, human or animal, previously thought of as respondents, may instead have the functional character of operants. The question as to which actions or responses are respondent and which are operant remains open. However that may be, *why* they are distinguished from each other is important. Respondents are organism responses that are elicited by antecedent stimuli. In that sense, they are reflex in nature. Usually they have been thought to include, among others, glandular or smooth muscle responses; that is, they are autonomically mediated. When a respondent is observed to occur, it is to be assumed that it was preceded by appropriate stimulation. If the respondent occurs, the stimulus was there. In contrast, operants for the most part involve striated or so-called voluntary musculature, although, as noted, that restriction appears less and less to be the case. Operants have a critical difference from respondents. Operants *may* be elicited by antecedent stimuli. However, they have the significant characteristic of also being subject to influence by consequences that follow their occurrence. When an operant is followed by a favorable consequence (positive reinforcer), there tends to be an increase in the frequency with which it subsequently occurs. Operants diminish in frequency if they are followed by aversive consequences or by the absence of positive consequences.

Examples should help to illustrate. A sudden drop in temperature leads to vasodilation, and one's extremities become warmer. That illustrates respondent action. The response of vasodilation was proceeded by and, in that sense, was under the control of the antecedent stimulus of temperature change. Given the stimulus conditions, the response was automatic. Contrast that with an operant. A housewife, perhaps while making a bed, experiences a sharp pain in her back, perhaps a muscle spasm. She straightens from her previously bent-over position, gasps, and puts her left hand to her back to hold or rub the site of the spasm. The shift in her body position, the gasp, and the gesture of moving the hand to her back are all operants. They involved striated musculature. They were subject to voluntary control in the sense that she straightened and did not twist, gasped and did not cry out, and moved her left and not her right hand, but in this case they occurred in response to an antecedent stimulus. Given the circumstances of the spasm, it could have been predicted with assurance those or highly similar operants would occur. They bordered on being reflexive. They do not quite merit that designation, however, because even if she were not prepared to do so before, the housewife could be brought to where she would not take those actions when similar spasms occurred in the future. However, through the systematic management of contingencies to those operants, or to operants incompatible with them, she could also be brought to engage in such protective actions when no spasms occur.

Suppose, for example, and it should not be difficult to imagine such a situation, the housewife had had much back pain in the past—perhaps a disc problem now resolved and producing minimal or no residual noxious stimulation. Suppose, further, making beds and similar heavy housekeeping chores had never been pleasant or rewarding for her. Her interests were in other pursuits. Finally, suppose that she has two teen-age daughters well steeped in helping with household chores. Given those conditions, when a spasm or some random pain stimulus from her back results in the protective operants and her daughters see the pain displays, they may step in. They may caution their mother not to do heavy work when her back hurts. They may take over to complete the task. When they do that, they have thereby delivered one or more potentially potent reinforcers. They have provided their mother with rest and the successful avoidance of pain. They have also provided the social reinforcer of displaying their regard, concern, and readiness to help, which is a not unrewarding event for almost any mother. These are likely to be positive consequences. In this arbitrary example, they may be contingent on occurrence of the pain behavior. If there is no pain behavior, there is no stepping in to help. If pain behaviors occur, help and rest systematically follow.

The learning effect is automatic. The pain behaviors may come to occur without being a spasm or some such noxious stimulus. It is not at all necessary to infer that the house-wife makes a positive decision to pretend that she has pain so that her daughters will take over a noxious task. It is true that she could make such a decision and implement it by the display of pain behavior. But it is equally true that, given the systematic contingency arrangement specified and re-peated over time, the housewife's condition-ing could indeed occur. She could become incapable of discriminating that there was no longer a pain stimulus in her back when confronted with visual or symbolic cues in-dicating bed-making behavior should begin.

The rudiments of these principles will receive more detailed presentation in suc-ceeding chapters. The important point for the moment is to note that operants have a sensitive relationship with the immediate environment in which they occur. They may increase or decrease in frequency according to how the environment responds to their occurrence. Using the empirically demon-strated principles of operant conditioning, behavior changes may be brought about by arrangement of consequences to operant be-haviors. Increase the rate or frequency of a behavior by arranging for systematic posi-tive reinforcement contingent on its occur-rence; decrease a behavior by arranging for nonreinforcement or for aversive or punish-ing consequences. This systematic manage-ment of contingencies or consequences has proved an effective way of helping people to change their behavior.

To repeat one implication of operant con-ditioning, behavior is sensitive to or respon-sive to—and in that sense, partially controlled by—the immediate environment in which it occurs. That is a most important point in the evaluation of chronic pain.

Pain behaviors are, for the most part, operants. They are the verbal reports, the winces and grimaces, the moans, the re-quests for medication or for assistance, the limp or guarded motion, the limiting or re-stricting of behavior to avoid anticipated pain. These are operants. There are, in ad-dition, the palmar sweating, the variations in heart rate, and the like, which, autonomi-cally mediated, also serve as indicators to the observer that pain may be being experi-enced. But, as noted, there is an increasing body of evidence to indicate that even those autonomically mediated behaviors are not immune to conditioning effects. They are capable of being influenced by consequence manipulation, as are the striated muscle re-sponses.

What this comes down to is that the oc-currence of pain behavior *may* indicate that there has been an antecedent stimulus that, in the context of chronic pain, may be aris-ing from the site of body damage. On the other hand, if the patient's environment has had the effect of providing sufficient posi-tive reinforcement for pain behavior (or insufficient positive reinforcement to main-tain alternative well behavior, or punishment for that well behavior, or all of these), it is entirely reasonable to consider that there may have been little or no antecedent nox-ious stimulation from body damage to pro-duce the pain displays.

Keep in mind that operants are capable of being elicited by antecedent stimuli as well as being influenced by or coming under control of environmental consequences. It is therefore possible in a given situation that the pain behaviors are occurring because of some mixture of antecedent pathogenic stim-ulation and contingent environmental con-sequences. Clinical experience suggests that most chronic pain patients show the mixed picture of pain behavior part of the time or in some degree under control of pathogenic stimuli and partially under control of en-vironmental consequences.

These matters will receive detailed con-sideration in the sections on patient evalu-ation and on treatment. The major concern for the moment is in regard to psychogenic pain. Conceptually, the different perspective proposed here is portrayed in Fig. 3, which is to be contrasted with Fig. 2. Again, the proportions allocated to sources of influence are arbitrary and schematic. Behavior is limited or constrained by genetic factors. In addition, a certain amount of behavior may reasonably be related to well-established

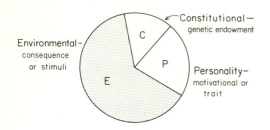

I. Observe "Illness Behavior" (Symptom)

2. Identify "Illness Behavior"- Consequence Relationships

3. Change Behavior by Principles of Learning

Symptom

?

Rx

Fig. 3. *Behavior influence factors—behavioral model.*

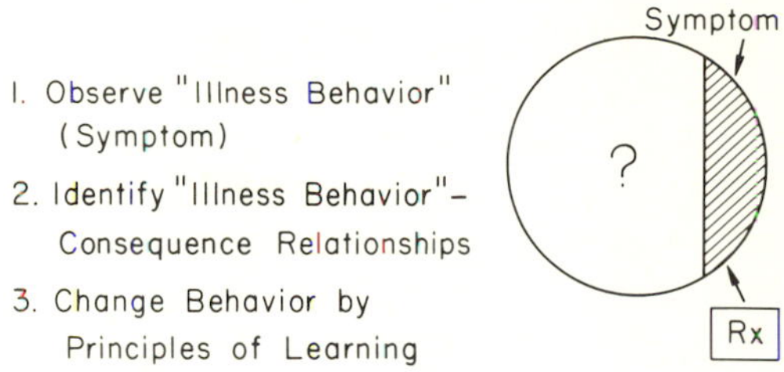

Fig. 4. *Learning model.*

high-frequency behaviors (a term that would appear more descriptive than personality traits, underlying motivation, or deep-seated attitudes) in the sense that they have a high probability of occurring in a variety of stimulus situations. Whether that means that they are indeed independent of the immediate stimulus conditions or that they have become conditioned to a wide range of stimuli is, for our purposes, of secondary importance. What is important is that behavior, including pain behavior, must be considered as highly sensitive to and influenced by the immediate environment, somewhat more so than seems ordinarily to be implied by traditional psychodynamic formulations of personality theory.

If the physical or medical diagnostic effort suggests a low relationship or a virtually nonexistent one between physical findings and pain behavior, the next step is *not* to infer that the pain is psychogenic and under control of some personality or motivation factor. The place to look is in the interaction between pain behaviors or alternative well behaviors and the systematic consequences in the patient's environment.

The issue here is not a mere intellectualized conceptual exercise. The position taken here is that much of the picture with many patients who have chronic pain is to be understood best not in terms of what the patient *has,* his personality or motivations, but in terms of what he *does.* It is the interaction between pain and well behavior and environmental cues and consequences currently on the scene to which one must attend to understand much of what heretofore has been called psychogenic.

The point is displayed schematically in Fig. 4. The learning model approach to analysis of a pain problem recognizes that the visible and audible manifestations of pain—the social signals of pain behavior—may be under partial or total control of environmental events. Evaluation will have to examine sequences of behavior (pain or well) and environmental consequences. If that evaluation reveals systematic relationships, treatment or management must be directed, at least in part, toward modifying those relationships, that is, toward the management of contingencies to behavior.

If one accepts the interpretation of data and the reasoning of this chapter, it would seem appropriate to discard the term psychogenic. The term implies mental control, personality problems, and motivational issues. It leads away from looking at patient-environment (including physician) interactions. It implies that the patient receiving the label is demonstrably different from people having physical findings related to their displays of pain. It also tends to lock the patient into a category: he has psychogenic pain. It is all too easy, therefore, to think about the patient as having only psychogenic pain.

A more functional pain evaluation question asks to what extent the pain behaviors are the reflex or automatic reactions to antecedent noxious stimuli arising from body damage or are operants occurring because of the reinforcing consequences by which they are followed. That formulation of the question corresponds to assessing the extent to which the pain behaviors function as *respondents* or as *operants.* Talking about whether a patient's pain is organic (physical, real) or psychogenic (mental, imaginary) flies in the face of the consistent evidence that *what the patient experiences is real to him or her.* The proper question is not whether the pain is real but, rather, the extent to which it is controlled by antecedent stimuli and occurs reflexly (is respondent) or is controlled by consequences (is operant).

The balance of this book will use and distinguish the terms respondent and operant pain. The two are not mutually exclusive. They can and do occur concurrently. The distinction is intended to direct attention toward the principal sources of control operative at a given point in time.

In closing this discussion of psychogenic pain and as an introduction to the alternative of a learning or behavioral model view of the matter, it is well to keep in mind that respondent as well as operant pain may benefit from a variety of behaviorally based interventions. In the case of respondent pain, it may prove to be true in a given case that there is no method available for reducing significantly the amount of noxious stimulation from the source of body damage. However, it is possible that one can intervene further along in the pain sequence to bring about some relief. Activation or distraction may diminish transmission by closing the gate. Increased activity may be promoted by contingency management techniques. The studied use of learning-based strategies may also inhibit the development of operant pain elements to the picture and thereby prevent future increases in the pain problem. Each of these will be considered later.

3 The acquisition of operant pain

This chapter will present a brief statement of operant conditioning principles and will then consider how those principles may account for some or occasionally virtually all of the pain displays presented by chronic pain patients.

To this point historical, theoretical, and empirical matters relating to pain have been reviewed. The clinical arena was entered in a limited way by considering psychogenic pain. The analysis of psychogenic pain pointed to flaws of logic in the concept and in the way it is applied. Empirically based challenges to the concept were also noted. It has been proposed that learning or conditioning factors must be taken into account.

In the review of psychodynamic accounts of how people may come to display pain when physical findings are limited or lacking, a number of plausible explanations for pain behavior without body damage were outlined, based mainly on clinical experience. Those accounts set forth in psychodynamic formulations can be sharpened. More precise statements or relationships between pain behaviors and the events that preceded them need to be made.

However plausible are the explanations or rationalizations as to why a person may have come to display pain behavior in excess of physical findings, they do not point to a clear and effective course of action. For example, when a finding of psychogenic pain is made and the ensuing action is to initiate psychotherapy, the pain problem is not often resolved. The record of psychotherapy as an effective method for treating psychogenic pain is unimpressive, particularly in view of the frequent number of patients who reject the referral and refuse to participate. They often see it as a misdiagnosis of their pain problems.

A second reason for a need for more precise understanding is that the search for antecedent historical circumstances or personality problems to account for the pain may divert one's attention from a spectrum of other potentially important factors. The current interactions, the here-and-now relationships between displays of pain or well behavior and environmental events influential on them, are often of greater significance. They may not bear close relationship to personality problems.

Relationships between behavior and environmental events that influence them are current and dynamic. Behavior is not fixed; it is ever changing. It follows that the analysis of a patient's chronic pain must take into account how pain behavior is being influenced, as well as how it was influenced toward its present form.

The objective of this chapter is to consider ways in which learning or conditioning may influence pain behaviors. It will be necessary to consider both the development of operant pain behavior, which is a matter of the patient's history, and the current environment in which he or she functions.

In the briefest of ways, the major underpinnings of learning have been referred to. Details as to the technology and operating principles by which to carry out contingency management programs will be reserved for Chapter 4. Further description of the major dimensions of operant conditioning is essential to the review of how people may develop operant pain. These will now be set forth.

The key principles are few in number and relatively simply stated. At the core is the operant-respondent distinction. *Respondents* have their specific stimuli and occur automatically when the stimulus is adequate. Respondents can therefore be said to be controlled by antecedent stimuli. *Operants,* in contrast, are responsive to the influence of the consequences that systematically follow their occurrence. Operants can and do occur as a direct and automatic response to antecedent stimuli, as is true of respondents. But, in addition, operants may come to occur because they are being followed by positive or reinforcing consequences. Conversely, their rate will diminish when positive reinforcement is withdrawn. Punishers or aversive consequences also weaken operants.

One way of summing up the foregoing is to consider that what a person does at any given moment, under any given set of stimulus conditions, is a function of the stimuli operative at the moment and the net or positive-negative balance of the consequences he perceives as accessible or not accessible. In the context of pain, for example, if a person is bombarded by peripheral noxious stimulation (the gate is open), respondent pain behaviors are likely to be emitted. There is adequate stimulation and an automatic response. If there is little or no peripheral noxious stimulation but pain behaviors are receiving effective reinforcement, those pain behaviors are also likely to be emitted. They now occur because of the reinforcing consequences to which they lead. If well behaviors are not reinforced and perhaps are punished, the pain behaviors are even more likely to be emitted. The alternatives to pain behaviors lead to aversive consequences (punishment or nonreinforcement). All three possibilities, respondent pain behavior, reinforced operant pain behavior, and punished or nonreinforced well behavior, may occur or exist simultaneously in any combination.

The next basic principle is that conditioning effects are temporary. Once established, operants are maintained only if they continue to receive reinforcement. The amount of reinforcement required to sustain them may diminish considerably, but if they are no longer reinforced, their rate will dwindle and ultimately reach zero.

The time-limited character of learning can be seen as both a plus and a minus, although, however one chooses to judge it, it is still an empirically supported fact. It may be seen as a plus in the sense that behavior is forever subject to change. We need never quit learning or changing our behavior. A patient need never come to feel stuck with some behavior (some operant) and that it cannot be changed. Given the proper conditions, change can and will occur.

The temporary character of operant behavior might be seen as a minus or a problem in the sense that those who would help a person change behavior must also be concerned with helping to provide the conditions necessary to maintain the change. The effective reduction in operant pain by withdrawal of positive reinforcers in a treatment setting will not automatically endure. Unless the contingency arrangements previously maintaining pain behaviors are changed, the old pattern will probably re-emerge. It should be noted, however that it is not necessary that the same pattern, type, and frequency of reinforcement used to bring about change in the treatment setting need to continue. All that is needed in the future is that effective positive reinforcement of the well behaviors is made accessible and that effective positive reinforcement of pain behaviors is not. Which reinforcers are used is not important; it is important only that effective reinforcement occur.

The third principle is that conditioning effects are usually specific to the stimulus conditions in which they arose. A behavior acquired in one setting is likely, initially, to occur only in that setting or in closely similar ones. A child first learning to read in school is likely at first to read less well, if at all, at home. Appropriately designed and reinforced practice at home soon brings comparable mastery there as well. But that generalization is not automatic or certain. A pain patient, on relearning to walk without a limp in the hospital setting, and who has rehearsed the new gait only in the physical therapy gymnasium, may display initially a tendency again to limp in other parts of the hospital or outside the building. That is to be expected. It does not indicate a motivational problem. Generalization of the new behavior to other stimulus conditions is probable if adequate rehearsal is provided under appropriately structured learning conditions. This principle concerns generalization. That topic will be defined and described in Chapter 4, and its tactical implications will be dealt with in Chapter 13.

The fourth principle is that stimuli present when reinforcement or punishment are occurring are capable of becoming reinforcers or punishers in their own right. They can become conditioned reinforcers or punishers. This is the other part of generalization. In the case of the conditioning of reinforcers, it means that it is possible to expand the network of effective reinforcement for a patient. As an arbitrary example for illustrative purposes, a previously long-inactive pain patient may be brought to an activity level permitting involvement in, say, a clerical job. Work previously may have been aversive or punishing, either because it was associated with exacerbation of respondent pain or because of socially aversive consequences that were indirectly supporting operant pain. The new working environment may be designed to enhance social reinforcement to the patient for his or her efforts. The beginning work efforts may be maintained primarily by arrangements that make rest contingent on performance. That interim arrangement may get things started. But social and other forms of reinforcement concomitantly occurring on the job may come to be adequate to maintain the work behavior, there and later in other settings.

Those are the basic elements. There are a number of variations in the arrangements of the elements that need to be considered. When reinforcement does not occur each time the behavior or action to be reinforced occurs, it is said to be intermittent reinforcement. There are several tactical considerations of importance in regard to whether reinforcement is continuous or intermittent, and, if intermittent, with what frequency it occurs and what time relationships it has to the behavior of interest. The issues concern what are called schedules of reinforcement. In this connection, the speed of reinforcement can also be a critical factor. Under certain conditions, it has been shown that reinforcement may *begin* to lose potency when the behavior-consequence interval exceeds about 0.6 second (Herman, 1973). In clinical settings one can rarely reinforce as rapidly as that. Promptness of reinforcement is important, however, particularly in the early stages of a behavior change program.

Finally, there is an additional set of tactical procedures having to do with the special case of establishing a new behavior (one not previously in the person's repertoire), or with increasing the frequency of a behavior presently occurring at a near-zero level, and with promoting its maintenance. The process is called shaping. The behavior to be acquired or increased is broken down into constituent parts. Successive approximations (that is, adding, bit by bit, these constituent parts) are reinforced until the whole is established. There is an analogue to shaping by which the new behavior is helped to be brought under control of complex stimuli or naturally occurring reinforcers. It is called stimulus fading. That process exposes the new behavior to increasingly varied and complex settings that may then serve to maintain the behavior while the stimuli and reinforcers used initially to establish the behavior are faded out of the picture.

A detailed illustration of shaping will be applied in Chapter 11 in regard to problems of distorted gait. A brief illustration here applied to the shaping of walking may prove helpful. The first element to be shaped might be weight bearing on one and then both feet and legs. A next element might be the alternating and reciprocal shifting of weight from one leg to the other. As each element is rehearsed it is reinforced until mastered. The next element is then added and reinforced to mastery, and so on, toward the target behavior of free ambulation without a limp. The process is, again, the reinforcement of successive approximations (elements added to elements) to the target behavior.

The process of stimulus fading concerns replacing the special stimulus characteristics of the training or learning environment (the treatment setting) with the patient's natural environment. This refers back to the third principle (conditioning is initially somewhat specific to the situation in which it arose) and serves as a reminder that it is important to broaden the conditions under which target behaviors are emitted so that they can become associated with and helped to be maintained by naturally occurring events in the patient's normal milieu.

The foregoing summary of operant principles should provide sufficient introduction to permit exploring ways in which operant pain may develop. There is another issue that needs to be brought into the picture before proceeding with the development of operant pain. A disease model style of looking at patient problems leads one to look at but one side of the coin: the illness events and what causes them. The illness is diagnosed in the sense of seeking to identify the causative agent. Treatment then seeks to eliminate that cause. People taking that approach often appear to assume that when the illness is removed, health or well behavior will follow. In the absence of illness, health prevails.

Illness behavior and health behavior are largely operants. Like other operants, they are also subject to the guiding influence of environmental contingencies. That in turn means that a critical factor in determining whether illness or health behaviors occur relates to the consequences or contingencies with which they are met. This is particularly true where the illness is chronic or long standing, thereby ensuring that there will have been ample time for systematic consequences to have their effect and for learning to occur.

Let it be supposed, for example, that a given patient is displaying indications of illness that are clearly under control of some form of underlying body damage—perhaps

an infection or a fracture. Many of the things he does in relation to his illness are operants. They involve striated musculature. They are potentially subject to voluntary control, but they are also subject to influence by consequences. In this case, they are occurring as an automatic response to the antecedent stimuli of the pathology. The post–myocardial infarction patient may move for some time in a guarded, hesitant manner. He does not engage in certain behaviors previously occurring with some frequency. The patient with a fractured arm, for a period of a few days or weeks, stops cutting meat with a knife and fork. Eating-related behaviors are, for a time, no longer a two-handed activity. The patient with fever and infection may recline excessively by his or her normal standards, may move gingerly, may gasp and moan, or may make frequent requests for fluids. In each case, not only was the patient doing certain things (operants) in relation to the illness or injury, but also the patient was not doing other things (also operants) previously having some frequency in the well-behavior repertoire. When treatment is effective, what happens next? What about the operants or well behaviors the patient ordinarily would have been displaying but which were prevented from occurring because of the illness? When the illness is gone, if those well behavior operants continue to receive the reinforcement that maintained them before illness, they probably will recur or be resumed if the period of disuse has not been lengthy. If the patient was engaged in certain well behavior activities (such as working at a job), he must have been receiving reinforcement for those activities, otherwise they would not have been occurring. Illness temporarily prevented their occurrence, but treatment made them again available. The patient, under those conditions, could be expected to resume pre-illness well behavior repertoire.

The problem is more difficult when a patient's environment is providing systematic reinforcement to illness operants (for example, pain behaviors), and it is even more so when that environment is punishing or failing to reinforce alternative well behaviors. If diagnosis missed the pain behavior-consequence relationships and aimed solely at an underlying pathogenic factor, treatment probably would have limited positive effect. It would not change the pain behavior-environmental consequence relationships. Lasting changes in symptom behavior could not be expected. When the patient's environment is failing to support well behavior, and maybe punishes it, treatment gains, however substantial, are also threatened and probably will not last even if briefly achieved. At the level of treatment planning, this means that the professional must be concerned with what the patient's environment will do if he gets better. There will be more concern about that issue later on when dealing with diagnosis or patient evaluation.

This issue is also important for goal setting and treatment planning.

In the behavioral analysis of chronic pain, it is essential to consider both sides of the coin. What are the environmental contingencies for pain behavior? Is pain behavior reinforced systematically and effectively? If that is the case, treatment must change those relationships. Concomitantly, what are the environmental contingencies for well behavior? Is it reinforced systematically and effectively? If well behavior is not being reinforced, it must be receiving either a deprivation of reinforcers or an aversive or punishing consequence. In either case, it may be that the patient's pain behaviors represent not the product of direct reinforcement but the indirect product of failure of reinforcement of alternatives. Pain behavior under the latter conditions can be seen as a form of avoidance behavior. It is behavior designed to avoid the undesirable consequences of being punished or of being deprived of reinforcement when well behavior is expressed. Treatment must also try to change that.

The discussion of ways in which learning may shape or guide either the development or the maintenance of a problem of chronic pain will consider both antecedent

or personal history (pre-illness events) factors and current circumstances bearing on the subject. It will also consider the direct reinforcement of pain behavior, indirect effects leading to avoidance behavior, and the degree to which the patient's environment reinforces well behavior.

To simplify the discussion, the material will be organized into three major categories. The categories are not mutually exclusive, nor are they observed necessarily to function singly and separately in the clinical context. They will be dealt with separately for expository purposes:

1. Direct and positive reinforcement of pain behavior
2. Indirect but positive reinforcement of pain behavior by avoidance of aversive consequences
3. Failure of well behavior to receive positive reinforcement

Each of these categories will be examined in relation to previous or personal history events of patients (an enterprise similar to the search for psychodynamics and their origins) and in relation to patients' current situations. As has been noted previously, histories tell something about where to look in the current situation for cues and consequences influencing the relevant behaviors, but that is not enough. To bring about change, the present behavior-consequence relationships must be changed. Moreover, the behavior-consequence relationships critical to the patient's pain problem often have their origins in the present and may be not be related in any important way to earlier experiences or to alleged personality, motivational, or emotional problems associated with those earlier experiences.

The intent of this section is to rationalize and illustrate how operant principles may work to develop patterns of operant pain. Environments provide naturally occurring behavior-consequence relationships that shape and change behavior. What are described here are ways in which these may occur. The descriptions are based mainly on my experience over 8 years involving several hundred behavioral analyses with chronic pain patients. Additional clinical experience has come through interacting with colleagues who were carrying out similar analyses. The descriptions given are not meant to be formal case descriptions as a kind of quasi-empirical foundation to the comments. The intent of this section, instead, is to help those unfamiliar with operant conditioning or contingency management procedures to better understand how they may work in vivo. That understanding should facilitate the use of operant principles as part of diagnosis or behavioral analysis of patients with chronic pain. It should also help amplify the procedures for setting up treatment programs presented in Section III.

Direct and positive reinforcement of pain behavior

History

Reference has been made previously to work by Merskey and Spear (1967), which showed that patients with pain complaints and no physical findings tended more than patients with somatic complaints, no pain, and no physical findings to yield histories indicating more frequent or lasting episodes of pain. One could think of this tendency to display more pain behavior now in relation to having experienced more pain in the past as a product of lower pain thresholds, lower pain tolerance, or as the recurrence of a long-standing emotional problem. It seems more to the point to consider this kind of situation in learning or conditioning terms.

As noted previously, pain threshold and pain tolerance are not necessarily related. Moreover, tolerance may refer only to ability to endure a particular and specific noxious stimulus, as measured by some kind of withdrawal or avoidance response. Tolerance may also refer to a broader range of behaviors in which the person communicates to the environment that pain is experienced at a level sufficient to interfere with a current activity. He may make an audible signal or engage in avoidance be-

haviors, such as reclining because moving hurts too much. In either case, the indicator that tolerance has been reached is the occurrence of an operant, a pain behavior. When the operant occurs, is it (and was it in the past) reinforced? When physical findings are present, the pain behavior may be functioning in respondent fashion, that is, it is under control of the noxious stimulus. But now a situation is being considered in which the physical findings currently are missing or insufficient to account for the pain behavior being displayed. That is also the situation reported by Merskey and Spear (1967): pain complaints but no physical findings. What happened in past years when such a person displayed pain behavior? If the pain behavior was then elicited mainly by antecedent noxious stimuli, the avoidance or protective behaviors taken in response would, if successful, have been reinforced by their successes. There is more about that later in this chapter. Regardless of whether protective or avoidance behaviors eased respondent pain, what effects did they have in the immediate environment? Did they elicit reinforcement from parents and other family members?

Everyone has seen a running youngster stumble and fall and then turn to the watching mother to look briefly before deciding whether to cry. If the mother seemed concerned enough, crying was more likely. If the mother, by her behavior, appeared to feel that crying was not indicated, crying was less likely to occur. The mother's reactions had the effect of promising certain consequences contingent on crying or noncrying. When the mother's manner appeared to signal that crying was all right, there was the implicit promise that crying would be reinforced. Crying is but one of a number of the child's pain behaviors that might be reinforced by a mother in that example.

Childhood illness, whether involving pain or not, is a likely place for conditioning to occur. Illness, of whatever type and level of severity, will involve some mixture of impairment and continued function. The question arises as to whether parental reactions discourage continued function and movement during the illness. They may by their actions make illness a dominating thing. Alternatively, parents may indicate that continued function, within prudent limits, is important. Function may be promoted and reinforced or discouraged and even forbidden. Clearly, if either of those alternative patterns strongly prevails to the detriment of the other, the child is likely to develop a strong illness behavior or a strong well behavior repertoire.

One of the interesting and important facets to these early training opportunities concerns the parent's—particularly the mother's—reinforcers. If the mother is much reinforced by indications from her child that the child is dependent on her, then the mother's nurturing and protective actions are themselves likely to be reinforced and strengthened. When the child expresses distress, the mother's protective action eases that distress. The child then displays lessened distress and thereby reinforces the mother for her intervention. That mother is more likely to intervene in a similar fashion in the future. If a mother is strongly reinforced by movement, progress, or independent function in her child, then that mother is more likely to promote those kinds of behaviors. In the latter case, her protective actions do not lead to reinforcement for her, whereas the promotion of function does.

This kind of reciprocal relationship in the behavior-consequence relationships between two people is also commonly observed in marital pairs in which one member of the pair has chronic pain or chronic illness. Just as in the mother-child examples, the responses of each serve to help maintain the behavior of the other. This is an important point. The major impact of parental or spouse support of illness-related behaviors by special attention, nurturance, or discouragement of activity occurs when these consequences are in significant degree contingent on the illness. If things are going well, there is less attention and nur-

turant concern. For some people, access to these consequences may virtually require some illness behavior.

It is not necessary to debate whether noxious stimuli were present in childhood illness and pain episodes. Pain could have been respondent, and undoubtedly it frequently was in everyone's childhood. The key question concerns what environmental contingencies the pain behaviors met. The more frequently illness and pain episodes occurred, perhaps by chance, the more opportunity there was for the pain behavior-consequence relationships to have their effect. If the consequences were in the direction of nonreinforcement of pain behavior, the subsequent rate or probability of pain behavior would be correspondingly diminished. However, if pain behavior was reinforced, it would be more likely to occur.

There is another facet to this issue to consider. Pain is often confirmable only by the visible or audible signal that pain is being experienced. When a child cuts a finger and the bleeding is visible, crying or some other display of distress is not surprising and gains confirmation by the sight of the blood. Environmental responses of maternal protective and reassuring behaviors are then to be expected, and we make little of that. However, if the noxious stimulus results from a bump or a barely visible or invisible bruise, twist, or strain, visible confirmation of the basis for distress is lacking. Under those conditions, signs of distress in the form of pain behaviors rely, for their authenticity and for influence on those around the person in distress, on the dramatic effect of the display. If the cause of the pain does not show and the pain display is of little intensity or persuasiveness, a mother is not likely to engage in attentive, nurturing, and protective behaviors (unless she is a mother for whom such behavior is strongly reinforcing). The pain behaviors may quickly fade, extinguished by lack of reinforcement. Another possibility, however, is that the intensity or dramatic impact of the pain display may instead increase. Crying may become louder. Limping or grimacing may become more pronounced. What consequences then follow? If the louder (more intense) pain signal is followed by protective mothering behaviors and all the social reinforcers that go with it, a kind of discrimination learning situation will have been set up. The youngster has learned that the social reinforcers of mother solicitousness are contingent on loud as distinguished from soft pain signals.

Some mothers provide insufficient mothering, solicitous, social reinforcing behavior toward their children. They may be too busy. They may not like children all that much or they may not enjoy coping with illness. They may have pain problems of their own, making the prospect of attending to another's pain problem unattractive. Whatever the reasons, a mother or father who is selectively responsive to distress signals in the direction of responding virtually only when the signals are loud or strong, but who does then respond with effective positive reinforcement to the loud signals, will have thereby contributed to shaping loud or highly compelling pain behavior displays. Social reinforcement from such a key figure as a parent, infrequently delivered and tending to come only in response to loud signals, shapes intense distress signal behavior.

Environmental consequences to childhood displays of pain or illness surely will have had some consistency. Whether the pain or illness displays by the child were direct responses to noxious stimuli (that is, respondent pain) or occurred when noxious stimuli were minimal is unimportant. The key issue relates to the kind of environmental responses elicited, and to the extent to which those environmental consequences were reinforcing and contingent on illness displays. When the environment was relatively nonresponsive, conditions for developing stoicism or more reluctance to signal pain could be said to have prevailed. That would also be true when louder signals of pain were not selectively responded to in effectively reinforcing fashion. The childhood environment in which pain behavior was effectively reinforced by solicitousness and special attention contingent on illness produces a rich repertoire of pain behaviors and a dearth of more stocial-type behaviors.

In passing, to keep this in perspective, the foregoing is not meant to imply that displays of distress in one's child should be ignored. The point is that parental response to pain and to nonpain displays can exert great influence, particularly if they are pain contingent. If that influence flows excessively toward reinforcement of distress or toward inadequate reinforcement of distress tolerance, the result is likely to be a behavioral repertoire well laced with pain behaviors.

It is interesting to note the frequency with which chronic pain patients with much illness or pain in childhood report either of two extremes. One is that during childhood there was a good deal of parental concern and readiness to take supportive action when pain or illness occurred. The other extreme is to characterize one or both parents as having been reluctant to respond to pain and to do so only when the pain seemed severe. In both cases, clinical experience indicates that parental nurturant behaviors often were pain or illness contingent.

There is another way childhood may promote readiness to display illness or pain later in life. That concerns modeling or imitation learning. As a matter of expository convenience, modeling has not yet been described. It can be dealt with briefly now, not because it is unimportant, but because the critical elements are simply stated.

Imitation or modeling plays an important part in human learning (Bandura, 1965; Bandura and Walters, 1963). We see or hear another's behavior and we may emulate it, all or in part. We may do so without being aware that we are. Ready examples of this are to be found in the acquisition of language by an infant. The child hears sounds and begins to imitate them. Another common example is the acquisition of complex motor skills. Golf or tennis are not readily mastered by reading or by hearing about how to perform. It is much more the case that the learner observes performance and then tries to imitate it.

The potency of modeling as a source and method of learning is determined in large part by the consequences that meet the modeled behavior. If the behavior of the model whom one observes leads to reinforcement, the observer is more likely to emulate the behavior. A model's actions that lead to punishment or lack of positive reinforcement are less likely to be imitated. For example, Bandura (1965) showed films to groups of children in which adults displayed various forms of verbal or physical aggression. In one film the models were punished for such behavior, in another they were reinforced, and in a third no consequences systematically followed. The observer children were subsequently tested to measure the amount of imitative behavior they displayed. Children who had watched the film in which aggression was punished subsequently made significantly fewer imitative responses than did either the children watching the reinforced or the no-consequence condition.

Of greater and more durable importance is the question of the consequences that meet the imitative behaviors adopted from the models. To draw on the preceding example, if the child now displays the modeled aggressive behavior, is that reinforced? If it is not, it probably will quickly fade, but if it receives effective positive reinforcement, its future course will be like that of any other operant.

The influence of modeling is all around us. One of the more obvious illustrations is with regard to accent of speech. The figurative example of the speech style of children from parents having New England or Arkansas accents was considered in the first chapter in the context of cultural influences on behavior. The child imitates the accents he or she hears. Moreover, if he were to do otherwise, as is the case when one moves from one area of the country to another that has a distinctly different speech style, he is likely to receive aversive consequences. He may be made fun of or, at the least, singled out by the raised eyebrows of the listener as somehow different. The environment of the young child and of the older person both models and shapes by selective reinforcement the styles and accents of speech, as well as any number of other behaviors.

Modeling becomes an issue of some importance in the behavioral analysis of pain. It is no coincidence that there appears to be a disproportionately large number of instances in which chronic pain patients come from homes in which chronic illness or chronic pain were modeled by parental figures. When that has been the case, the two key questions are, (1) What were the consequences to the model when pain or illness behavior was displayed? and (2) What were the consequences to the observer (in this instance, the maturing child) when, after a parental illness or pain episode, imitative behaviors were displayed? Stoical parents are likely to raise stoical children. The parents have modeled little pain behavior, and when it was displayed by the ill or injured parent, it was not likely to have been reinforced contingently by the spouse. Furthermore, the same contingency relationships are likely to have prevailed when progeny of the marriage displayed pain behaviors. In contrast, histrionic parents shape histrionic behavior in their children. They model it, and, in doing so, they also model or demonstrate that such behavior does not receive aversive consequences, at least within the home, regardless of whether it is directly reinforced. When histrionic behavior is displayed in relation to pain or illness in their children, that too is less likely to be punished and may receive selective, contingent positive reinforcement.

It follows from the above that modeling can influence operant pain. It also follows that the behavioral analysis of a problem of chronic pain should examine the question of whether illness-related behaviors were extensively modeled in the patient's earlier years and, if so, the consequences they met.

Current reinforcement

Interactions between patient pain behavior and family responses will be considered first, because they relate directly to the immediately preceding section.

There are many ways in which family response to pain behavior may be directly reinforcing. Perhaps the most direct is the situation in which the concerned attention of wife or husband is discriminantly different when pain or distress is being displayed, and that special kind of attention is contingent on pain or illness. There may be attention and intercommunication when there is no pain, but it may be different in ways that are important to the patient. If it is the husband who has the pain problem, his wife may ordinarily be relatively nondemonstrative of concern and affection. But she may become much more pointed and intense in her expressions of interest and concern when her husband is ill.

One of the early patients to undergo behavioral analysis of chronic pain and a subsequent treatment program based on operant methods was a man in his 40s who had been incapacitated for nearly 20 years, including throughout the duration of his marriage by what came to be seen as operant pain. His wife worked to augment the income he derived from the illness-related insurance funds he received each month. Each working evening, she would return to her husband who had spent much of the day reclining in his bed before the TV set, which had been moved into the bedroom. She would prepare dinner and then bring the dinner into the bedroom where they would eat side by side, he sitting up on the bed and she at a TV tray beside him. So far as could be determined from her account and his, she tended to express much concern and solicitousness during meal times, as well as on other occasions. On infrequent occasions, relating perhaps to a vacation trip to some other area or a visit by relatives, he would mobilize himself enough to get out of bed to eat at a table. When he did that, he did not receive special encouragement and solicitousness. To the contrary, his wife tended on those occasions to express doubt that such behavior was to his benefit and to chide him for engaging in what she perceived as taking risks. Her solicitousness and nurturing approval was, in substantial degree, contingent on his emitting such pain behaviors as remaining in bed. The pattern was mutually reinforcing. When he reclined and received her support and protective attention, he was not only expressive of gratitude to her, but he also displayed reduced signs of pain. He only reclined. He did not moan or grimace, grasp his back, or request medication. In those ways he reinforced her protecting behaviors for, as she saw it, her efforts were successful. Conversely, on the rare occasions when he made it to a table to eat, he was, by her account, a visible and audible picture of pain. His movements were guarded. He grimaced. He often rubbed his painful back. He openly expressed doubt that he would be able to last out the meal. When her admonitions to be prudent and return to bed prevailed and he did so, she was rewarded by immediate reduction in his pain behaviors, and he was rewarded by termination of her nagging him to be careful and by a resumption of her affectionate concern.

The foregoing is an extreme example, although not, in substance, a rare one. In the course of a behavioral analysis of the problem, the question is asked of both patient and spouse as to exactly what happens when pain is displayed. More often than not, the first response is, "Nothing." That usually means that the spouse does not systematically take a particular affirmative action such as rubbing the sore back, bringing medication or a heating pad. Under detailed questioning, however, one often finds that there are subtle but consistent shifts in attention contingent on pain displays. The pain-ridden wife walks across the room without displaying pain and her paper-reading husband does not look up. When she limps, holds her back, or gasps while walking, his attention is diverted to her, and he watches and perhaps makes a solicitous comment. One patient, a wife for whom medical evaluation indicated much operant and minimal respondent pain, reported that her husband would always look away when she first displayed pain. He had long resented the intrusion of her pain problem on their way of life, and he had felt her pain was "exaggerated" or "all in her head." Moderate signs of pain systematically led him to look away, a pattern which probably initially had prevented him from making a hostile comment to her. The looking away pattern had only limited durability. If she continued to manifest pain, his good manners, basic concern (and probably some guilt over having resented it when she suffered) led him to turn to her and offer to help. He would bring her medication or step in to take over and complete the household task in which she had been engaged. He was reinforced for such efforts by her open expressions of gratitude (thereby easing his guilt) and by an ensuing reduction in pain display. She was reinforced by termination of his withdrawal (by turning away) and by his direct help. The interaction of the two had provided a discrimination learning task in which she had become conditioned to louder pain displays. He had helped to condition her by his differential response to brief as compared with extended pain displays.

There are, of course, frequent instances in which direct and obvious reinforcement occurs contingent on pain by the affirmative help of a back rub, bringing the heating pad, bringing of medication, or the like. In addition, in more subtle form, the wise spouse may try to divert the attention of the hurting mate by changing the subject or by launching into an attention-demanding conversation, such as by asking questions about the day's activities. That, too, is a form of special and pain-contingent at-

tention. If no pain behavior were displayed, there might not be such active attention.

It should be borne in mind that in the kind of interactions just described, conditioning can progress to where the pain behavior itself need not be displayed. It need only be anticipated by the observer. That may be sufficient to trigger the reinforcing consequences. The example of the wife who brought dinner to the bedroom illustrates. Her husband did not need to display pain behavior for her to do that. All that was required was that she had experienced enough earlier episodes in which pain behavior had been displayed for her to continue the eating-in-the-bedroom arrangement. Under those conditions, she could be said to be engaging in avoidance behavior. Being solicitous toward him successfully avoided or postponed his displays of pain behavior. Moreover, if asked whether pain was occurring in her husband, she would almost certainly say "Yes" in all sincerity, when all that occurred were behaviors previously preceding pain displays.

Inasmuch as what is reinforcing to one person may not be reinforcing to another, gaining an account of the interactions in a home setting between patient pain displays and spouse responses does not always reveal an obviously reinforcing relationship. Some spouses are, for example, reinforced by seeing their mates become angry. The expression of pain behavior may anger the spouse and cause him or her to leave the room. That, too, can be reinforcing to some people. Suggestions for how to explore these questions further will be dealt with in the section on patient evaluation. The initial key issue is to see if there is a particular response or set of responses by the spouse that are pain contingent. Once that is established, if it is, the reinforcing properties of these responses can be explored.

The kinds of illustrations presented here can of course occur in interactions with other family members than the spouse and with people outside the family circle. The maintenance of a significant amount of operant pain behavior by people outside the family would almost certainly require either that the family was also helping to maintain the pain behavior or that there was an unusual and systematic amount of interaction between the patient and the person(s) outside the family. If evidence for that was not found, it would indicate that the pain behaviors were not under control of direct environmental reinforcement, except in the ways shown in the next two sections.

Support or maintenance of chronic operant pain by attention or social responsiveness in one of its forms is not found frequently in single adults. Ordinarily, there does not seem to be sufficient access to selective attention to maintain operant pain. The exceptions seem mainly to relate to a single person who has a close and frequent contact with another person, as in a courtship or the perennial bachelor still living with his mother. There are, of course, other ways in addition to attention by which operant pain may be effectively reinforced, as will be discussed in the balance of this chapter. A behavioral analysis of an unmarried chronic pain patient can often be shortened, however, by exploring quickly for close and frequent interpersonal contacts with other than a spouse. If there do not appear to be such relationships, that aspect can be discarded.

Compensation. The topic of monetary compensation when illness occurs has received much attention in regard to chronic pain. One hears in clinical settings the term *compensationitis* used as an informal diagnostic label.

Compensation can function as an effective reinforcer. It may increase the rate of the behavior on which it is contingent and, when withdrawn, may result in a reduction in that behavior. Monthly paychecks help support a host of behaviors in many of us. But compensation is by no means automatically an effective reinforcer, and its dispensation will not automatically have that effect. A number of other factors need to be taken into account before one can infer that a given patient's pain behavior is under control of the monetary reinforcers derived from compensation.

In the first place, from a purely technological perspective, compensation in the form of monthly checks is delayed reinforcement. The greater the interval between occurrences of the target behavior and the reinforcer, the less the impact of that reinforcer. Working in the other direction is the fact that the patient will have had years of rehearsal at elaborate chains or sequences of behavior, spread over 30-day intervals, that gradually had come to be maintained in significant part by monthly paychecks. Prior experience is capable of having minimized the loss of effectiveness of a 30-day delay in reinforcement. However, the fact of the delay ensures opportunity for other behavior-consequence relationships to occur in much shorter and more efficient time cycles either to alter the relationships between behavior and compensation checks or to help maintain it. In short, the delay of compensation reinforcers makes it likely that interim behavior-consequence relationships can have great influence. To illustrate, a husband with pain and on compensation receives the monetary consequences once each 30 days (or whatever the interval may be). If his wife is reinforcing pain behavior and failing to reinforce well behavior, operant pain is likely to develop and be maintained. But if the wife is not reinforcing pain behavior and is reinforcing well behavior, she does so well within the time cycle of the compensation check. She is therefore in a position to exert considerable influence on the situation if her reinforcement is systematic and effective.

It is easy to oversimplify the compensation issue. The fact of compensation does not by itself provide a sufficient basis for inferring that the patient's pain behavior is under control of those monetary reinforcers, although it could be. It works the other way as well. That is, it also follows that withdrawal of compensation could not be expected automatically to lead to a reduction of pain behavior, although that could happen, too. The spectrum of other factors that influence the rate of pain and well behavior ought also to be considered in relation to the question of the importance of the patient's compensation to the maintenance of operant pain. Is pain behavior receiving contingent reinforcement in other ways? Is well behavior being punished or going unreinforced? Is pain behavior successful avoidance behavior, that is, does it effectively avoid otherwise aversive consequences? Clearly, a number of precise behavior-consequence relationships need to be examined before concluding that compensation maintains the patient's pain behavior.

One way of assessing the role of compensation for a given patient is to explore the importance of compensation to the spouse. There are two commonly encountered patterns in clinical settings. In one, the patient is the major or only breadwinner, and the spouse is not capable for one reason or another of becoming an effective substitute wage earner. Under those conditions, compensation is likely to be a critically important reinforcer to the spouse as well as to the patient. Interview with the spouse may reveal that he or she is mindful of this fact and is strongly reinforcing in regard to compensation. The check, then, seems more likely to be a major element in the picture. However, the spouse may be discontent with the compensation check, perhaps feeling considerably more could be earned by working. Or, in ways relating to the so-called Christian ethic, there may be reluctance to accept non–work-contingent money. That spouse therefore fails to reinforce reliance on the check and promotes alternative behaviors. The check is then probably less of a factor.

The second common example works in the other direction. Compensation relating to pain may be coming not to the major breadwinner but to the working wife. In that case, interview may reveal that the compensation funds are of little importance to the household, and other sources of maintaining reinforcers to operant pain need to be pursued. Obviously, compensation to the secondary breadwinner may also be important to both and may receive mutual reinforcement.

Perhaps the most important product of the clinical experience thus far accumulated with these behavioral methods as regards the matter of compensation is the observation that many patients previously identified as hopeless compensation cases have proved to be able to achieve considerable treatment progress. The presence of compensation in the picture should not be taken as an automatic deterrent. The opportunity to intervene with behavior-consequence arrangements that have the greater potency of immediacy (versus up to 30-day delays) should not be overlooked.

Iatrogenic reinforcement. Physician attention, like family attention, may reinforce pain behavior. There are at least two additional ways in which the health care system may provide direct, positive, contingent reinforcement for pain behavior. These are in addition to the several indirect sources of reinforcement that may become available as a consequence of actions of the physician or others in the system, and which will be dealt with later in this chapter.

Medication. Medication is capable of being a potent reinforcer, depending on how it is handled. Attention has been called to this matter in earlier publications (Fordyce, 1973, 1974; Fordyce and associates, 1968, 1973). The magnitude of the problem is reflected in the enormous funds expended annually on medications and in the frequency with which one encounters in the clinical setting chronic pain patients who are addicted or habituated to analgesics. In my experience, addiction or habituation appear in something over 50% of chronic pain patients.

Pain medications usually are not administered to resolve the pain problem. They are intended to ease suffering while the pain problem is being resolved or, if it is not to be resolved, to minimize suffering during the life of the pain problem. The second and related intent is to reduce interference in normal function from pain so that an optimal level of daily pursuits can be maintained. These objectives are not always clear to the patient. Prior experience with the health care system will have tended to develop patient expectation that medication itself offers a solution to medical problems. As a consequence, the patient is likely in some degree to perceive pain medication as leading toward both relief and resolution of the problem. Stated in behavioral terms, medication offers hope of gaining access to the reinforcers associated with both feeling better and with being well. It is not surprising that many patients act to promote the use of analgesics and narcotics by their physicians.

A detailed examination of the physician-patient or, depending on the particular circumstances, the health care delivery system–patient transactions in regard to pain and analgesics reveals some interesting behavior-consequence relationships. It is well recognized that indiscriminate or overly ready use of pain medications is ill advised. The risks of addiction, habituation, and toxicity are too great. The traditional protective strategy is to deliver them only when there is clearly a need; otherwise they are to be withheld. That arrangement, the traditional *prn* regimen, is plausible. Intuitively it makes sense. But it fails to take into account the powerful influence that contingent reinforcement arrangements have on behavior.

The patient on a *prn* regimen receives medications contingent on indications that they are needed. If no pain is reported or observed, they are not provided. If need for medication is demonstrated, they are delivered. How is need demonstrated? *Need* can in this context be operationally defined as the display or expression of pain behaviors, of operants. Contingent consequences to those operants include the medications. If the patient communicates to his environment in sufficiently pursuasive fashion that he is experiencing pain and there is therefore a need for an analgesic, the

systematic consequence is the analgesic. But he must signal the pain. He must engage in some pain behavior. The consequence is contingent on that.

What is the effect of the analgesic consequence? It is likely to produce some element of relief of pain and some element of an improved feeling of well being. The effect need not, of course, be limited to pain relief. The effect may, for example, only relieve anxiety, or it may, in the case of a depressed patient, provide an increase in the available pool of energy. All that is important in helping to make the medication a positive reinforcer is that it makes the patient feel better in some way. The influence of analgesics and narcotics on feeling or emotional states other than pain per se is of increasing relevance when the patient has concomitant emotional problems. That issue comes to the forefront when the evidence from evaluation indicates that there is much operant pain and, further, that what is perceived by the patient as pain may instead be anxiety, depression, or whatever. In those circumstances, the medication need not touch pain at all to provide a reinforcing sense of feeling better.

It may well be that the more the patient's pain behavior is operant pain under control of environmental consequences, the more likely medication, delivered as needed for pain, serves as a reinforcer to further maintain operant pain.

There is another side to the coin. Patient signals to his or her physician that pain is felt and that relief through medication is needed occur in the context of a social transaction in which the consumer expects and even demands help. Concomitantly, the purveyor, the physician, is cast into the role of the source of help or relief. He is expected, as well as requested, to provide relief. Should he fail to do that, in the patient's eyes, treatment may well be viewed as having failed. Failure to provide relief leaves the physician facing several possible aversive consequences. The patient may be angry and berate him. The patient may continue to press for medication, perhaps in an obnoxious or incessant manner. Treatment has in a sense failed. The patient often next seeks help elsewhere. The physician is of course well aware that pain medication does not resolve pain problems, but that knowledge does not relieve him of the aversive consequences that may follow when he withholds the medication.

It should be evident that the *prn* regimen provides fertile soil for the development of a high operant level of requests for pain medication, regardless of whether one chooses to label that as habituation or addiction. A tight relationship has been set up. The reinforcer occurs contingent on the pain or sick behavior. Moreover, when the reinforcer is delivered, both parties to the transaction, patient and physician—to say nothing of family members—are often effectively reinforced. The patient gets relief. The physician also gets some relief, the relief of temporarily fewer demands for medication and of temporarily fewer displays of what easily could be seen as failure

of treatment. The physician also receives some monetary reinforcement for the medication regimen, and, for some, that too will influence medication dispensing behavior.

The interaction of high medication intake and addiction with functional impairment is illustrated by the case record reported in Fig. 5. The patient was in his late 40s. After a number of years of success at a highly skilled trade, disc problems emerged, for which surgery was indicated. That treatment was not successful. Over a period of approximately 15 years he received 13 surgeries for his chronic back pain and a succession of *prn* medication regimens. He was highly addicted to narcotics at the time of admission. Fig. 5 reports changes in medication intake in response to the pain cocktail regimen described in Chapter 9. To illustrate relationships with activity level, the number of 200-foot laps he could walk without pause for rest is shown for the same time span as the pain cocktail regimen. When walking reached 6000 feet, it was held at that ceiling to provide additional time for other

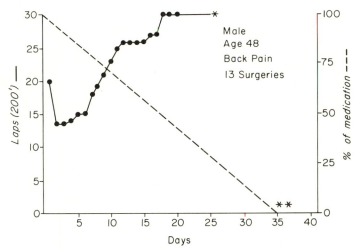

Medications at Admission : 1.Talwin 45mg. 2.Thorazine 150mg.
3.Valium 20mg. 4. Dolphine 40mg.
5.Chloral Hydrate 500mg.

* Laps held at 30 to permit time for other activities
** At day 35 all meds. zero except number 5 : 300mg/day

Fig. 5. *Walking distance and changes in medication intake.*

activities. The numerous surgeries produced irreversible impairment, restricting employability. In addition, 15 years on the sidelines made re-employment a practical impossibility. He became one of the legitimated retirement people discussed in Chapter 5. But he ceased pursuing further medical and surgical solutions, reduced medication intake to palliative levels, and resumed, on a limited basis, recreational and social activities.

It is the very patient whose pain behaviors are more likely to be under substantial control of environmental consequences than of antecedent stimuli from body damage who is more likely to get into this bind. That type of patient has a higher probability of associated emotional distress, which gains concomitant relief from the medication.

Viewed in behavioral terms, the *prn* regimen can be seen as an efficient method for producing the very effect it was designed to minimize. Pain-contingent medication works to increase control of pain behaviors by environmental events rather than tissue damage and to increase medication demand.

One might well question why it is that not all chronic pain patients on *prn* regimens are addicted or habituated to pain medications. There appear to be several forces working in the other direction to oppose habituation and addiction and to reinforce alternative behaviors. Many chronic pain patients have respondent and not operant pain. For such patients whatever medications are used may not produce significant ameliorating effects to their distress and thus would not function as effective positive reinforcers. In that situation, medication may be contingent on pain behavior, but it is not a positive reinforcer. It could therefore not be expected to increase the subsequent rate of the operants it contingently follows: pain behaviors. Another example of the failure of medications to function as effective reinforcers is found in many pain patients who are also restless and who may gain more pain relief

from movement (for instance, pacing the floor) than by reclining. The side effects of pain medications in the direction of tranquilization may be aversive rather than reinforcing. Clinically, it appears predominantly to be the restless, self-demanding patient who is more likely openly to voice concern about addiction and to express more reluctance to take analgesics. Tranquilization is not, for such a person, a reinforcer.

A second force working against habituation or addiction may be the behavior of the physician. By his verbal accounts, he can call into play aversive consequences relating to habituation, addiction, and toxicity, as well as the limitations of analgesics as problem solvers. His effectiveness in this regard can be augmented by the demonstrated failure of the medication to resolve the pain problem.

The likelihood that a *prn* regimen will promote habituation or addiction is enhanced by the reciprocal reinforcing relationships in the process. The patient's displays of pain behavior are reinforced by medication and the attendant changes in feeling state. The physician is reinforced by temporary termination of the expressions of hurting and the requests or demands for medication.

The frequency of habituation and addiction stand as persuasive testimony to the failure of *prn* regimens to solve the problem or, conversely, as testimony to their power to make matters worse. The regimen is not certain to work to the patient's disadvantage, but it well could. Be that as it may, a learning model approach to chronic pain suggests alternative ways of handling the medication issue that provide for different pain behavior-environmental consequence relationships. The evidence thus far accumulated supports the inference that they are effective (Fordyce and associates, 1973). They will be described in detail in Section Three. Fig. 6 reports average changes in medication intake in a series of thirty-six consecutive chronic pain patients across the inpatient phase of treatment using the pain cocktail regimen (Chapter 9). The patients averaged 42 years of age and 2.7 major surgeries for their referring pain problems. Their diagnoses varied, but they all had in common what appeared at the time of admission to be significant elements of operant pain in their respective pictures.

A behavioral analysis of medication regimens has pointed to one way that a pain problem having its origins in body damage (that is, respondent pain) can come under operant control by virtue of the methods used to treat it.

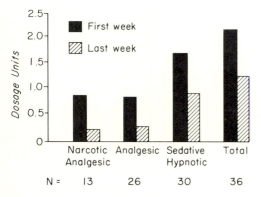

Fig. 6. *Changes in medications during inpatient treatment.*

Exercise and activity. A second major way in which medical treatment may inadvertently serve to establish or promote operant pain concerns the manner in which rest occurs in relation to pain behavior. As in the case of pain medication, one finds clinically that rest and inactivity play a pervasive role in many pain problems. It is of more than passing interest to note the frequency with which chronic pain patients who are observed or reported to spend much time reclining or resting show consistent trends toward the need for increasing amounts of rest, in spite of little substantial indication that the body damage from which the pain arose is itself worsening. In a sense the picture is similar to that noted in regard to medications. In both cases, when consumption of medication or of rest has been high, the trend seems almost always to be in the direction of the need for increasing amounts of those consequences to maintain the patient. When a pain problem has existed for an extended period and rest or medication has been tried but has failed to provide a solution, it is time to consider alternative analyses of the situation. A behavioral analysis of the situation appears to provide useful leads.

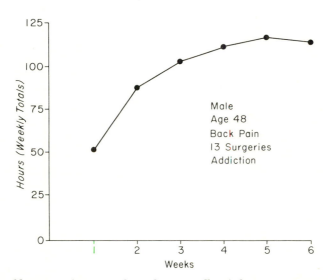

Fig. 7. *Weekly uptime (sitting and standing or walking) during inpatient treatment.*

One could reason that rest or medication regimens may have successfully avoided even more severe pain. One test of that question would be to show that *reduced* medication or rest helped. In selected cases, that has been the finding as reported in Fordyce and co-workers (1973). That is, medication and rest were systematically reduced. The result was decreased, not increased, pain behavior and increased, not decreased, activity level. The patient described just above who had received 13 surgeries further illustrates the point. Fig. 7 describes the change in his general activity level as measured by diary records (a procedure discussed in Chapter 6) reporting distribution of time among sitting plus standing or walking (uptime) and reclining. As noted before and as shown in Fig. 5, while medication intake was diminishing, specific exercises such as walking were increasing along with time measures of general activity.

Before proceeding, a moment should be taken to restate an important part of the definition of a reinforcer. This topic is dealt with in detail in the next chapter and has been touched on previously. For now, let it be remembered that a consequence or event can be said to be reinforcing (positive reinforcement) if, subsequently, the rate of the behavior on which it is contingent increases. Conversely, if the alleged reinforcer is withdrawn, if the operant on which previously it was contingent indeed diminishes in frequency, it is correct to conclude it was a positive reinforcer. The definition is circular. If it works, it is a reinforcer. If it does not influence the behavior on which it is contingent, it is not a reinforcer. The test is always empirical. The behavior changes in rate or it does not.

The reason for introducing this elaboration on the definition of positive reinforcers at this point is that rest (time out from activity) deserves careful examination in reinforcement terms in the context of chronic pain. As noted earlier, some patients recline or rest when they hurt, whereas others move or pace. The contrast provides an excellent illustration of how to define positive reinforcement. If rest did not provide some relief to the recliner, he would not continue to use it as a remedy. If pacing did not provide some relief to the pacer, he would not continue to use it.

If there is, for example, a disc problem, movement may quickly trigger severe pain. The patient then reclines and is reinforced by the subsequent easing of pain. Reclining helps. The relationships among movement, pain, reclining, and easing of pain, in that example, are probably simple and straightforward. The pain can be seen as respondent and the rest or reclining, although operant, is maintained specifically by the helpful effect it produces. Social reinforcement plays little or no role. Similarly, spasm relating to muscle tension is sometimes effectively eased by movement. The spasm is respondent. The operant of pacing is maintained by the effects or consequences it leads to—relief.

The problem in this arises because rest has other effects as well as those of easing pain. Rest virtually ensures that ongoing activity will be interrupted. Rest provides time out. The housewife ceases to make beds, vacuum rugs, and scrub floors. The employee does not go to work. There is interruption in or restriction of many social activities. It becomes a matter of central importance to determine whether those changes in behavior, which are a by-product of rest, receive other positive reinforcers in addition to whatever pain-relieving qualities they have. The patient who rests and thereby also gains access to other positive reinforcers risks the development of operant pain.

The housewife who dislikes heavy housework is potentially doubly reinforced when pain occurs. Rest eases the pain, and rest may lead to the assumption of the arduous task by another family member. The employee by resting successfully avoids a job crisis with which he or she feels unready to cope or simply avoids going to a dissatisfying job or of interacting with unpleasant co-workers. Some people do not enjoy socializing. Staying home has advantages for them.

The next step in the analysis is to consider what happens when rest or time out continues to occur with some frequency. Do reinforcers in addition to the easing of pain continue to be available? Are household chores done by others, or do they perhaps receive benign neglect? Or, instead, do they pile up to be done only by the patient? Does absence from work receive monetary reinforcement in the form of wage replacement funds from insurance or compensation? If time out does gain access to sustaining reinforcement, at least an element of operant pain can be expected as part of the diagnostic picture.

Notice that in the arrangements just described, the reinforcers for time out or rest sometimes are contingent on pain behavior. Perhaps the only way the housewife receives help with heavy chores is if she demonstrates to her environment that she is unable to do them. The pattern of pain-contingent reinforcement may also apply to the other examples. Reinforcers accessible by rest or time out have the technical requirements for being effective. They may increase the behavior they follow, and they may be contingent on those behaviors.

These examples were begun in the context of situations in which physical findings were there to be found. That is of course not a requirement. A transitory peripheral pain stimulus might initiate rest and termination of activity; such behavior subsequently to be reinforced by the payoffs of time out as well as by pain relief. Physical findings that were major elements in the picture at the outset of the pain problem may be resolved or reduced. The effect of successful treatment is to remove both a pain stimulus and, concomitantly, a potent reinforcer that has been contingent on pain behavior. If the disc problem is effectively resolved by, say, surgery or traction, subsequently the rest is no longer reinforced by pain relief. However, it is likely that treatment will not have had its day until

a period of time has passed, time in which rest was occurring in contingent relationships with whatever consequence it met. Reduction of the pain stimulus and removal of pain relief as a reinforcer may not have altered the other contingent relationships. Rest still may pay off in other ways. Pain behaviors under those conditions may continue after successful treatment, or they may resume after a period of time. But, of course, now the patient has operant rather than respondent pain. Notice that the change is not in the behavior itself. The pain behavior may continue to look and sound the same. The change is in the contingency relationships (the reinforcement). Instead of pain relief, it is time out from some aversive activity that maintains the same pain behaviors.

The same basic relationships can apply to the pacer who moves rather than reclines when pain comes. Pacing or movement may interrupt ongoing or projected activities and thereby produce time out. This is seen clinically, although not as frequently as the recliner pattern. For example, a reluctant card player agrees to go along with the eager spouse to a card party but must periodically arise from the card table to move, shift position, or pace to ease pain. Repeated sufficiently, it is not long until social approval is attached by those present to terminating the card game. More frequently, however, pacers are reinforced by activity, just as recliners are reinforced by inactivity. It logically follows that the pain behaviors of pacers are less frequently under control of time out as a reinforcer.

The topic of time out is the focus of the next section and will be related to pain problems in a number of additional ways. For the moment, the concern is with rest as a reinforcer and with the hazards of iatrogenic promotion of operant pain through injudicious use of rest as a prescription.

Rest is usually prescribed or recommended in either of two ways. One is to prescribe a fixed interval of rest, as in an order of 10 days of bedrest or 72 hours of traction. The second pattern is to make it the equivalent of *prn,* that is, take when needed. When the pain arises, rest to stop it. Or, if one senses that the pain is about to arise, rest to avoid it. In the first example, rest may or may not be pain contingent. If termination of the prescribed period of rest is contingent on the patient's report as to how he or she feels, rest is pain contingent. If, after 10 days of bedrest, pain is reported and the prescription is extended, rest is indeed pain contingent. However, it may be decided beforehand that 10 days of rest is all that should be necessary, either to resolve the problem or to give rest an adequate trial as a solution. At the end of the 10 days, rest is withdrawn as a prescribed consequence to pain behavior without regard to the patient's reported pain level. It is then not pain contingent.

The second pattern (taking rest when needed) seems to be used more often. Rest is prescribed and is terminated or extended mainly according to what the patient reports. In that arrangement, rest is pain contingent. Similarly, the patient may be encouraged to work to tolerance. That is, when engaged in pain-relevant activity or exercise and pain arises, increases, or is anticipated as being imminent, stop to rest. Tolerance, in this context, does not necessarily imply working beyond the onset or marked increase of pain to the point of its being intolerable to endure. That use of tolerance is unlikely to be prescribed except perhaps by the most spartan of physicians. To the contrary, a situation is set up for discrimination learning. The patient's task is to detect pain, its increase, or its imminent appearance. When he or she does so, the remedy of rest is then to be applied. Rest is pain contingent. More precisely, rest is contingent on discrimination of a cue. The cue may be mild or severe pain, but it may also be only the anticipation of pain. It is entirely possible that the patient, in all good faith, may rest because of pain when there has been no

pain but only a cue that previously indicated pain was likely soon to come.

It should be evident that these arrangements risk promoting operant pain. The risk is particularly high when two conditions for learning are present. One is that rest gains access to reinforcers in addition to those immediately associated with pain relief, such as time out from unpleasant activities. The second is that rest is pain contingent, for that ensures that the other reinforcers are also pain contingent. Just as in regard to medication regimens, activity or exercise regimens are capable of promoting and sustaining a pain problem. They may bring the pain behaviors under control of systematically reinforcing environmental consequences by making the reinforcers pain contingent.

A remedy or counter-strategy to the foregoing problem will be set forth in detail in Chapter 10. It can be noted at this point that there are simple strategies regarding the format of medication and exercise regimens by which to help forestall development of operant pain and, where it has already developed, to begin reversal of the process.

Indirect but positive reinforcement of pain behavior (avoidance learning)

Much of our behavior results from avoidance learning. We behave or act in certain ways because to do otherwise would lead to aversive or punishing consequences. We act to avoid those consequences.

Behaviors that effectively avoid aversive consequences are thereby reinforced. Avoidance behavior that pays off by successfully avoiding an aversive consequence is more likely to be continued. Each time it pays off, it is automatically reinforced. More than that, under certain conditions, the avoidance behavior needs to be successful only some of the time to be maintained by what is then intermittent reinforcement.

It is often necessary that there be only

periodic glimpses or traces of the aversive consequences to maintain the avoidance behavior. If enough conditioning or learning has occurred, they do not need to be present at all, so long as cues that previously signaled the imminent appearance of the aversive consequences now occur. This is an important point in regard to chronic pain behaviors. Once established, a protective or avoidance-of-pain behavior (for instance, a limp or a restriction of amount of bending, lifting, or walking) may continue to occur consistently at some later time when there is little or no respondent pain.

A common example will illustrate how the process of avoidance learning works. A driver commutes to work each day by a certain street. Suppose that like so many drivers, he is inclined to border on and not infrequently exceed the speed limit. One morning he gets a speeding ticket. That aversive consequence results in slower driving that day and perhaps for a few other days, as well. The effect on his driving is not likely to be durable and pervasive if he previously was a consistently fast driver. However, at the particular spot at which he received the ticket he is likely to continue to slow down for a much longer period of time. It is not necessary that he observe the police car each morning to continue the avoidance behavior of slowing down. The cues that remind him of approach to the spot are sufficient. But now let it be supposed that he slips or forgets one time and gets a second ticket at about the same spot. One can be confident the avoidance behavior of slowing down in the vicinity of that spot will be persistent, regardless of whether he slows down in other areas of the city. He continues with great persistence to avoid a police car in the absence of visible signs. He is likely to continue to experience twinges of apprehension (and perhaps guilt) when he sees that he is approaching what is, for him, "ticket corner." Cues previously preceding the ticket (for example, approaching the corner or twinges of guilt or apprehension)

are sufficient to maintain the avoidance behavior virtually indefinitely. More precisely stated, he may emit the avoidance behavior for hundreds of trials without additional direct reinforcement.

Avoidance behavior, once established, can be persistent. Avoidance behavior appears to play a major role in chronic pain. The behavioral analysis of a chronic pain problem requires careful attention to the matter of avoidance behavior. The chronic pain patient seems often to develop a buffer zone of protective or avoidance behaviors. At first, when the body damage factor was present and active, the protective behaviors avoided or minimized the respondent pain. A limp or compensatory posturing became more comfortable than the normal gait or posture and was therefore reinforced each time it was rehearsed. Experience with the pain, which was coming from some physical damage, may have taught the patient that walking more than 300 yards or three city blocks resulted in pain. Therefore, when walking, the approach to the 300-yard mark became a signal to stop to rest to avoid the pain, which would occur were one to continue. What was experienced subjectively may have been the pain, although in fact it was only anticipated. Keep in mind that, once the avoidance behavior is established, it is no longer necessary to experience the respondent pain for the avoidance behavior to occur. Such automatically occurring body cues as the amount of exertion or fatigue associated with walking 300 yards may have become conditioned cues. Those cues may elicit the same pain behaviors that in the early history of the problem occurred only when 300 yards had been exceeded and the noxious stimulus arose from the site of body damage; that is, there was respondent pain.

In the illustration just described, what the patient experiences at the approach to the 300-yard mark is the same as or highly similar to the respondent pain that was experienced earlier when 300 yards was exceeded. The result is a convincing display of pain behavior based on the honest experience of somatic distress but relating instead to cues that previously preceded pain. If it were the case that the body damage factor had previously been resolved and there was no respondent pain, those pain behaviors could be seen as strictly operant pain.

One of the clearest examples of this phenomenon in my experience concerned a lady in her late 60s who had had a vulvectomy to arrest a carcinoma. The surgery was successful, but over the next 4 years a gradually worsening pain problem developed, associated with the operative site. Multiple and thorough examinations at the time of referral 4 years after surgery suggested that there was much operant and, at most, minimal respondent pain. The patient had an extensive repertoire of pain behaviors, including many avoidance behaviors, of which I shall focus on but one. She could walk about 400 to 800 feet without interruption to rest. The patient, her husband, and other family members reported that it was her consistent pattern to begin walking but, when the 400- to 800-

foot mark was approached, to dissolve into tears and thereafter to require physical assistance to move. This pattern was confirmed in directly observed walking trials within the treatment setting. Walking to tolerance, she never exceeded 800 feet. Every visible and audible indication she displayed suggested that she experienced severe pain after a certain amount of walking. However, concomitant with the walking trials, she was placed on a fixed bicycle and requested to work to tolerance: she was to stop when the bicycle riding produced sufficient pain (or weakness or fatigue). She had not ridden a bicycle since her pain problem began. In fact, so far as could be determined, she had had almost no experience on a bicycle. Whatever there had been had occurred more than 50 years previously. Across two sessions per day for about a week, she never failed to reach 1.5 miles on the bicycle and sometimes went beyond. In this unrehearsed activity, with no opportunity for having acquired cues anticipating pain, she consistently exceeded 7500 feet, as compared with 400 to 800 feet of walking. Fig. 8 portrays her per-

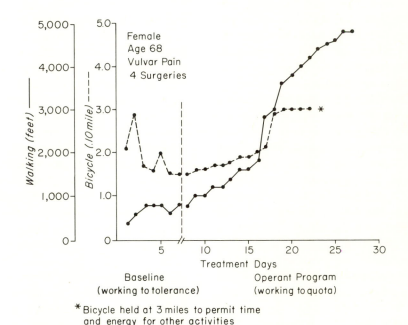

Fig. 8. Exercise tolerance as a function of task familiarity.

formance at these tasks during working to tolerance (baseline trials) and subsequently when rest and attention were programed contingently. The mechanical advantage of a bicycle hardly seems sufficient to account for the discrepancy, particularly when one remembers the pain related to her vulvar area. It was concluded that the pain behavior she displayed when she had walked nearly 400 to 800 feet was an operant that occurred in response to cues previously indicating that pain would occur were she to continue. Her pain behavior had come under virtually total control of environmental cues.

Much behavior is carried out to avoid aversive consequences. It might be asked why the protective or avoidance behaviors of pain patients do not always persist after the pain problem has been resolved. There are two naturally occurring circumstances that serve to limit avoidance behavior. Krasner and Ullmann (1966) point out that a behavioral repertoire based solely on avoidance behavior is not likely to persist long. One reason is that the aversive consequences that the avoidance behaviors are designed to avoid need to occur periodically, or persuasive or compelling cues that they might occur need to be perceived. If the fast driver no longer sees police cars anywhere, his selective slowing down behavior will probably fade to near zero. But there is a second and probably more important consideration. When the avoidance behaviors occur, what are the direct consequences they encounter? Are the avoidance behaviors themselves directly reinforced? Does the environment of the patient respond in such a fashion as to help to maintain them? If avoidance behaviors meet reinforcing consequences in addition to avoiding the aversive event, they are likely to be maintained. If they do not receive reinforcing consequences, they probably will fade unless intermittently reinforced by occurrence of the aversive events or cues relating to them, which they were designed to avoid. Similarly, avoidance behaviors may avoid more than one set of aversive events.

A limp may avoid pain and may also avoid having to go to a dissatisfying job. In such a situation the avoidance behavior may be maintained after resolution of the pain problem by the indirect reinforcement of its successes at avoiding other aversive consequences.

The point can be illustrated in regard to a limp that serves originally to ease a hip or low back pain. Early in the history of the pain problem the limp is consistently reinforced by easing or avoiding pain. But let us suppose the physical or organic element is resolved. The limp is a more energy-costly way of moving about. As such, it has potentially aversive characteristics in itself. To limp is to become more fatigued and to be less able to move around as freely or as far as before. The person with the limp will probably periodically try walking without the limp to test whether pain will occur. By attempting to walk normally, he saves time and energy and is thereby reinforced. If the pain does not recur, or if it occurs in much reduced intensity, the limp may be abandoned. It is not only that the avoidance behavior is no longer necessary but also that the avoidance behavior itself led to some aversive consequences: fatigue and restriction of activity. Suppose, however, that the limp led to reinforcing consequences contingent on the limp. When the limp is observed by family members, special solicitousness may be expressed. The limp may be a signal that pain medication is indicated, with whatever feelings of well being they may produce. Under those conditions the limp may lead systematically to reinforcing consequences otherwise not available. The limp receives positive and contingent reinforcement. It is now no longer necessary for pain to occur. The limp may be maintained by environmental consequences that follow it.

The major points about avoidance learning can now be summarized:

1. Avoidance learning represents behavior that successfully avoids or minimizes aversive consequences.

2. Avoidance learning is common and persistent.
3. Once established, cues previously anticipating the aversive consequences may themselves take on the aversive properties and serve to help maintain the avoidance behavior.
4. Once established, avoidance learning may require minimal reinforcement to be maintained. Maintenance will depend on whether the aversive consequences are still present *or* the avoidance behavior is itself directly or indirectly reinforced.

Pain behavior as avoidance behavior

History. The greatest congruence between traditional views of psychogenic pain and operant pain is found in this section. Relationships between operant pain and personal, emotional, or mental problems are likely to reflect avoidance behaviors acquired in earlier years. The essential element is that the pain behaviors effectively avoid some present or anticipated aversive social, emotional, or interpersonal consequence.

The objective for the moment is not to catalog or review all of the ways in which emotional problems have been related to pain but rather to build a word bridge between those traditional views and a behavioral perspective. Therefore only brief examples will be used to illustrate. There are many other possible examples. The traditional perspective usually labels pain–personal problem relationships as the conversion of a problem of anxiety, for example, to somatic form as pain. Another pattern is to see a person with some body damage and much pain behavior as having excessive self-concern, which in turn elicits intense and persisting bodily preoccupation and hypersensitivity to pain. Such a person is said to have low pain tolerance. These so-called somatic expressions of emotional problems seem more parsimoniously to be described as avoidance behaviors. Similar formulations have long been recognized by psychodynamicists who call attention to

secondary gain. The symptom pays off by reducing anxiety or some other emotionally aversive consequence.

The essential elements of avoidance behavior are found in these kinds of examples. An aversive situation, respondent pain, exists. A protective action develops that avoids or minimizes the pain and thus is reinforced. Concomitantly, there is some kind of emotional or interpersonal problem, perhaps fear or anxiety regarding a present or anticipated consequence. The avoidance behaviors developed to minimize the pain serve also to avoid or minimize the fear or anxiety. The fearful child who is ill remains in bed and eases the somatic distress of his illness but also avoids or minimizes fears experienced on the playground or at school. The pain or illness behavior of reclining is reinforced by reduced somatic distress. Concomitantly, those same pain or illness behaviors also successfully reduce the fear and again are thereby reinforced. Such an arrangement, maintained for a lengthy interval and receiving additional positive reinforcement from parents, could become persistent. More to the point, the child could be expected to find it most difficult to distinguish between somatic distress and fear. The cues that preceded the fear situation could take on the aversive properties of, for example, the somatic distress associated with a fever or a painful bruise or sprain or whatever somatic event made up the physical illness. Given enough rehearsal and enough systematic and effective reinforcement, all the conditions of avoidance learning are present. The pain or illness behaviors come to occur in response to *either* of two sets of cues: pain and illness or fear. Either set of cues may elicit the pain behaviors, and the victim is not able to discriminate. The ensuing avoidance behaviors (conversion symptoms) may persist indefinitely, depending on the consequences they meet.

It is important to remember that avoidance behaviors may need only intermittent reinforcement. However, avoidance behaviors that persist over long periods are probably receiving some current reinforcement in addition to the avoidance of the pain or the fear that existed years before. That current reinforcement may be direct, as in positive reinforcement by family members when pain behaviors are displayed. The current reinforcement may be indirect. Pain behaviors may lead to time out from some currently present or anticipated aversive consequence, as distinguished from the aversive consequences operative years before when the pattern was being established. The reinforcement need not be in the form of successful avoidance or minimization of currently present respondent pain. Avoiding some other aversive situation would serve just as well as a reinforcer (Reese, 1966).

Suppose a patient presents himself to his physician with a complaint of low back pain. Physical findings are minimal or lacking altogether. The principal pain behaviors are verbal descriptions of the site, quality, and intensity of the pain; frequent requests for medical assistance and for analgesics; and restriction in activity. Movement is guarded, and much of the day is spent reclining. An actual case will illustrate. Onset was several months previously after a wrenching of the patient's back in an accident. It was a return of a previously existing back pain problem, which had been quiescent for several years. There had been two or three previous episodes, each of several months' duration. Each had gradually been resolved with conservative management. The patient was age 46 and had received three surgeries for back pain. He had recently been promoted in the executive hierarchy to where he was interacting extensively with a domineering, caustic boss. Earlier in his life his caustic and domineering father had laden him with much work responsibility. Performance never won approval. The father's usual response to a completed task was to criticize performance and to lay out the next task. Illness had been one of the few ways in which the patient had escaped parental

criticism and then only when the illness appeared to be severe. This kind of pattern is familiar enough, and further historical details are unnecessary for the illustration to be made. Following are the key elements:

1. There is a history of illness leading to restricted activity *and* to time out from the highly aversive criticisms of the punitive father. Therefore the avoidance behaviors designed to ease illness also eased anxiety or fear.

2. The recent back wrenching yielded some respondent pain—perhaps a great deal, perhaps only minimal and time limited. In either case, cues were present that led to the avoidance behaviors of restricting activity.

3. Concomitantly, because of the recent promotion resulting in an increase in exposure to caustic authority, conditions for additional reinforcement for the avoidance behaviors were present.

In that kind of situation, the patient can be expected to experience pain. He could also be expected to be (and in the actual case, was) unaware of pain behavior-job status relationships. For him, it was back pain and nothing else.

Reinforcement for avoidance behaviors was current. The patterns of avoidance behavior developed in earlier years were now elicited when pain cues occurred. Restricted activity and the network of associated pain behaviors were being maintained primarily by successful avoidance of punitive father figures now in the form of a boss. It was avoidance behavior. It developed earlier but now occurred because of present cues and was maintained because it avoided current aversive events. Fig. 9 portrays the extent of his impairment before and after treatment as measured by distance walked without interruption and by weekly uptime (sitting and standing or walking) totals. In addition, he progressed from addiction to analgesics to palliative levels.

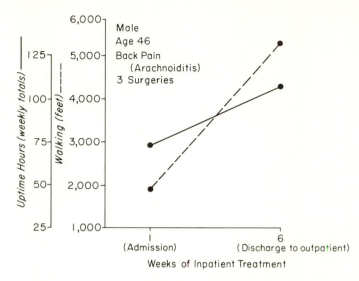

Fig. 9. *Walking and uptime changes in operant treatment.*

The present. There are no learning or reinforcement principles to add in this section. The central issue still concerns the reinforcement of pain behaviors by avoiding aversive events in the environment. These aversive events are unrelated to the pain per se, but they are prevented from occurring by pain behaviors. There are innumerable possible examples, but this is not a book on mental illness, mental hygiene, personality, or psychiatry. Three kinds of illustrations will be presented because they occur frequently and may prove of special interest to those working with chronic pain.

There are many common and straightforward illustrations of avoidance learning relating to events of the present. It has been said by some that a woman presenting a complaint of vague lower quadrant abdominal pain should be assumed to have sexual difficulties until proved otherwise. In my experience, the observation is not without merit. A number of cases have been encountered in which the abdominal pain had proved most persuasive to a number of treatment facilities and had resulted in one or more surgeries, without a resolution to the pain problem. One feature of the pain behavior was that it prohibited

or severely restricted frequency of intercourse. If the woman found intercourse aversive (independently of any issue about pain), pain behavior would be reinforced by time out from intercourse. The potential for that arrangement exists in marriage. There can be repeated and not infrequent reinforcement by time out from intercourse. In several such cases, successful treatment consisted of weaning from the medications, a gradually paced increase in overall activity level (by physical therapy exercises and the like), and sexual counseling or retraining of the marital pair. This is illustrated by the case reported in Fig. 10. Changes in one of the exercises specifically impaired by her lower quadrant pain (hip extensions) are portrayed. There was greater restriction on the right than the left side. After a series of working to tolerance or baseline trials, a contingency management program emphasizing rest and attention as reinforcers increased her tolerance for the hip extension exercise bilaterally, as well as for a number of other exercises. Concomitantly, the marital pair were introduced into sexual counseling. This was transferred and continued to a successful outcome in their home community. Intercourse ceased being aversive, and

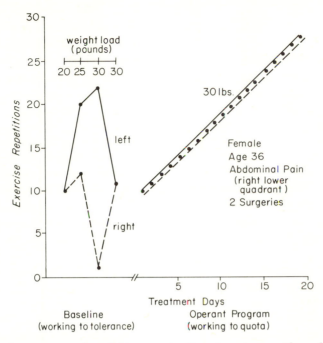

Fig. 10. *Changes in weight pull hip extension (impairment as avoidance behavior).*

the avoidance behaviors reduced in treatment disappeared. They were no longer reinforced.

The key element in this kind of situation usually can be explored by determining what the patient would do that is not presently done if there were no pain. A closely related but not identical question that adds additional useful information concerns what the patient is not now doing because of pain that used to be done. Activities reduced or eliminated by the protective pain behaviors may be aversive. If any of them are aversive, conditions for maintenance of pain-related avoidance behaviors exist.

A second kind of example is sometimes encountered that is really not conceptually different from the first. A patient may have a performance deficit for any of a number of possible reasons. (In the preceding example, difficulty with intercourse could be seen as a performance deficit by husband or wife or both.) Activities likely to risk exposing the performance deficit will be potentially aversive. Pain behaviors may

buy time out from those activities. That often discussed social institution, the wife's headache, is sometimes a case in point. One patient, a young and attractive married woman, had an upward-striving husband who did much business entertaining. His wife was a great potential asset in those endeavors. However, she had limited education and had come from a lower-class family. She developed marked feelings of social inferiority when her husband's entertaining forced her to converse and socialize with people somewhat more educated than herself. Her headaches became increasingly frequent as her husband's efforts to entertain business associates increased. Evaluation indicated much operant pain and led to treatment that could focus on desensitizing her to social interactions.

As a third illustration, vague and persisting pain problems in older patients are sometimes found to be avoidance behavior problems. The arteriosclerotic patient or one who has had a minor stroke may have a significant memory impairment. That memory difficulty may not be apparent to those around the patient except in certain memory-taxing activities. Given the subtle cortical deficits, the special demands on immediate memory functioning associated with card playing make that activity aversive. Pain, wherever its locale, may lead to time out from card playing and thereby successfully mask or avoid the embarrassing and status-threatening memory deficit. It is striking to observe how often the older patient with pain problems will display, under appropriate examination, some form of intellectual deficit relating to cortical impairment. Pain is a less socially aversive symptom than brain damage or memory loss.

Similar patterns have been observed in relation to Huntington's chorea, multiple sclerosis, and other diffuse and progressive neurological conditions. For example, one patient with Huntington's chorea presented vague abdominal wall pain, which prevented working at a highly intellectually demanding kind of work. The evidence indicated that the cortical deficits emerging with advance of the disease were the aversive events for which pain behaviors provided time out. In a case of multiple sclerosis, the highly socialized lady had sustained partial loss of bladder control,

resulting in occasional minor bladder accidents and the ever-present risk they would occur again. She gradually developed pervasive, vague, shifting pain problems that left her unable to attend the frequently scheduled social affairs she and her husband had long been involved in and which presented the risk of acute embarrassment. Moreover, a vicious cycle evolved. She withdrew more and more. Activity level dropped as pain behavior climbed. In her case it was possible to reduce the bladder accident problem by a combination of minor surgery and bladder management training. It was essential, however, to restore activity level and to reduce social (in this case, her husband) reinforcement of her pain behaviors. Fig. 11 describes some of the changes brought about in the activity level of this severely disabled lady.

The underlying principle in these last examples is that pain behavior earns time out from a previously valued activity for which there is a recently developed performance deficit. That should be contrasted with the earlier avoidance behavior examples in which there was time out from what had long been an aversive event or activity. Chronic, progressive illnesses and advancing senility are common sources of

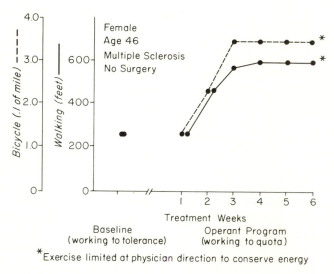

Female
Age 46
Multiple Sclerosis
No Surgery

Baseline
(working to tolerance)

Operant Program
(working to quota)

*Exercise limited at physician direction to conserve energy

Fig. 11. Per session average walking and bicycle riding (impairment partly avoidance behavior).

emerging performance deficits that now make heretofore reinforcing activities aversive.

Pain that is not clearly explicable and that accompanies a progressive illness presents the possibility that it is a problem of operant pain as avoidance behavior.

Nonreinforcement of well behavior

Strictly speaking, this third and final segment of the development of operant pain is but another example of either or both of the preceding sections. That is, pain behavior may occur because it receives relatively more reinforcement than well behavior. This may be true either because it is directly reinforced or because it avoids even more aversive consequences. However, making the distinction of the nonreinforcement of well behavior calls attention to an important conceptual issue. It reminds us that illness and health are not reciprocals. It redirects attention to the importance of establishing effective well behavior as well as diminishing illness. In the long-standing pain patient, this issue is nearly always a central element in the picture. Ignoring it leads to treatment failure or to only time-limited treatment successes. Because of the conceptual similarity to preceding sections, illustrations can be limited.

History

One obvious illustration is the person who has grown up with a history of limited opportunities to achieve successes or who has many skill or performance deficits. Being well and engaging in the daily pursuits of most people will not so often have led to effective reinforcement. Such a person can be expected to develop an extensive repertoire of behaviors designed both to avoid the aversive consequences of failure and to elicit positive reinforcement from the immediate environment. Such a person may, for example, have adopted the role of the carefree, careless, irresponsible village ne'er-do-well. If practiced long enough, such behavior may lead others to lessen their demands and expectations, "because of course he would mess it up anyway." The person might have adopted a reclusive, hostile, isolated style designed to keep people (and their performance demands) at a distance. But he might also have developed a vast illness repertoire. Weakness, ease of fatigue, hypersensitivity to pain or stress, and a readiness to get sick in the face of demands may describe much of the behavioral repertoire. In each case there is relative nonperformance of culturally expected tasks or roles. In each case, were those tasks to be attempted, prior conditioning has taught the person that aversive consequences associated with failure or inadequate performance were likely to occur *and* that the buffer zone of protective pain behaviors leads to less aversive consequences. Pain or illness behaviors may lead to additional positive reinforcement in the form of special attention and the like.

In addition to performance deficits, there is another important source of failures of reinforcement of well behavior. The immediate environment may respond to pain behaviors with consistent and even militant prohibitions on activity or well behavior. This issue has already been considered in the context of the direct reinforcement of pain behavior. It was pointed out how family members may specifically encourage and selectively reinforce resting or other forms of pain behavior. Similarly, physicians may, by the form of medication regimens or the prescription of exercise and rest, inadvertently contingently reinforce pain behavior. All that needs to be added at this point is to note that these family and health care system responses often go beyond the reinforcement of pain behavior. They may include systematic and sometimes vigorous constraints on contrary activity or well behavior. The patient may be admonished to take it easy and be criticized if he does not comply.

Physician recommendations regarding rest and activity restriction need careful thought. The patient often cannot well judge what is a reasonable length of compliance. The end point of rest, as well as the beginning, needs to be spelled out and criteria identified. The point is illustrated by the case of a 16-year-old boy. He came with the complaint of low back pain that had persisted for nearly a year and for which bed rest and a highly reduced activity level had been prescribed. The boy festered at the inactivity but complied, receiving further encouragement no doubt from the militant insistence of his parents that he follow physician orders. Despite his restlessness, his movements were guarded. He either experienced pain on movement or, more likely, anticipated that he would. Evaluation indicated that whatever physical finding had warranted the bed rest and restricted activity nearly a year before was no longer present. Precise current tolerance limits for walking were needed as part of an operant conditioning-based treatment program. To that end, he was asked to climb flights of steps until pain, weakness, or fatigue forced him to stop. He was reassured that the stair climbing would not produce body damage. On the first stair climbing trial he completed fifty-five flights of thirteen steps up, and an equal number down, with only momentary pauses to catch his breath! In each other exercise he performed from the outset at approximately equivalent levels. So far as could be judged, his pain behaviors had been maintained for some months almost solely by the prescribed prohibition of activity, that is, the withholding of reinforcement for well behavior by physician and parents.

There is another set of factors bearing on the nonreinforcement of well behavior. Family members of a pain patient may find that the patient's pain behaviors yield time out from aversive activities for them. If the patient is inactive, the spouse may effectively avoid aversive activities. The possible examples are countless and need not be catalogued here. A few case illustrations will be presented to suggest the range of possible patterns.

One lady in her late 40s had had multiple back surgeries but the pain persisted. Much medication was taken. There were frequent calls for physician assistance. Activity level at home was severely curtailed, requiring her husband to do the heavy housework and help prepare meals. Emancipated daughters also came in periodically to help out. Physical findings indicated modest pathology, mostly resulting from the surgeries. Evaluation of the total situation indicated that the husband was a complex mixture of sullen resentment at the interference in their lives from her pain and of rather militant readiness to offer medication and encouragement to take it easy when pain behaviors were displayed. The latter behaviors on his part were more than mere solicitousness and husbandly concern. He made it clear that he was not ready to limit or reduce his overprotective behaviors. On further exploration, it developed that the husband had a secondary impotence, based on some problems of his own and not on neurophysiological deficits. These dated from the same general time period as when his wife's pain problem (initiated by a fall at work) had begun. He was a restless and active man and resented the constraints on camping and fishing that his wife's pain problem entailed. But he also found that her pain limited or reduced the frequency of intercourse. She had long been a more enthusiastic sexual partner than he. She made not excessive sexual demands but, for him, more than he desired. There is little to suggest he in any significant way produced the pain problem. But the evidence indicated he helped to maintain it by militantly and selectively reinforcing activity constraints within the home.

Another female patient was her husband's second wife. His first wife had died of a myocardial infarction while engaging in heavy lifting after a long siege of back pain. His second wife developed back pain secondary to an accidental fall. Physical findings after the first few weeks were minimal, but a pervasive pain problem

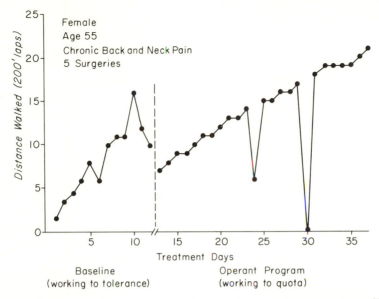

Fig. 12. *Increased exercise tolerance with termination of nonreinforcement for well behavior.*

gradually developed. Movements were guarded and most of the day was spent in bed. This lady had previously been active. Behavioral analysis of the patient's pain behavior and environmental responses to it indicated that her husband was militant in constraining her from activity. He seemed to have an almost phobic fear that his second wife would also die if she exerted herself, particularly in the presence of some back pain. He went so far as to padlock the basement door so she could not carry laundry to the laundry room! A great deal of retraining was required to change his overprotective behaviors. She rapidly blossomed into a high activity level within the hospital. But a number of evening and weekend passes with structured rehearsals on his part were required to develop his skill and readiness to reinforce activity. Fig. 12 describes the rapid and steady change in her ability to walk without interruption for rest when reinforcement was withdrawn from her pain behavior and rest and attention became contingent on performance. It will be noted from Fig. 12 that baseline or working-to-tolerance trials began to show increased exercise tolerance. The upward trend of

baseline trials is often encountered. Fig. 12 also illustrates two instances of failed quotas. That point is dealt with in Chapter 10.

One occasionally encounters adolescent males with chronic pain. When that happens and physical findings are vague or minimal, the behavior of the mother should be reviewed. Some mothers delay emancipation by shaping and dedicatedly reinforcing illness or pain behavior. This pattern has also been observed in a handful of instances in relation to the perennial bachelor whose mother continues to look out for her son's bad back.

There are innumerable other illustrations one might encounter. The key point is to recognize the importance of the family and the immediate environment to the chronic pain problem. In an earlier part of this chapter it was noted that one often needs to determine what actions or behaviors the patient is no longer practicing because of the pain, or what the patient would practice if there were no pain. The same pair of questions should be asked of the spouse. What does the spouse no longer do because of the patient's pain problem? What would the spouse do that is not now done, were the pain problem to be resolved? Those questions provide entry into the issue of whether the patient's pain behaviors provide time out to the spouse from otherwise aversive events and thereby lead to contingent reinforcement of pain behavior and nonreinforcement of well behavior.

The special case of depression

Clinically, it is the exceptional chronic pain patient who is not depressed. Empirically, the pervasiveness of depression in patients with chronic pain was documented repeatedly in both Chapters 1 and 2. In the analysis of the concept of psychogenic pain, psychodynamic formulations of how pain and depression may be related were presented and discussed. The concept of depression itself, when viewed in behavioral terms, appears to have special characteristics that need additional consideration in relation to the development and evaluation of operant pain and, later, in relation to treatment. A necessary prelude to doing that has been the presentation of operant principles. We can now consider this important feature to the clinical picture of chronic pain.

Depression may be seen as having several possible roles in regard to chronic pain. The uncomfortable and functionally impaired pain patient is saddened by his or her plight; he or she is depressed. In that instance, the depression is a result or product of the pain problem. Another possibility is that prior associations between depression and pain result in cues or stimuli for one producing the other as well. In that instance, depression is an accompaniment to pain as a consequence of previous conditioning. Depression and perhaps other members of the broader response class of distress are effectively elicited by pain stimuli. Alternatively, it may be cues or stimuli to depression that also elicit pain responses or behaviors. In that instance, pain is a result or product of depression. Insofar as the patient identified the problem as pain (and not depression), the

patient may be said to be misperceiving.

Each of the three possibilities cited represents the presence of something: an emotional state of depression, regardless of whether it is perceived by the patient as such. Psychodynamically the presence of the emotional state of depression is likely to be viewed as a product of guilt, withheld or internalized anger, or sense of loss. There has been considerable study of depression from behavioral perspectives (Ferster, 1966; Lazarus, 1968; Lewinsohn and Atwood, 1968). Those analyses suggest yet another way of looking at depression, one which appears to have particular relevance to chronic pain.

Depression may be seen as a state of deprivation of reinforcement. The key element is the *absence* of something, effective positive reinforcement. The clinical manifestations of depression (for example, sleep disturbance, loss of appetite, or retarded performance) are incidental, as are the alleged or inferred causes of the depression. The person who has suddenly lost his or her spouse by death or divorce has also suddenly sustained loss of access to many if not all of the reinforcers previously sustaining marital-related behavior. As a consequence, he grieves. If either the death or the divorce had been of gradual onset, alternative sources of reinforcement likely will have at least begun to be secured and, if those efforts were at all successful, the reinforcement deprivation would not have been so great. The grieving would then be correspondingly less severe.

Even the depression presumably related to withheld or internalized anger seems to fit this paradigm. When the anger is not expressed, whatever reinforcement previously derived from expressing anger does not become available. At the same time, it is not likely that successfully withholding anger will itself receive immediate and effective reinforcement except in unusual circumstances. People with whom one is angry are not likely to be effective social reinforcers for the nonexpression of anger. Perhaps, in addition, the lack of expression of anger is often only relatively true. The less-than-openly angry behavior may still be easily perceived by others. It is not then likely to receive positive social reinforcement from one's milieu.

The chronic pain patient usually, although not always, sustains a deprivation of reinforcement if the pain problem is severe enough to interfere with daily activity. The amount of functional impairment relating to the pain problem usually measures the amount of reinforcement deprivation. That is, the patient is cut off from some activities in which he previously engaged. Those activities had been receiving reinforcement or they would not have been occurring. They now cannot occur, or they occur in reduced frequency or form. Their sustaining reinforcers are lost. The longer the history of the problem and the greater the interference in the premorbid behavioral repertoire, the greater the deprivation of reinforcement and the greater the amount of depression to be expected.

There are two exceptions. One is where the functional impairment does not result in a deprivation of reinforcement because the activities no longer performed were aversive or nonreinforcing. In that case, there is no loss of reinforcement, and so there is no depression. The second exception is where alternative sources of reinforcement have emerged and adequately replace the deficit. That kind of exception might be illustrated by the pain patient whose family provides ample and effective positive reinforcement of pain behavior.

Diagnostically, the behavioral view of depression has several implications. Foremost is the expectation that depression probably will be present, whether clinically apparent or not. If it is not present, there is the further diagnostic implication that the patient's pain problem is not costing the patient very much. That, in turn, as will be discussed in Chapters 5 and 6, has implications for the behavioral analysis of the total problem. There is also the issue of pain and depression having interchangeable characteristics. That is not specific to behavioral perspectives, but it does serve as a reminder that, diagnostically, pain and depression are sometimes mistaken one for the other.

The behavioral view of depression takes on special pertinence in regard to treatment planning, as well. The best general statement of it is that treatment will need to provide for access to effective sustaining reinforcement for posttreatment behavior. That issue will receive considerably further treatment in later chapters. The point, however, takes on a special shape when it is remembered that depression is often accompanied by retarded activity level. Activity level must then be increased to provide access to sustaining reinforcement. One cannot work or play well enough for it to pay off with adequate reinforcement if performance is lethargic or retarded. Both energizing medications and systematic efforts at increasing exercise and physical activity level are often important features in the operant-based treatment of chronic pain.

4 Techniques of behavioral analysis and behavior change

This chapter describes methods and procedures for behavioral analysis and for carrying out contingency management programs. The key principles underlying these procedures were described in the preceding chapter. The working rudiments can now be set forth in more detail. The behavioral analysis of a patient's pain problem requires more than passing familiarity with these concepts, as does laying out effective treatment programs.

This section of the book is the first to deal directly with the technology of changing behavior. A few comments regarding ethical and moral issues are in order before proceeding further into this topic.

Behavior modification, including, particularly, operant conditioning, has by now gained considerable acceptance, even by many who viewed it initially with varying mixtures of alarm, disdain, and disbelief. The rapid expansion in use of these methods during the past decade into a widening circle of settings has generated some acceptance by sheer weight of momentum and precedent; additionally, results stand on their own feet. However, these methods, like all other forms of intervention in the helping professions, must be accountable in the ethical and moral standards by which we function.

In books of this type, the ethical and moral standards of those who propose a procedure, and of the procedures they propose, usually are viewed implicitly as acceptable until indications to the contrary become evident—or, at any rate, seem to in some critical eyes. In the case of behavior modification, however, it seems appropriate to add comments about ethical and moral issues, not because the procedures are fraught with unethical or im-

moral perils, but because of the frequency with which people express questions in those directions when the methods are first encountered.

It goes beyond the scope of this book to deal in detail with ethical issues. A few brief comments will be made to outline the more critical aspects of the issues and to respond to them. Further discussion of these issues may also be found in Berni and Fordyce (1973) and in Ulrich and associates (1966).

First of all, operant methods are sometimes characterized as *manipulative*. Every professional intervention, of whatever orientation, style, or technique, is potentially manipulative, whether it be surgery, exhortation, prayer, massage, medication, or whatever. The degree to which it is carried out in a fashion fairly termed as manipulative will depend on the adequacy of the communication between therapist and patient. If objectives, methods, and, as well as possible, an explication of alternative methods and their anticipated outcomes, have been discussed and agreement to proceed is mutually arrived at, there is little need for concern about manipulation. *Manipulative*, in this context, appears to refer mainly to applying a method or producing an effect on or about a patient without his or her knowledge that that was underway. In the medical context, the use of placebos is a common example. A response to the manipulation issue can be brief. By all means explain to the patient before beginning what one proposes to do and how it is to be done. Proceed only when there is agreement that this is the program he or she wants to follow.

The second most common ethical or moral issue seems to be the assertion sometimes made that these methods dehumanize or that they are insensitive. That is a more difficult problem to deal with because it depends so much on "whose ox is being gored." To argue that for behavior to be influenced by consequences (an empirical observation that has been confirmed beyond counting or challenge) is dehumanizing, is to argue from a view of humans that does not conform with facts. The real thrust of *that* position would appear to be that the critic would *prefer* that behavior not be influenced by consequences, or that, if behavior were not influenced by consequences, people would be different (that is, "more human"!). That argument is not unlike arguing against the law of gravity. One may not like it, or one may prefer that it worked a different way, but to argue that it is not so is fruitless.

The second part of this issue is related to insensitivity. This issue has been raised repeatedly by those of the traditional psychodynamic persuasion. The merit of the argument that the methods of behavior modification are used in an insensitive way by a given practitioner will depend on the specific instance. If, as one suspects is usually the case, the insensitivity issue is raised because the practitioner is observed to proceed (or it is anticipated he may) without discussing and planning with the patient, then there is no disagreement here. It has already been stated that full knowledge and consent should be reached before proceeding. If, however, it is claimed that the methods are intrinsically insensitive, then, indeed, whose ox is being gored?

The connotation of insensitivity in this regard appears to claim that the methods fail to take into account adequately some of the sensitivities of the person. That is a curious argument, one which appears to be rather vulnerable. It is found lacking on at least two counts. One is that traditional personality theories can properly be seen as characterizing people as relatively insensitive, for the major thrust of those personality theories is that behavior is guided from within; that is, it occurs somewhat in-dependently of the immediate environment. Stated another way, one's personality shields him to some degree from the influences to which he presently is exposed. That proposition would appear to indicate as much *in*sensitivity as sensitivity, for it claims that people have *less* sensitivity to their environments.

The reverse of the coin is to note that the nucleus of operant conditioning proceeds from the fact that, as humans, we are indeed highly sensitive to what is going on around us. Our behavior consistently reflects that sensitivity by being influenced by it. The statement is not that we are crushed or dominated or led by the nose by the environment, but we are influenced. That is hardly insensitivity.

Such a brief consideration hardly deals with all potentially relevant ethical or moral issues. Hopefully, it fairly defines an acceptable and defensible position.

There are a number of considerations to be weighed in deciding how much detail is essential to the purposes of this book. Too brief a presentation risks promoting superficial or premature attempts to apply contingency management procedures in working with chronic pain patients. On the other hand, readers might be provided with more than they want or need to know about the subject. Many medical practitioners, for example, will, in the course of their practices, use the concepts and methods described far enough to arrive at tentative diagnostic decisions. A quick or rough behavioral analysis of the situation, perhaps carried out because physical findings were questionable, may indicate the possibility of considerable operant pain, and lead to referral to practitioners specializing in the analysis of behavior. Similarly, if in whatever fashion it is determined about a patient that there is a significant amount of operant pain or that the respondent pain present could perhaps be alleviated by systematic increases in activity level, referral may be made to a facility prepared to carry out such procedures. A balance needs to be found in regard to the amount of detail and depth to be provided.

The strategy adopted here is to set forth the essential rudiments but with limited discussion and illustrations in this chapter. Illustrations and more depth of consideration will automatically derive from later chapters dealing with behavioral analysis of pain as part of the diagnostic process and with sections on treatment methods. Additional description and illustrations in chronic illness settings may also be found in Berni and Fordyce (1973).

Brief illustrations of major points will be offered from time to time. These will be based, for the most part, on case applications with which the author is familiar, either as the engineer or consultant to the application in treatment settings, or as drawn from behavior change projects applied directly to patients in a training hospital or clinic setting and carried out by students (resident physicians, physical and occupational therapy undergraduate students, predoctoral and postdoctoral psychology interns, and graduate students in nursing and rehabilitation counseling) under his direction or that of colleagues. In the interest of brevity of presentation, no effort will be made to provide all salient aspects of case examples. Only elements essential to illustrate the point at hand will be presented.

What is behavior?

Behavior means action. It is something a person does. Ogden Lindsley (1969) has said, "If a dead man can do it, it isn't behavior!" by which he means, as a figure of speech, that a dead man might be conceived of as feeling sad, but he cannot cry. He might think, but he cannot add a column of figures or write an answer. He might feel restless, but he cannot walk. The term *behavior* in this context refers to observable, countable action. Those are the phenomena that one seeks to change when embarking on a contingency management program with a patient (Reese, 1966).

Consider the example of obesity and overeating. The behavior of concern is eat-

ing behavior: loading a fork with food and conveying same into the mouth. One might say about a chronically obese, chronically overeating person that he or she is self-destructive or rejects the self-concept that is usually thought of as normal and consciously or unconsciously participates in activities that have the effect of masking or destroying the normal self by overeating. Such statements, or any number of possible variations, are attempts to explain or understand the behavior of overeating. But the behavior is still overeating. A contingency management approach might initially look for cues and contingencies in the environment that appear to maintain eating behavior or that fail to reinforce acceptable alternative behaviors. Assuming such relationships were pinpointed, it might then proceed to modify some of those contingencies toward the end of reducing the rate or frequency of eating behavior. More specifically, the target, in a given case, could well be reducing the number of mouthfuls of food ingested per day. That is behavior.

Chronic pain provides a multitude of examples, many of which will be the focus of treatment methods set forth later. Pain as behavior consists of the pain behaviors or displays of pain. The patient grimaces or limps or asks for medication. One possible set of explanations for such pain behaviors is the presence of body damage. In a given case, another explanation may be that the pain behaviors—the operants—have come under control of environmental contingencies. If treatment proceeds under the guidance of that latter diagnostic conclusion, it focuses on trying to reduce grimacing, reduce limping, and reduce requests for medication, as well as whatever other pain behaviors the patient has that influence the environment and are influenced by it (Fordyce and associates, 1973).

The objective is to help the patient change what he does, his behavior.

Pinpointing behavior

The behavior change process requires precision. One must be specific about what behaviors are to be changed. The power of contingency management depends on initially precise relationships between bits of behavior and consequences that follow.

It is not enough to set one's goal with a given patient as that of helping the patient to get better or to reduce his pain problem. The program must be broken down into specific behaviors to be changed; for example, reduce medication intake, increase walking, or decrease reclining. Unless that is done, the effectiveness of the contingency relationships set up to help the patient will be muffled to a point at which the wrong behaviors may be reinforced and the target behaviors may fail to receive reinforcement.

Behavior is influenced by the consequences it touches (that is, consequences that are immediately contiguous in time), and so touch they must. To be effective, a consequence must be contingent on occurrence of the behavior to be increased, *and* in early phases of the behavior change process it must be delivered immediately. Those time relationships can and should be loosened later in the process. If the specification as to what behaviors are to be reinforced is fuzzy or too broad, reinforcement can only be aimed at the general vicinity of the target and may only occasionally touch it.

To illustrate, consider a pain patient who, as one of his pain behaviors, walks with a pronounced limp. It will be assumed that, whatever its origins, the limp now occurs because of the environmental consequences that have been following it. Walking in the physical therapy gymnasium might be prescribed as part of treatment. The reinforcers programmed to increase activity, let us say, are rest and therapist encouragement. That is, *x* amount of walking immediately leads to *y* amount of rest and to praise by the therapist. But here is a mixed bag of behaviors. Activity or walking is to be increased, but limping —as a pain behavior—is to be decreased. If the patient walks enough to meet a treatment quota but does so with his limping action, the subsequent rest and therapist attention touch both walking and limping. Those are usually effective reinforcers and could be expected to strengthen walking *and* limping. More precision is needed.

One remedy is to separate walking from limping, at least where rest and attention or praise are programmed as contingencies. The walking quota can be changed to "number of steps without the limp." Initially, that might be only one, two, or a handful of steps. Even so, the program begins at a point within the patient's reach. He can, let us say, walk two steps before he must limp. A brief period of rest—a pause between steps—and therapist praise now occur immediately after two nonlimping steps. That arrangement permits the reinforcers to engage with or touch the behavior to be increased, nonlimping walking, and not the behavior to be decreased, limping.

This kind of careful scrutiny is essential in behavior change programs.

Changing behavior

Changing behavior by contingency management is a precision enterprise. The starting or entry point—identification of the behavior to be changed—must be precise. The complexity of that task is reduced considerably when it is recognized that almost every behavior change problem can be analyzed into one or a combination of these three possibilities:

1. Some behavior is not occurring often enough and needs to be increased or strengthened.
2. Some behavior is occurring too frequently and needs to be diminished in frequency or strength or eliminated.
3. There is behavior missing from the patient's repertoire that is needed and that therefore must be learned or acquired.

It is easier to pinpoint what behaviors to change and to work toward bringing that about when the problems are analyzed in those terms. A ready illustration of this guiding framework is often found in patients with chronic low back pain. For the sake of the illustration, let it be agreed that the workup indicates considerable operant pain and a corresponding dearth of effective well behavior. Let it be supposed further that the patient demands and takes much pain medication and besieges his immediate environment with visible and audible indications of distress (grimacing, moaning, or compensatory posturing), that he spends much of the day reclining before a TV set, and that he has a long history of ineffective relationships with co-workers, as a consequence of which employers have found it easy to let him go, however effective was his work output.

To bring that set of problems down to manageable size, one can determine what should be increased, decreased, or eliminated, and what should be added to the patient's repertoire to fill significant gaps to ensure adequate well behavior. Clearly, the roster of pain behaviors needs to be decreased. That is, reinforcement needs to be withdrawn as a systematic consequence to (1) requesting pain medication, (2) taking pain medication, (3) grimacing, (4) moaning, (5) compensatory posturing, and (6) daytime reclining (or TV watching). These are the ways in which the patient's world is informed that there is a pain problem and that may therefore elicit contingent attention. There are likely to be yet other pain behaviors, but these are enough to make the point.

The second issue concerns behaviors to be increased. For simplicity of illustration, the choices will be arbitrary. The type of list is defined by the particular circumstances of a particular patient. It might be decided that the list of behaviors to be increased includes the following:

1. Walking (with minimal or no limping)
2. Deep knee bends
3. Pelvic tilts
4. Stair climbing (with minimal or no limping)
5. Situps or letbacks
6. Carrying objects across a room (of gradually increasing weight)

7. Conversations with people in which there is no visible or audible indication of pain

Each of these is an operant. Each is a behavior that, as mastered and performed, moves a pain patient toward freedom of action and motion. They are useful and sometimes essential to a more successful way of life. To paraphrase the point, the patient's objective in life may not be to do pelvic tilts, but if he can do them, he will be able then to do other things that go to make up his objectives or lead to them. In this context, they are behaviors to be increased.

The final question concerns behaviors to be shaped or added to the patient's repertoire. Survival at work may be seriously compromised by inability to relate with co-workers, which is a deficit arbitrarily inserted into this example. To ignore that problem would be to ignore the limited reinforcement such a person may receive for otherwise effective well behavior. Those limitations may be a result of uniformly adverse interpersonal relationships. Analysis of his interpersonal interacting behaviors may reveal a self-centered conversationalist who ignores others, overrides them, or is consistently critical of them. Those all could be seen as behaviors to be decreased. But, in a given case, it might instead be concluded that the behavior that is lacking is that of giving social reinforcement to fellow conversationalists and fellow workers. In the strictest sense, the patient presumably knows about such behavior, and, in that sense, it is in his repertoire. But by observation of his social interactions one may note that the social reinforcing behavior rarely occurs. It therefore qualifies as a target for shaping, that is, for breaking down "socially reinforcing others" into a series of specific elements or examples and selectively reinforcing their occurrence. Such a list might include the following:

1. Establishing eye contact and smiling while listening to others.
2. Prefacing an interruption with a

comment indicating that the one to be interrupted had been listened to.

3. Praise or approval-type statements in response to others.

Such a list might take any of dozens of forms. The point is that each element of this list and of the preceding two lists is an operant. It is an observable, countable behavior to which, therefore, it is possible to arrange that effective reinforcers touch its occurrence.

Organizing a patient's program into the categories of behaviors to be increased, decreased, and acquired can be helpful to patients, their families, and the health care professionals working with them. It helps everyone to maintain a focus on the target and to develop more skill and precision in keeping reinforcing consequences contingent on only the behaviors they were designed to reinforce.

Increasing or strengthening a behavior

Positive reinforcers increase or strengthen the operants they follow. Strengthening of a behavior is to be expected when an effective positive reinforcer is made contingent on and is delivered as a consequence of the behavior to be increased. Arranging that such potentially effective reinforcers as rest become contingent on amounts walked should have the effect of increasing or strengthening walking behavior. That is, the patient will come to walk longer and farther. The qualifications of *effective reinforcer* and *contingent* are further elaborations of the technology regarding reinforcers. These will be dealt with later in the chapter.

There is another point that has particular importance for chronic illness, including chronic pain. When it is observed that a behavior is not occurring at expected or desired levels of frequency or strength, it can be assumed that the behavior is not being reinforced or is not in the patient's repertoire. A chronic pain patient observed not to be moving around much probably receives little reinforcement for walking. If walking exacerbates pain, it is no sur-

prise that he does not walk much. Physical findings may, however, provide a basis for doubting that modest amounts of walking lead to increases in pain. This is a different matter. Walking that is unlikely to produce respondent pain is surely going unreinforced, or such alternatives as sitting or reclining are being reinforced, or both. For the moment the former will be considered: the patient's environment is failing to reinforce walking behavior.

It probably would not be difficult to increase walking within the formal treatment setting for a patient for whom the pain behaviors, including in this example much reclining and little walking, can reasonably be labeled as operant pain. But the workup suggests that the patient's environment inadequately reinforces walking. It would therefore be important to rearrange family responses to walking and nonwalking behaviors to ensure that walking will be strengthened and maintained.

Increasing the strength of a behavior often involves decreasing reinforcement of less desirable alternative behaviors, which are also incompatible with treatment objectives.

Decreasing or weakening a behavior

There are three ways to diminish or weaken a behavior. One is to punish the behavior by delivering a noxious stimulus immediately after its occurrence. That is a true statement that has practical, ethical, and moral limitations. Behavior stopped or interrupted by punishment tends only to be deferred, not eliminated. Aversive conditioning, as it is called when noxious or aversive stimuli are used to interrupt a behavior and inhibit its occurrence, rarely is clinically useful except under special circumstances not germane to the problems dealt with by this book. Aversive conditioning will therefore receive no further consideration here; it is put aside for ethical, legal, moral, and pragmatic reasons.

A second way to decrease or weaken a behavior is to let it no longer be followed by positive reinforcement. Effective reinforcement that has been occurring contingent on the behavior to be decreased, when withdrawn, usually results in a fading and ultimate disappearance of the behavior. The process is called extinction. It should be noted that the withdrawal of reinforcement usually leads initially to a brief upsurge of the behavior before fading begins.

A third way to decrease or weaken a behavior that often proves effective is simply to reinforce effectively a behavior incompatible with the one to be reduced. To repeat an illustration used earlier, one way of reducing reclining is to withdraw the reinforcers that have been maintaining that behavior. An alternative method is to attach effective reinforcement to walking, for walking is in a sense incompatible with reclining.

Particular attention should be paid in evaluation to the question of what reinforcers, delivered by whom or in what way, and in what schedule, are serving to maintain operant pain behaviors. If the patient is lying down more than he needs to, somebody is doing something wrong. Reclining behavior may be directly or indirectly reinforced. Walking may be punished. Walking may fail to receive positive reinforcement. That kind of information plays a vital role in designing an overall program for a patient. There must be a clear grasp of what behaviors are to be changed *and* what reinforcement arrangements in the patient's life need to be changed. Otherwise, treatment gains will fade away.

Counting behavior

One cannot determine whether behavior change has occurred unless it is known how much the behavior was occurring before and how much it occurs after efforts at change. Statements by patients that they feel better (or worse) do not suffice. Patients may say they are better or worse for many reasons, only some of which relate to the state of their health or to the frequency of pain and well behaviors. But more than that, one cannot determine

whether a given plan of contingent reinforcement is having a beneficial effect unless it is possible to make precision observations about the rate of the target behavior and the delivery of reinforcement contingent on it.

The importance of being specific about what behaviors are to be changed has been emphasized. It is essential to have quantifiable units of the target behavior to accomplish that. For that there is the *movement cycle.*

A movement cycle refers to a completed unit of a behavior. A cycle begins with the start of the behavior and ends when the person is in a position to repeat the behavior. For behaviors having a relatively low frequency or rate, the movement cycle should be virtually the smallest measurable unit. Behaviors having a considerable frequency permit movement cycles to be combined into larger units.

Consider the example of walking. If a patient has been essentially bed-bound or has been walking but a few steps at a time, the movement cycle at the outset of a behavior change program designed to increase walking should be the advance of both feet. That is, "left-right" is the movement cycle. The patient would not be in a position to repeat walking behavior when only one foot has been advanced. He is ready to repeat when the second foot comes forward. The limited walker requires a movement cycle of each pair of steps, left and right.

Suppose a patient begins at or achieves a walking distance of several hundred feet before pain, weakness, or fatigue interfere and result in stopping. It would be arduous and unnecessary to count each pair of steps. Instead, a course may be measured in the physical therapy gymnasium, in a corridor, in the patient's house, in his driveway, or wherever. Patients will take about the same number of steps each time they traverse the course. The exceptions to that are too trivial to bother with. The movement cycle can now become the number of laps. A lap could be either one way over the course or a round trip. It is unimportant which, so long as the choice is used consistently.

A shift from a smaller unit (for example, left-right pair of steps) to a larger one (for example, 200-foot lap) can be made as treatment progresses.

A movement cycle must be complete, or patients and observers will be confused and make important counting errors. If one were counting doing situps in the physical therapy gymnasium, the movement cycle would be prone to sitting to prone. It is not prone to sitting. Only when the prone position has been resumed may another situp begin.

Another example will be considered to be sure that there is clarity on this point. It is often useful to assign chronic back pain patients the task of operating a hand-powered printing press in the occupational therapy room. It is a temptation to measure performance by counting the number of minutes of work. Minutes are not movement cycles, nor are they operants. Furthermore, minutes do not have specifiable behavioral referents. Stating that someone has worked 10 minutes tells nothing about how much was done. Units of measurement must be in terms of the target behavior; in this case, number of pulls on the hand press, at such and such a level of weight or resistance. A pull, in this case, means to pull the lever forward and to let it return to the starting position from which it could again be pulled forward.

There is another reason for counting behavior. One must know the starting point before behavior change can be assessed. This is called the *baseline*. A behavior in the patient's repertoire that is to be increased or decreased should first be observed and counted to determine its frequency or rate at the outset of treatment. To return to the example of walking, once it is known that the patient can and does walk, say, a few dozen steps or more before stopping, the option of using laps on a measured course is probably the easiest method. The length of a lap should be *less* than the distance the patient is walking at

the outset. If the patient walks approximately 60 to 100 feet before stopping, laps should be something less than 50 feet, perhaps 25 feet. The patient is provided several opportunities to walk to tolerance to demonstrate how much he or she can walk. The number of laps walked is the baseline. A single baseline trial is insufficient to yield a reliable value. There is no fixed formula. Baseline trials should continue until a pattern seems fairly clear, and that is rarely fewer than four trials.

One can determine whether behavior change efforts are having an effect only when the baseline has been determined by direct observation. Those baseline observations should be made *before* setting up contingent reinforcement. Otherwise, there is no way to determine whether changes that occur are related to the contingent reinforcers or to some other effect. This is not a mere sop to scientific methodology. If change is not occurring and there was no baseline, futile methods may persist needlessly. If change is occurring but is related to effects other than the selected reinforcers, subsequent use of those reinforcers to help change other behaviors will probably be wasted effort.

There is one more measuring or counting point to be made. The counting of movement cycles must include both the number of movement cycles and the relationship of that number to some unit of time. It is of limited and sometimes grossly misleading value to say about a patient that he walked 2000 feet. What is meant? Did he walk 2000 feet last week? Is that his cumulative total since entering the program? Did it take him three walking sessions of varied duration to achieve that total? Or did the patient walk 2000 feet in this morning's physical therapy session? The interest is in the frequency or *rate* of the behavior, that is, how much it occurs over some specifiable unit of time.

Difficulties with the concept of movement cycles and counting behavior are reported often enough to warrant additional illustration.

In defining behavior, the example of eating and obesity was mentioned. Helping a person to change eating behavior requires that the baseline of current eating behavior be established. Movement cycles could be swallows or mouthfuls of food. When one has swallowed, he can then prepare again to swallow. It is a complete movement cycle. In the case of mouthfuls, the movement cycle would be: load fork, convey to mouth, empty into mouth, return fork to the plate. Completing that sequence puts the eater in a position to repeat.

Both swallowing and the concept of mouthfuls, as defined, have some freedom to vary in size. That means there will be some imprecision. The same could be said for the left-right sequence in walking. The steps may not be equal in length. In the practical case, however, the therapist is dealing with behaviors that will, in the course of events, be repeated dozens and perhaps thousands of times, but with restrictions as to how much it is possible to vary. This source of variation rarely provides basis for alarm or concern. Counting them over several sessions usually provides an adequately stable baseline.

A more pointed example of movement cycles and baselines in the context of operant pain is found in patient verbalizations about pain. What is the movement cycle, and what is the baseline? On one occasion, a patient might say, "I now feel a sharp, lancinating pain running down my back and leg into my toes." Another time, he might say, "My back hurts." A third time, he might moan, gasp, and say, "Oh!" Are those movement cycles, and are they equivalent? Theoretically, one could count the number of words or even the number of syllables! Experience indicates that to do either would in most cases be overkill. Brief observations of each patient almost always reveals a pattern of single pain statements or longer narrative discourses. The former is easily defined. The movement cycle is simply one statement about pain. In the case of the more voluble pain patient, it may be necessary, initially, to be a bit arbitrary and lump discourses of varying lengths into a statement about pain without a change of subject. As will be illustrated further later on when dealing with training family members, one of the easier and seemingly more practical ways to handle this problem is to ask the spouse to list the ways in which pain is displayed or conveyed to others. This approach usually outlines fairly well the typical pattern of pain behavior verbalizations as movement cycles.

Before proceeding to the topic of reinforcers, a brief recapitulation should help keep these concepts clearly in mind.

1. Behavior is action. It is observable, countable movement.
2. To change behavior it is important to be precise about what behaviors are to be changed. Behaviors to be changed can be categorized as follows:
   a. Behaviors occurring with insufficient frequency, which need to be increased or strengthened.
   b. Behaviors occurring too frequently, which need to be reduced in frequency or eliminated.
   c. Behaviors not in the repertoire or occurring at a near-zero rate that are needed and therefore must be learned.
3. A prerequisite to changing behavior is to know how often it is occurring, that is, the frequency per unit of time. To count, one must have a unit or movement cycle. A movement cycle begins with the start of the behavior and ends when the person is in a position to repeat.
4. Assessment of behavior change requires a baseline counted in movement cycle terms to permit assessment of change.

Reinforcers

The one sure way to determine whether something is a positive reinforcer is to observe whether, when programmed appropriately, the result is an increase or decrease of behavior. The suspected reinforcer, when delivered contingently, should make the target behavior occur more frequently. Withdrawal of the reinforcer as a systematic consequence to the target behavior should bring the rate down. There are no inherent reinforcers. Their definition is circular. A consequence is a reinforcer if it works. If it does not work, it is not a reinforcer. The important point about all of that is that one should not assume that a consequence that is expected to have positive reinforcing effects will indeed have those effects. It is essential to observe and to measure to determine the effectiveness of a programmed consequence as a reinforcer.

In human service settings, the potential reinforcers likely to be of interest to a contingency management program are learned or acquired. They are consequences previously experienced that have come to have reinforcing properties for that person. In most cultures, money is often an effective reinforcer. However, the Australian bushman, exposed for the first time to a modern setting, is not likely to consider a dollar bill, or one of larger denomination, as much of a reinforcer. It is not something for which he is willing to emit behaviors.

Attention and socializing are reinforcing for many people. Others actively shun those activities.

It is important to keep in mind that a contingency management program, at its outset, makes some educated guesses about what reinforcers to arrange, but the program cannot assume that those guesses surely will be correct.

The first requirement for a reinforcer, then, is that it must be *effective*. When programmed in proper fashion, it must change that person's behavior.

The second requirement for a reinforcer is that it can be *controlled* or made contingent. A reinforcer that cannot be controlled should not be used.

Control of a reinforcer means that it occurs or becomes available when and only when it is supposed to. Reinforcement used to increase a behavior should occur and be accessible to the person only after the behavior to be reinforced and not at other times as well. To decrease or eliminate a behavior, the reinforcer that previously was sustaining that behavior must never occur when the behavior occurs.

Suppose a pain patient has the objective of increasing walking. Rest has been chosen as the reinforcer. Walking is prescribed as one of the exercises at physical therapy time. The basic procedure is that the patient is to walk a specified number of laps or round trips along a 100-foot corridor in the treatment area. After completing his quota of laps he may rest. However, the therapist is too busy. She is double scheduled, working simultaneously with another patient. She cannot directly observe the early walking sessions. Or, perhaps she is a bit careless and uses the patient's walking time as an opportunity to grab a cup of coffee. She does not observe. The patient walks a few laps, which is about half of his quota, and stops to sit and rest for a few minutes before going on. Rest is then not contingent on the target behavior, the walking quota. The reinforcer has not been controlled. The amount walked daily is not likely to increase. The remedy is simple. Rest, the reinforcer, is made contingent on meeting the quota. The patient is instructed that walking quotas refer to uninterrupted walking. Rest becomes available as soon as the quota is met. The therapist observes the early trials to be sure the pattern is being followed. She may be able later to reduce the amount she needs to observe.

Consider now the reverse situation. A reinforcer is to be withdrawn to diminish a behavior it has been maintaining. The preceding illustration can be extended to make the point. Suppose the same pain patient had long been vocalizing pain and when he or she did so, those nearby would encourage rest to ease the pain. Attention followed by rest are, in that arrangement, contingent on vocalizing pain. If there is no audible signal of pain, there is no encouragement to rest. The treatment plan is to withdraw that special attention as a reinforcer contingent on pain behavior. When, during physical therapy walking sessions, the therapist hears gasps or complaints of pain, unlike the family, she ignores them. She does not respond by encouraging rest. But suppose the therapist is inexperienced and particularly solicitous. She may think that her attention and solicitousness will provide extra motivation to help the patient improve. When she hears gasps and pain complaints, she offers the patient her special encouragement and reassurances: "Why don't you rest a moment and then you will feel well enough to do more?" Attention as a reinforcer has not then been withdrawn as a systematic consequence to complaints of pain. It is not controlled. The remedy lies in getting that therapist to let her special attention become work contingent and not pain contingent. She is to tune out or ignore pain complaints and to provide reassurance and attention at the moments when the patient is walking free of vocalized pain.

The issue of control of reinforcers takes on special importance in health care settings because it so heavily involves the question of whether the patient can be treated on an ambulatory or outpatient basis or will require at least some time in a more structured inpatient environment. This issue will receive more consideration later on. It is an important question. If pain behaviors are being maintained by reinforcers in the natural environment, in one way or another those contingent relationships must change. The patient need not always be withdrawn from the environment that is providing the wrong patterns of reinforcement. The essential thing is to change these reinforcement patterns. To ignore the issue is to court treatment failure. If the key reinforcer cannot be withdrawn as a systematic consequence to a behavior to be reduced, the behavior will probably not diminish.

There is a second important aspect to reinforcer control. A reinforcer that has been arranged to become contingent on occurrence of a particular behavior must indeed be delivered when that behavior occurs. A reinforcer that cannot be delivered after the behavior should not be used. The immediately preceding example can again be used to illustrate the point. If therapist attention is to be the programmed reinforcer, the therapist must be present at the critical times to deliver it. Delays in reinforcement delivery from, say, double scheduling can destroy treatment effectiveness. Similarly, rest as a reinforcer requires that the patient be able to and allowed to rest immediately after the behavior to be increased. Therapy schedules are self-defeating if they rush patients into the next exercise when one quota has been met. They have failed to let the potentially potent reinforcer of rest do its best work. They have not made the programmed reinforcer available. A similar problem may arise on a hospital ward. The treatment plan may include reliance on some form of professional attention as a reinforcer, contingent on activity without pain behavior. That reinforcer is not likely to prove effective if the nurses are too busy to attend to the patient with proper selectivity. A programmed reinforcer must indeed be available for delivery at the proper times.

A third requirement of reinforcers is that they must be capable of being delivered *promptly*. Delay of reinforcement weakens the effect. As noted in an earlier chapter, there is evidence that delays of as little as a second may have a discriminable reduction in effectiveness. That is not to say that reinforcers must be delivered within a second to have effect, but their effectiveness may wane rapidly with delays in delivery.

The issue of promptness of reinforcement is particularly important in the early stages of a behavior change process. Once the process is well underway, considerably greater flexibility in reinforcement patterns and timing will emerge. At the outset, however, promptness is of critical importance.

Many common illustrations of this point can easily be recognized. The extreme negative case is illustrated by noting how little effect a first grader receives from encouragement to study so that he will have a successful career later in life. The 20-year delay in that behavior consequence relationship is of course fatal. Similarly, in the mastery of a complex skill, prompt and frequent reinforcement is essential in the early stages. The new tennis player is not effectively reinforced by the prospect of being competitive at some future date. The wise instructor breaks a learning task into small components, an example of shaping, and richly reinforces performance of each bit. The situation is analogous in regard to the chronic pain patient. Reinforcement of the early stages of exercise performance by the promise of future well being is simply not effective. The delay is fatal. There need to be interim reinforcers that can be delivered promptly to begin the process of increasing activity level.

Characteristics of reinforcers can now be summarized as follows:

1. *Effectiveness.* A reinforcer must influence the rate of the behavior on which it is contingent. If the behavior rate does not change, change the reinforcers.

2. *Control.* The reinforcer must occur or become accessible contingent on the behavior to be increased. Or, in reducing a behavior, the reinforcer must be noncontingent, that is, it must not occur when the behavior occurs. A reinforcer that cannot be controlled should not be used.

3. *Promptness.* A reinforcer must be delivered promptly after the behavior it is designed to increase.

Selection of reinforcers. In 1959, David Premack pointed out a fact about reinforcers that is of inestimable value in simplifying and organizing thinking about how they are to be selected. Premack noted that high-frequency or high-strength behaviors can be used to strengthen or increase the rate of behaviors of lesser frequency. That has come to be known as the Premack Principle. To paraphrase the Premack Principle, something a person shows he likes by doing frequently may be programmed to increase

the rate at which he does something presently occurring at too low a rate.

Most mothers grasped the Premack Principle long before it was formally published. Those who have not, will wish they had. The youngster who resists studying or homework or doing some assigned chore encounters a working application of the Premack Principle when his mother stipulates that TV becomes accessible when—and only when—the homework or chore is completed. Watching TV is almost always a high-strength or high-frequency behavior of youngsters. Programming TV to be contingent on such a low-strength behavior as study or mowing the lawn helps the subsequent rate of the target behavior to increase. Conversely, if the youngster happened not to care for TV, making TV time contingent on performance of some undesired chore would have little effect. For such a youngster, TV watching has a rate comparable to lawn mowing and would therefore be an ineffective reinforcer.

The Premack Principle proves to be of such great utility that additional examples should be noted to ensure utilization of this ingenious tool. Smoking is a high-strength behavior to a heavy smoker but not to a nonsmoker. A club joiner or a salesman is likely to find reinforcement in the attention of or interactions with people, as indicated by the amount of time spent interacting with them. In the context of chronic pain, one of the most important illustrations of the Premack Principle concerns what people do when they hurt. Some people rest or recline. That kind of pain patient finds rest and reclining to be effective reinforcers. Other pain patients get up to pace or to change body position when pain increases. That kind of pain patient is not likely to find rest an effective reinforcer, but activity or movement might be. This application of the Premack Principle to chronic pain will receive much use in the operant program described in Section Three.

No behavior change project need be dropped for the lack of a positive reinforcer. The Premack Principle ensures that some high-strength behavior exists in every situation. If there is difficulty, it is not likely to be in the finding of a reinforcer but in arranging to make it prompt and contingent.

Natural versus exogenous reinforcers. Reinforcers are usually thought of as rewards or incentives. Rewards or incentives are events that tend to occur only under special conditions. They are not always a natural part of the situation. Reward or incentive programs usually do entail special arrangements. The reinforcers are then exogenous to that situation. There is a place for exogenous reinforcement in behavior modification, but it is often not a big place. It is usually easier and more effective to work with reinforcers that occur naturally in the setting. Events that are already present and need only to be programmed in a prompt and contingent manner serve as well as or better than elaborate special incentive arrangements.

Virtually all of the illustrative examples presented thus far in this book have used naturally occurring reinforcers. Rest, time out from some activity, or attention have been the prime examples. These will receive more elaboration in the next few pages. In addition, in treatment settings or in the home environment, one can identify naturally occurring events that can be programmed to become effective reinforcers to help a patient change behavior.

Suppose one were trying to help a chronic pain patient to complete an exercise sequence each morning and afternoon. If merely requesting the patient to do so suffices, fine! But if that were enough, there would be no problem. Instead, let the patient be one who promises to perform but does not do so. What does the patient do frequently? Perhaps it is to watch TV. TV watching is a natural part of the situation. According to the Premack Principle, it meets the criterion of being a potentially effective reinforcer because it is demonstrably a high-strength behavior; that is, the patient watches a lot of TV. TV can be programmed to become contingent ("no exercise, no TV"). Scheduling details can be worked out to ensure that TV becomes available promptly after exercise, or a delayed reinforcement plan, using a token or point system, as discussed in a later section of this chapter, can be designed.

The issue of natural versus exogenous reinforcers is primarily a logistical one. It is simply easier and more convenient in most instances to use naturally occurring reinforcers. One occasionally hears scare talk by people uninformed about behavioral methods to the effect that the methods require providing elaborate and special reinforcement. The methods require precision. They require knowledge about how to use them. They do not require much in the way of special kinds of reinforcement.

Rest or time out as a reinforcer. Rest or time out is virtually the ultimate in both the practical application of the Premack Principle and the use of naturally occurring reinforcers. Time out is something we all take—and not necessarily in relation to aversive activities. The enthusiastic hiker on a mountain trail periodically takes time out to rest on a log beside the trail. The interested, stimulated worker takes time out for a coffee break. Rest or time out in that sense is ever present and always potentially arrangeable as a reinforcer to help someone change behavior.

Time out is also thought of as a break from an aversive, unpleasant, or arduous task. The central element of avoidance learning was time out or avoidance of some aversive event. Used in that way, time out also meets the criterion for an effective, high-strength, naturally occurring reinforcer. Moreover, it can often be made available promptly, when needed.

Thanks to the Premack Principle, time out becomes one of the most versatile of reinforcers. It adds enormous flexibility to any behavior change process. For example, consider a patient who is reluctant to complete a series of exercises. What he wants for the moment is rest, not potentially painful exercise. He recognizes that the long-term gain of exercise is to his advantage, but that more remote consequence lacks the power to offset his immediate reluctance. It is a far more simple process than at first it might seem to arrange his program so that he earns and gains access to time out from exercise by exercising. Setting initially modest quotas, well within the curtailed performance level of the patient, provides the essentials for the contingent relationship. Completion of the quota automatically leads to end of that session and therefore to rest or time out from the aversive activity. Quotas can then gradually be increased. It works. Specific illustrations of this application will be provided later, in addition to those already presented.

Attention as a reinforcer. Attention, programmed selectively, can be a powerful tool to help people in a behavior change program, to say nothing of the purveyor of such services. Attention is sometimes mistakenly thought of as merely something adults give to children, and therefore the person who is influenced by it must be childish. That is nonsense, as is apparent on even slight reflection. Attention in this context refers to the social responsiveness of one person to another. Social responsiveness plays an active and integral role in interpersonal communication at virtually every level of human discourse.

Consider what happens in a conversation when the listener consistently avoids eye contact. The speaker quickly becomes aware of this. The speaker likely will feel less inclined to converse. Alternatively, he or she may make special effort to re-establish eye contact by taking some kind of attention-gaining action, such as raising or lowering the voice, making a hand gesture, or speaking more rapidly. The protracted absence of eye contact is quickly felt as less social responsiveness and the strength of the conversational bond is correspondingly diminished. The person who consistently avoids eye contact when conversing will find himself or herself an unfavored conversational partner.

Notice in the eye contact example that the amount of nonresponsiveness was slight. There may have been ample conversational response. Body posture, for example, may have continued to be oriented toward the conversational partner. And yet the impact of such a subtlety as lack of eye contact could be noticeable. A more active or pronounced style of nonresponsiveness has correspondingly greater impact. A listener in a conversation who turns his or her head away, shifts body position to be oriented away from the conversational partner, or blithely interrupts with comments on another subject, quickly turns off the conversation. Social reinforcement has been withdrawn from the speaker's conversational behaviors. Their subsequent rate in that setting will quickly dwindle.

The reverse kind of illustration is equally apparent. Some people develop particular skill at being good listeners. The term means that they are effective reinforcers of conversational or discussion efforts. What is it they do? They maintain eye contact. They smile or nod or gesture appropriately to indicate interest and attention. They make comments designed to reinforce the speaker's conversation. In short, they are effectively reinforcing.

People who are responsive to or sensitive to others are hardly childish. Attention or social responsiveness play important roles in our daily lives. They are significant environmental consequences. As such, they influence behavior.

Add to the source of attention a dimension of prestige or of special importance, and the impact of attention as a reinforcer increases. Virtually every practicing physician is well aware of that; perhaps most aware of all is the family physician. The attention of the physician is important to the patient. One example of this is the frequency with which family physicians and others find patients in their caseloads who come repeatedly for help with obviously synthetic complaints. A complaint or symptom is necessary to justify the office call. The patient works to earn the physician's attention by generating illness complaints and by going through all the ritual of making and keeping an appointment. That behavior is often effectively maintained by the few minutes of undivided attention it receives.

To the patient, each element of the health care team is likely to have this special importance in some degree. Chronicity of illness virtually ensures that this will be the case. The patient must keep returning to the system for help. His or her whole way of life may be involved in the illness and its various ramifications. The actions and responsiveness of the system and the professionals in it are not taken lightly.

Virtually without fail, attention or social responsiveness programmed in a contingent fashion to help a patient meets the criteria for a reinforcer. It is nearly always effective. It is capable of being controlled, although not always easily. It can almost always be delivered promptly. It is naturally available, and the potential supply is virtually limitless. Moreover, satiation for attention, if it ever occurs, is likely to be short-lived.

A few illustrative applications of the constructive use of contingent attention are now in order. Keep in mind that these examples will be applied to patients identified as having significant amounts of operant pain, limited amounts of respondent pain, and who have entered into a thoroughly explained operant-based treatment program. Let it be supposed that a given chronic pain patient, when approached at his or her bedside on morning ward rounds, consistently greets the physician with complaints of pain. Reassuring nods, comments, or gestures would constitute physician social responsiveness or attention contingent on pain complaints. But suppose they are withheld. Eye contact is maintained but the physician's facial expression and manner is neutral and noncommital. At the end of the description of complaints, he or she may say, "I see," or "I understand," but in matter-of-fact tones. There is then a brief pause, perhaps 1 to 3 seconds, after which the physician asks, "How many laps did you walk in the physical therapy gymnasium yesterday?"

The same patient goes to the occupational therapy clinic to increase back exercise by working at a loom with weights attached. The quota is six rows at that point in the program. After four rows, the patient stops, puts a hand to the sore back, gasps in pain, and tells the therapist he cannot continue. The therapist does not reassure. She does not encourage further effort. She shrugs her shoulders, records the amount done, and says, "I'll see you this afternoon." She then walks away. She has successfully avoided letting her attention be contingent on pain behavior. Conversely, had the patient completed the quota of six rows without displays of pain behavior and interruption in performance, she would have recorded the performance and said something like, "Hey, that's great. The project is coming along well, and you're doing a nice job."

Continuing on with the same patient, in the evening on the ward the nurse brings medications. Her approach is greeted with visible or audible signals of pain, such as moaning, holding the back, or gasping in relief that the medications have finally arrived. The nurse is businesslike and noncommittal. She does not reassure. She does not try to change the subject or deflect the patient's attention from the pain. She is socially nonresponsive. She delivers the medicine and leaves. Had pain behaviors ceased when she approached, she would have delivered the medications, and, if the interval of no pain behavior continued, she would have taken a moment to chat briefly with the patient about almost anything except pain. Had there been no pain behaviors when she approached, she would have immediately begun chatting.

The sensitivity of patients to the attention of health care professionals is illustrated by Fig. 13, which shows changes in a patient's display of pain behaviors under different conditions of staff responsiveness and nonresponsiveness. The objective in this case study was only to demonstrate relationships between pain behaviors and professional staff responsiveness (Patout, 1973). The procedure followed was first to establish the

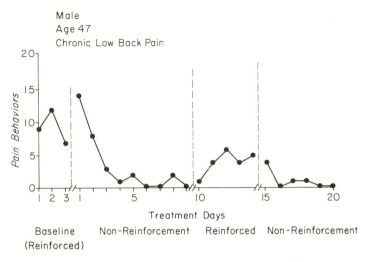

Fig. 13. *Effects of professional attention on pain behavior.*

baseline of patient pain behaviors (grimaces, moans, pain-related statements) in the company of professional staff. The baseline values across 3 days are shown in the graph. The staff then withdrew their attention as a consequence or reinforcer to the pain behaviors. This was accomplished by stopping if at all possible to chat briefly with the patient when he was observed at some activity without displaying pain behaviors. Conversely, if pain behaviors were observed by whichever team member approached, that professional continued on to other things, if possible, without interacting with the patient. If the patient displayed pain behaviors while interacting with a staff person, that professional was as neutral and noncommittal as practicable and would leave to do other things at the earliest practical opportunity. That phase of the study is shown as "nonreinforcement." It lasted 9 days. Under the regimen the daily rate dwindled rapidly to near-zero levels. To establish more surely that the change was related to staff responsiveness, a period of 5 days of a more traditional responsiveness and interest in patient pain behaviors was instituted. This phase, shown as "reinforced" on the graph, led to a rapid increase in pain behaviors, although not to the levels of the baseline period. The nonreinforcement regimen was then reinstituted. Pain behaviors quickly returned to near-zero levels and remained there for the duration of the study.

The shifting of attention as a systematic social consequence from illness to non-illness behaviors is often difficult for health care professionals to do. They are so practiced at being attentive and especially alert to indications of illness or distress that they find it difficult at first to adopt a noncommittal posture and manner. Recognition that illness-contingent attention is one of the more powerful ways our environments promote and maintain chronic pain behaviors helps. It also helps to recognize better how powerful one's attention is as a source of influence on patient status and progress. That powerful influence must not be misused. It must be used to the patient's advantage. Noncontingent or pain-contingent attention, when practiced by the health care professional, deprives the patient of a potentially helpful treatment tool. With friends like that, who needs enemies? Careful staff preparation is essential to the use of these methods.

Schedules of reinforcement. Schedules of reinforcement refer to relationships between occurrence of a behavior and the timing and frequency of its reinforcement. If a behavior were reinforced each time it occurred, it would be a continuous schedule. Reinforcement delivered less frequently is intermittent.

A great deal is known about the effects on behavior of different reinforcement schedules. Ferster and Skinner (1957), for example, report systematic observations for a total of 70,000 hours of recorded behavior and more than a quarter of a billion responses. The evidence from their work and that of others indicates striking consistency in the relationship between the rate and persistence of behavior and the kinds of reinforcement schedules it has met. The consistency is found across species, including man, across behaviors, and across settings.

There are practical and realistic constraints within the complex environments of treatment settings that automotically limit the precision of reinforcement scheduling. Were that not the case, it would theoretically be possible to increase considerably the effectiveness and rapidity of behavior change that one might help a patient to bring about. Those reality constraints that limit precision also permit and require dealing with reinforcement schedulng with less precision than might be applied in a laboratory setting.

There are certain general principles to keep in mind about the scheduling of reinforcement. The first is that continuous reinforcement (for each occurrence of the behavior, there is a unit of reinforcement; the schedule is 1:1) is an effective way to establish a new behavior or to re-establish an old behavior that has not been occurring. To *start* a behavior, reinforce it as frequently as possible, that is continuously or on a 1:1 schedule.

The alternative to continuous is intermittent, of which there are four patterns. Reinforcement may occur after several repetitions of the target behavior. It is a *fixed ratio* schedule when a specified number of repetitions of the behavior must occur before reinforcement occurs. Immediately after delivery of the reinforcement there is a pause. The pause will be longer if the ratio is higher; FR 40 (40 repetitions between reinforcements) produces a longer pause

than FR 10. The pause is nearly always followed by a sudden resumption of the behavior, which then tends to persist until the next reinforcement occurs.

In a *variable ratio* schedule, the number of repetitions necessary to produce reinforcement varies around some mean or average, which is the overall ratio. Variable ratio schedules produce the highest and most consistent levels of performance or output. That is so because they differentially reinforce rapid responding and do so in an unpredictable pattern. The more rapid the response, the sooner the reinforcement will occur.

Piece work in job settings illustrates ratio schedules. The more responses that are emitted, the greater the reinforcement.

The alternatives to ratio schedules are interval schedules. The target behavior may receive reinforcement after passage of a fixed interval of time. It is a *fixed interval* schedule. Alternatively, reinforcement may occur after periods of time that vary around some mean; these are *variable interval* schedules.

Fixed interval schedules tend to produce low rates of behavior. The longer the interval, the lower the rate. Further, immediately after reinforcement there is a pause and then a gradual resumption of the target behavior, which accelerates to its peak just before the end of the interval and the next occurrence of reinforcement.

Variable interval schedules also produce lower rates of behavior than do ratio schedules. The longer the average interval, the lower the rate. Variable interval schedules produce a steady rate.

Interval schedules, although producing a lower rate of behavior, tend also to produce more durable behavior. That is, when reinforcement is withdrawn, the behavior persists longer before ceasing altogther than is true of ratio schedules.

Working for a fixed monthly salary illustrates a fixed interval schedule.

So much for the basic vocabulary about reinforcement schedules. The practical implications in the treatment of chronic pain will be dealt with now. It was noted previously that the realities of treatment settings limit the precision with which reinforcement schedules can be applied. That is perhaps both a blessing and a vice. It is unfortunate in that particularly formidable or difficult behavior change problems do not proceed as expeditiously as might be expected, were treatment environments more systematic and consistent. It is a blessing in the sense that one finds it both possible and not difficult to set up behavior-consequence relationships in treatment settings that are effective in spite of the inherent lack of precision in the situation.

The first point to remember is to reinforce as close to a continuous schedule as possible in the earliest stages of a program when the behavior to be increased is new or has been occurring previously at a near-zero level. The militant application of this point in the early stages makes for considerably less work and more success in later stages. Conversely, carelessness in reinforcement at the outset both threatens chances for success and increases considerably the ultimate amount of time and effort that will be required to gain an acceptable outcome.

The next point to remember is that reinforcement should progress toward a *diminishing* schedule. As more and more of the desired behavior is emitted, it should receive less and less reinforcement. The common initial response to that proposition is horror or skepticism. But consider it in a bit more detail. Most of what people do is on an intermittent reinforcement schedule—ratio, interval, or both. Paychecks arrive once each month, which is a fixed interval schedule. Salesmen make periodic sales on a variable ratio schedule or perhaps a mixed variable ratio and variable interval schedule. But what about the issue of a diminishing schedule as progress occurs? Notice what happened when you entered school. The amount of work you were expected to produce to achieve an "A," or "B," or whatever, steadily increased with the passing terms and years, although the

reinforcers remained the same. "See Dick run" might have earned an "A" in first grade but it took two Shakespeare plays and a bout with Chaucer to gain an "A" in high school. Essentially the same reinforcers were programmed, but considerably more behavioral output was needed to earn them. Most employers do not expect as much output the first month on a new job as they expect several weeks later when the job is better mastered. Even the jogger puts himself or herself on a diminishing ratio schedule. In the early stages of a jogging program, it may be 100 yards of jogging before a walking or sitting interval. Later, as stamina builds, it becomes 200 and then 500 yards, and so on. More effort is required and expected before the reinforcer becomes available.

It is perfectly reasonable to expect a patient to do increasing amounts of an exercise for a given amount of reinforcement in the form of rest. The increments in exercise are a mark of improvement or progress.

The next point to remember is that ratio schedules should first be used when moving to intermittent reinforcement. Reliance on interval schedules in the early stages of a hospital treatment setting is unwise. The problem is that passage of time between reinforcements does not automatically ensure that the time interval will have been adequately filled with behavioral output. A physical therapist who is to reinforce a patient for doing sit-ups by coming around every 5 minutes to offer praise, encouragement, may find that the patient was sitting quietly waiting for her instead of exercising. Her plan had not made reinforcement exercise contingent but time contingent. Start with a continuous schedule. Move toward a ratio schedule of diminishing reinforcement. Only later, when the patient has made considerable progress, is it prudent to rely on periodic (variable interval) therapist reinforcements.

A case example will illustrate how the process may be carried out. The patient was in her mid-40s. Her pain problem be-

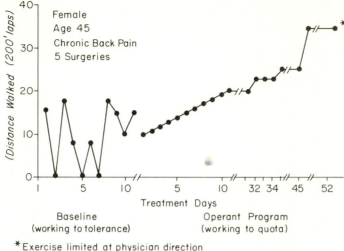

Fig. 14. *Walking quotas as diminishing ratio schedules.*

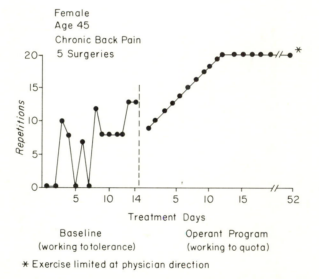

Fig. 15. *Exercise (letbacks) quotas as diminishing ratio schedules.*

gan with an accidental fall while at work on a clerical job some 15 to 20 years previously. Her back pain had led to five surgeries but with only brief periods of relief of pain and functional impairment. In addition, secondary to surgery, she had a neurogenic bladder and incomplete bowel control. The behavioral analysis of her problem indicated there was much operant pain in the picture. She was admitted for the operant program. Among other elements of the

treatment program, a series of exercises was prescribed. We shall concern ourselves with two, walking and letbacks. During the first several days after admission the patient was requested to work to tolerance on each exercise, stopping whenever pain, weakness, or fatigue caused her to want to stop. Those initial sessions are known as baseline trials. Those and subsequent treatment sessions are reported in Figs. 14 and 15. During some of those sessions she was unable to perform at all. Her performance began to stabilize, and the general level of her current ability to complete these exercises emerged. At that point treatment began. Baseline values were averaged. In the case of walking laps (200 feet each), the baseline average was 10 for eleven baseline trials, 13 for the eight trials in which she performed at all, and 14.5 for the last four trials when performance showed signs of stabilizing. Inasmuch as she appeared ready to achieve ten laps consistently, an initial walking quota of that amount was set. Lap quotas were raised at the rate of one per day until late in the program when the rate of increase was reduced and ultimately stopped as the target daily walking level was approached. Stated another way, rest, one of the programmed contingent reinforcers, became available only when increasing distances had been walked. It was a diminishing ratio schedule. Fig. 14 describes her performance in the walking exercise. The letback exercise was handled in the same manner. During fourteen baseline trials (two per day for 7 days) she performed erratically. At first she failed to perform at all. Subsequently she became more consistent. The fourteen baseline trials showed an average of 5 repetitions per session, 9.5 for those trials in which she performed at least 1 repetition, and 10 for all trials after her last total failure to perform. The first treatment quota was set at 9, with daily increments of one repetition with, minor variations until the target level of 20 per day was reached. Fig. 15 describes her performance during baseline and treatment trials. The fixed ratio schedule for rest was initially 1:9. The schedule was reduced each day by 1, that is, 1:9, 1:10; 1:11, and so on. Concomitantly, although scheduled with less precision because it was virtually impossible to do otherwise, therapist attention was also on a diminishing schedule. Therapist praise and responsiveness came at the end of each performance when a quota had been met. That attention therefore occurred on a diminishing ratio schedule. The patient accomplished increasing

amounts before receiving the special therapist attention.

There is one more point to be made about the matter of reinforcement scheduling. It is important to consider what happens to the need for reinforcement when the patient leaves the treatment setting with all of its special arrangements. A difficult behavior change would hardly be worthwhile if there were no reasonable prospect that the change would endure after the patient leaves. It is a key issue, which has already been touched on in several ways. It will receive further consideration when procedures for promoting generalization of treatment gains are discussed.

A brief statement of operant rudiments was made in Chapter 3. It was pointed out then that stimuli or cues present when a behavior is being positively or negatively reinforced will tend to take on the coloration of that reinforcement. Those cues will tend to become positive or negative reinforcers in their own right. That means that additional sources of reinforcement (positive or negative, depending on the program) are potentially available. It is necessary for the patient to have access to these new potential reinforcers. The process of shifting to these new reinforcers is helped when they occur in the relative absence of the original treatment reinforcers. That is one of the fortunate by-products of diminishing reinforcement schedules. Intermittent reinforcement helps make it possible for other reinforcers to take over to maintain the target behavior. The process is called *fading*. The stimuli and cues that made up the treatment setting and the reinforcement arrangements are systematically faded.

An arbitrary example should help illustrate this important and useful point. The example will be oversimplified for ease of illustration. Suppose a patient has long suffered pain when walking, so long and so much that many unpleasant (learned) associations exist about walking in his town or on his job. Those stimulus situations have taken on unpleasant connotations. It will be assumed that the pain behaviors, whatever their origin, have largely become operant, controlled now by rest or attention instead of the previously active but now resolved organic problem. The patient undergoes an essentially successful inpatient-based operant program that results in, among other things, uninterrupted pain-free walking in excess of a mile. As in earlier examples, the beginning stages of treatment presented nearly continuous reinforcement by therapist attention and by rest after initially minimal amounts of walking. Reinforcement schedules were gradually lowered. Stated another way, walking quotas were gradually raised while holding reinforcement constant. The concern now is to establish and maintain the walking where it counts: at home, in town, and on the job. Ideally, this will be done with naturally occurring reinforcement requiring minimal or no special arrangements. The strategy to follow is to provide for essentially pain-free rehearsal of walking at home, in town, and, eventually, on the job if reemployment is one of the treatment goals. This is accomplished by such procedures as first having the spouse come in to walk for brief intervals with the patient, making it a point to be nonresponsive to pain behavior and to be an effective social reinforcer of the walking. That can be accomplished by promoting and sustaining interesting conversation while walking. Next, there are initially brief but gradually expanding visits home and to the town. Each visit is to include currently well-tolerated amounts of walking in the target environments: home, town, job setting. As the amounts of walking increase, the specially arranged reinforcers of rest and attention are decreasing. Concomitantly, the patient is being exposed on a pleasant and pain-free or pain-minimal basis to gradually increasing amounts of the cues and stimuli naturally present in the environments to which he will return. Those naturally occurring environmental events may then take over as sustaining reinforcers. The diminishing reinforcement programmed as part of treatment makes it possible for other, naturally occurring sources of reinforcement to have effect. Treatment arrangements fade away, and the natural environment can then resume asserting itself. There is no guarantee that will happen. But that is what effective posttreatment planning is all about: the search for effective sustaining reinforcers by which treatment gains can be maintained. That problem is the topic of Chapter 13.

Delayed reinforcement (token or point systems). It is often desirable and perhaps necessary to delay reinforcement. The reinforcer to be used may not be available until hours after performance, or using it immediately might be disruptive. Visiting time, TV time, or even simply time in one's own bed on the ward might have been programmed as reinforcers. They cannot readily be used after each bit of exercise. Physical therapy cannot be interrupted to permit a visit or 30 minutes of TV or a quick 10 minutes in bed on the ward. The remedy is to go to a token or point system. Reinforcement should occur promptly. Assume that TV time has been added to rest and therapist attention as part of a reinforcement plan for meeting walking quotas. The therapist provides the patient with a brief interval of rest before proceeding to the next exercise, although not a return to the ward to rest in bed. She also records performance and is socially responsive to it. In addition, however, she delivers a poker chip which, by previous arrangement, has been designated as negotiable for 30 minutes of visitor time or of TV time. The token bridges the time gap between morning exercise and evening visiting or TV watching. It is a token or symbol of a reinforcer that is to become available at a later time.

Everyone who earns money is on a token system. Job behaviors are emitted. They are periodically reinforced, either as ratio schedules for piece work, as commissions, or as interval schedules for salaries. In either case, the money is a token. Money is not inherently a reinforcer. It has taken on reinforcing properties because it can be traded in for things desired. It is a token symbolizing the impending availability of desired reinforcers.

Token systems have many advantages. Their use, however, often should wait until the program is well underway. The token may not be enough in the early stages of behavior change to bridge the time gap between behavior and reinforcement. In the example used above, rest and therapist attention were integral parts of the program. Only after initial progress should the token arrangements be added. Experience with chronic pain patients suggests that token systems can and often should be used, but not too soon in the process.

One advantage of a token system is that it permits one to relate a single reinforcer to several target behaviors. A set of exercises in the physical therapy gymnasium and yet more in the occupational therapy clinic all can be related to a single reinforcer by use of token or point systems. The size or difficulty level of the tasks need not be equivalent. The example of a patient with walking quotas of ten laps and situp quotas of eight was described on p. 92. In that example, completion of a quota led to rest and attention. Meeting quotas might also have earned some number of tokens, which, in turn, were negotiable for evening TV time. A patient might perform well in walking laps but begin to lapse on situps, with no apparent neurophysiological reason for the performance discrepancy. It would then be time to suspect that the reinforcement schedule for walking is better than for situps. A simple adjustment might be made to provide two tokens for completing situp quotas but only one for walking quotas.

Token systems provide another kind of flexibility to behavior change programs. They make it possible to relate a number of reinforcers to a single or to a complex set of behaviors. In the illustration just discussed, tokens might have been tradable for visiting time, for TV time, and for time in bed. Yet other reinforcers could be added to the list, such as time off the ward in the evening to go to the hospital cafeteria or hours out of the hospital on a weekend pass.

There is of course no inherent reason why a token, per se (such as a poker chip) need be used. Recording on a graph or in a notebook the amount performed and the points earned provides the essentials. The rate of exchange should be spelled out to both patient and staff. It is important to be systematic. Tokens earned and then spent on the programmed reinforcers must be retrieved, or appropriate recording of the expenditure must be made. Tokens will rapidly lose their value if that is not done carefully. Failure to retrieve tokens is the equivalent of making them noncontingent.

Just as with any other reinforcers, tokens must be contingent on the behavior to which they were programmed. Many health care professionals are so sensitive to and sensitized by the problems and difficulties of patients that they find it difficult to make reinforcement contingent. A patient may approach a performance quota but not achieve it. Some therapists will then make the understandable but unfortunate mistake of reinforcing the patient because of the partially successful effort put forth. They assume in doing so that the reinforcer, now delivered on a noncontingent basis, will somehow motivate the patient to try harder next time. Noncontingent reinforcement will hinder rather than help patient progress. Sometimes, for a reinforcer to be effective, the patient must first experience that it is not automatically available. It must indeed be contingent on performance.

Generalization

It is fruitless to help a patient to change behavior in a treatment setting if the change does not persist into other settings and other times. The issue is to help a behavior to generalize from one setting or time to another. Generalization (Baer and Wolf, 1967) refers to the extent to which behavior occurring in one setting broadens in scope or occurs at other times and in other environments.

A pain patient who comes to walk about freely and to perform exercises vigorously in the treatment setting needs also to move about freely in activities of similar physical demand characteristics at home or on a job. The patient's free movement should broaden in scope to include activities related to but not identical with the exercises that served as the medium of treatment. Free movement should also occur in a variety of other settings, in the home, job, and community. It should generalize to other environments. Finally, the free movement needs to persist across time. The patient should still be moving freely 6 months and 3 years hence.

Generalization should be an integral part of treatment planning. The generalization or the maintenance and spread of performance is not a problem of the patient and his motivation. It is not enough to claim that dwindled performance after treatment stems from lack of motivation. Such a posture forgets that behavior is maintained by consequences, not by something called motivation. That dictum in turn means that if the system is serious about wishing to help patients to change behavior, it needs to be equally concerned with what can be done to maintain the changes brought about.

There are three strategies for helping to maintain performance by bringing about generalization. One is to program the patient with techniques of self-control. The patient is taught methods by which to set up and carry out incentive or reinforcement programming plans. A second method is to provide the patient's environment with special assistance to enhance effective reinforcement for the maintenance of performance. The third is to carry out the learning or conditioning process in such a way as to optimize the opportunity for naturally occurring reinforcers to take over to maintain the target behaviors. These will be considered in the order mentioned.

Self-control. Self-control means that the patient becomes his or her own behavioral engineer. There are virtually limitless possible ways in which this might be done,

but a few representative examples should illustrate.

Suppose that a pain patient who previously had a limited activity level, particularly in regard to walking, bending, and twisting, has been brought to a fairly high activity level. The problem is to get that free movement to continue, to occur elsewhere, and to broaden to include more kinds of activities. The patient is taught the working-to-quota strategy. He or she learns how to set baselines based on beginning tolerance limits and then to set initially lower quotas. The quotas are to be raised at a preset rate, not on a pain-contingent basis. In that fashion, the patient himself is programming rest as a work- or activity-contingent reinforcer.

Suppose another patient lacks sufficient incentives or reinforcement to keep moving. The patient is equipped with a supply of graphs and rehearses how to record and graph his or her own performance. Graphs, particularly when displayed where others can see them, are often effective stimulators or reinforcers. The graphs may reinforce the patient directly by depicting progress. The graphs may also remind friends and relatives to provide activity-contingent social reinforcement. Now the patient is devising methods for programming friends to be better reinforcers.

Suppose the same patient returns to employment, only to find that fellow workers, fearful that the back pain problem will recur, are protective and solicitous. When the patient moves or lifts, they may look worried or may caution the patient to take it easy. They may be attentive and reassuring if the patient appears to be fatigued or in pain. The problem is for the patient to try to get those around him or her to change their reinforcing behaviors. That might be undertaken in any of several ways. At first co-workers may be asked not to be solicitous: "Thanks, but it isn't needed." Should that not suffice, more direct action may be needed. One way would be to teach the patient to exercise selective attention according to whether the fellow worker was reinforcing the right or the wrong behaviors. When solicitousness was being expressed to the patient, the patient might shrug shoulders, comment only, "No problem," and say nothing further. But when nonsolicitous behavior was expressed, as when the co-worker offered encouragement for effort or made no comment when fatigue or pain was displayed, the patient could make a particular effort to stimulate conversation or otherwise socially reinforce the reinforcer. The patient may be able also to generate further self-reinforcement for these self-control efforts by keeping a count that reports the hopefully diminishing solicitous behaviors of others.

The topic of the development of self-control behaviors is far too complex to receive complete consideration here. It is important to know that the methods exist. If the methods for promoting generalization set forth in the following sections do not seem sufficient, self-control methods should be explored. The methods are difficult to carry out, but, when done effectively, they yield great cost benefit and provide much flexibility in the support of performance.

Programming the environment to maintain performance. Special reinforcing arrangements in the patient's environment are sometimes necessary to sustain performance. That environment may be failing to provide sufficient, naturally occurring reinforcement. Special efforts to program people in that environment to be more effective reinforcers may also contribute by helping them to stop reinforcing the wrong behaviors.

Programming reinforcement into an environment is conceptually simple because it is the same as any other contingent-reinforcement arrangement. Tactically, it is often difficult to do. The problems are obvious. There is the question of whether one can gain access to the people who are failing to reinforce properly and who are perhaps actively reinforcing improperly. Family, friends, and co-workers are all potential targets for these efforts. The logistics of spending enough time with them to change their reinforcement behavior may make this a costly enterprise. It is usually not enough simply to inform them what they ought to be doing. As noted before, information tends to be a low-power way of changing well-established behavior. A brief period of what amounts to skill training or supervised practice may be required. Who in the health care team is going to do that?

Tactical methods for reprogramming family members and others will be described in detail in Section Three and so will not be dealt with here.

Reprogramming the environment of the patient to help generalization encounters another kind of problem. The special reinforcement arrangements themselves are usually not arduous or difficult, once the method is mastered. It is sometimes difficult to find reinforcement for the reinforcers. What consequences are to maintain effective reinforcing behavior? For example, a husband may have helped to achieve a satisfactory level of consistency of social nonresponsiveness to his wife's pain behaviors and to be reinforcing of appropriate activity on her part. But to do those things may not be sufficiently reinforcing to him to be maintained. He was not doing them before treatment began. Why should he change? Signs of progress in a wife's activity level and toward reduction of her pain problem will not inevitably be reinforcing. It may be necessary to help the two of them to find things they can do together that properly involve her newly restored activity level and that are mutually reinforcing. Continued access to those activities may provide sufficient reinforcement to maintain the husband's reinforcing behaviors. This matter of working with patient and spouse regarding posttreatment activity planning will be considered further at several later points in the book.

Gaining access to naturally occurring reinforcers. The natural way is the easy way. In the course of daily living everyone meets a variety of naturally occurring reinforcers that maintain much of his or her behavioral repertoire. Rest, attention, praise, success, money, fun, and companionship are all natural parts of our worlds. We interact with those consequences in more contingent ways than often is recognized. They are effective reinforcers. They help to maintain our behavior. Usually the most practical and desirable method for promoting generalization is to work toward providing access to those and other naturally occurring sources of reinforcement. That is the most flexible and simple way to help a person to maintain performance.

It would be difficult to overstate the importance of this point. Each of us has lengthy and complex chains of behavior we routinely carry out to gain access to reinforcers that are an inherent part of our environments. To play on the cliche, "Some eat to live, and others live to eat." Some of those of the latter category work hours on end at perhaps unpleasant jobs to have caloric orgies at the dinner table in the evening. Others stick with essentially unrewarding jobs because they provide enough money to permit weekend skiing, elk hunting in the fall, summer vacations, etc. In this context, money is a naturally occurring reinforcer that provides flexibility of reinforcement. Money provides access to any number of other naturally occurring reinforcers.

The key element in using these naturally occurring reinforcers is to make them contingent on the behaviors increased in treatment. In the example of the pain patient who has been helped toward more walking, bending, stooping, and lifting, those activities are usually required before one can get to a movie, a card party, or a big dinner. If the activities were not required in a given case to do those other things, they should be programmed to become so. The new plan is to walk instead of driving to the movie. The card party should be preceded by appropriate amounts of preparatory housework. The pleasant evening conversation about the day's activities should

be reserved for a stroll rather than while sitting. In each instance, a naturally occurring reinforcer has become, at least in part, contingent on an activity targeted for increase in treatment.

One essential to treatment planning is to identify reinforcers in the environment of the patient that may be expected to help maintain performance. As treatment moves along, patient and spouse should be involved together in exploring how to gain access to those reinforcers and how to arrange things such that they become appropriately contingent. An effective treatment program for chronic pain (whether aimed at operant or respondent pain) should be concerned with posttreatment planning regarding employment, social and family activities, and recreation. This is not to suggest that treatment should try to tell people what to do with their time and their energies. Treatment planning should take into account what they already do or have done and what they might do within the limits of their own choices that will help to maintain treatment gains.

It is often not enough simply to identify what these posttreatment activities will be. Special efforts may be needed to facilitate access to them. The lonely widow with back pain is not going to realize effective social reinforcement from visiting a Golden Age Social Club if she lacks transportation. The work-oriented pain patient for whom re-employment is a suitable part of posttreatment activity may require vocational guidance into a new kind of work or additional skill training at the old job to better ensure effective reinforcement from that job.

These are the dimensions of generalization. Tactics by which to implement them will be dealt with in Chapter 13.

How to monitor and evaluate a behavior change program—or, what am I doing wrong?

A few practicing rules of thumb in how to judge whether changes are needed in the behavior change program should prove helpful.

Rule 1: If the behavior is not being counted, the system will not work.

Rule 2: Effective positive reinforcers, delivered promptly and contingently indeed increase the rate of the behavior they follow. If the behavior rate does not change, there must be one or more of the following problems:

a. *The target behavior is imprecisely or improperly defined.* It may not be in the patient's repertoire (teaching him to flap his arms rapidly will not lead to flying). Perhaps the target behavior has not been specified precisely enough to permit reinforcement selectively for it and not for other behaviors. Perhaps patient or therapist or both are unclear as to what is expected.

b. *The planned reinforcers are not truly reinforcing for that patient.* Is the reinforcer selected truly an incentive for which the patient is willing to strive? Is the behavior to be decreased or eliminated in favor of the target behavior continuing to be effectively reinforced? If so, behavior change will be inhibited.

c. *The reinforcement scheduling is improper or inconsistent.* (See Rules 3 and 4.)

Rule 3: Never never ask or expect a patient to do something he or she cannot do. It follows that quotas of exercise or of the waiting period until next medications must be based on observation of patient performance. They should not be based on expectation or desired performance levels. Let the patient show how much of something can be done before setting a quota. If a patient rarely performs to earn the reinforcement, the schedule is probably too demanding. Too much is being expected. The quota is too high, or the amount of reinforcement is too low, or both. When there is little or no performance at the outset, lower quotas or raise reinforcement, or both. A rough rule of thumb is that a good starting point is no more than an 80% performance of what one already has observed the patient do in baseline trials. If that does not lead to enough work to earn the scheduled reinforcement, lower the quota.

Rule 4: If the initial performance to earn the reinforcement is followed by waning performance, the problem is probably a form of satiation. The reinforcement schedule is probably too rich. A therapist or some observer may be reinforcing, regardless of whether quotas are met, that is, noncontingently. It may instead be that the schedule provides excessive reinforcement for the amount of behavior to be emitted. Check to be sure that reinforcement is being delivered properly. If it is, try lowering the rate of reinforcement.

SECTION TWO
Evaluation

The first section provided the grounding for Section Two. Section Two begins the process of applying behavioral concepts and methods to chronic pain. The first step in that process is to identify the kinds of problems for which these behavioral methods offer promise of help. This topic is explored in Chapter 5 by considering the range of possible treatment goals pertinent to chronic pain for which behavioral methods may be used. The material discussed in Chapter 5 is concerned with bridging the gap between two systems: traditional medical or disease-oriented care and behavioral or learning-based approaches. In a sense, Chapter 5 attempts to analyze medical problems in behavioral terms.

Chapter 6 is concerned with the behavioral analysis of chronic pain. It has long been recognized that behavioral methods are relatively easy to use. The greatest difficulty competently prepared professionals encounter in helping patients with these methods is in identifying what behaviors need to be changed. That task is often far more complex than at first it might seem. A careful and skilled behavioral analysis of each patient's situation is essential. Chapter 6 describes questions that need to be explored to determine whether a patient's problem includes significant elements of operant pain. There is also some consideration of the role of psychological testing in regard to chronic pain. This focuses on the most commonly used instrument, the Minnesota Multiphasic Personality Inventory.

The final segment of Section Two is concerned with patient selection. There are any number of reasons why patients found to have significant amounts of operant pain may not be candidates for operant-based treatment. Chapter 7 explores these issues.

5 Treatment goals

This chapter relates behavioral concepts to the health care system. Treatment goals to which behavioral methods apply are described, and the rationales behind them are explained.

In the Introduction and in earlier chapters the concept of pain was not defined, nor will it be defined now. The respondent-operant distinction was drawn, and pain *behavior* was defined. A conceptual point bearing on the definition of pain and relating to treatment goals needs to be considered before proceeding. A question is often raised in the context of treatment goals as to whether pain and pain behavior are the same. If one is changed, should there also be concern about the other? In the context of this book, the question basically is whether the reduction of pain behavior has modified the patient's pain.

There are two answers to the question, each at a different level of discourse. One answer is that the reduction of operant pain behavior reduces a patient's pain to the extent that what the patient perceives as pain has come under control of learning or conditioning factors. It is not necessary to differentiate or categorize the origins of the pain problem at onset, unless to do so also defines the extent to which it is currently respondent in character. Many pain problems are maintained by contingent reinforcement, when the originating body damage has disappeared or substantially abated.

This first answer to the question may be stated another way. Suppose that a patient has audible and visible displays of pain, has spent much of the day reclining because movement hurt too much, has been taking analgesics or other pain medications with regularity, has frequently approached the health care system for additional help, and has been enlisting the assistance of others to minister to the pain. Subsequently, let it be supposed that a treatment program effectively and lastingly reduces the rate of each of those pain behaviors to zero or to a notably lowered frequency. It is concluded here that the pain problem has improved. If some of those pain behaviors have diminished in rate of occurrence, there is some improvement; if all have diminished, there is more improvement.

Some will argue, ". . . but you haven't done anything about the 'pain'; only something about the way it is displayed or reported." That view assumes that there is some currently active level of respondent pain. If that is true, the criticism is probably valid. However, as will be touched on later, operant conditioning methods may also reduce in some degree the subjective intensity of respondent as well as operant pain. The major emphasis of this book, however, is on operant pain behaviors and other associated behavior, the principal targets of the behavior change process. This brings us to the second answer to the question of whether reduction in pain behavior means that there is also a reduction in pain. The answer is, of course, that there is no answer independent of the particular definition of pain one is using. When a patient is helped to do more while requiring less ongoing treatment and those effects seem destined to persist to the lasting benefit of the patient, it is for others to worry, if they so desire, about whether the patient has undergone any beneficial change in pain.

The immediately preceding philosophical aside was made at this point because of its special pertinence to the setting of treatment goals. We can now proceed with that topic.

The pain-related problems for which behavioral concepts and operant conditioning methods can play a significant role only occasionally involve the direct reduction of a disease or body damage process. More often the focus is on problems that are essentially by-products of disease or trauma. This difference requires some alteration in traditional approaches to treatment goal setting.

Here is the interaction between two rather different systems or perspectives, behavioral and medical. They need each other and belong together—at the very least in a close working relationship. But conceptual and procedural differences between the two make for some complications in fitting them together.

The health care system is in considerable degree organized along disease model lines. Jurisdictions have evolved mainly in terms of bodily systems (such as neurology and cardiology) or of disease or malfunction processes and methods for dealing with them (for example, rheumatology, anesthesiology, and orthopedic surgery). There are enough exceptions cutting across these categorization lines (such as, pediatrics and gerontology) to make the description an oversimplification. Nonetheless, in the main, medicine and health care aim at identifying and treating disease and body damage states along type-specialization lines. The divisions of labor within that process have emerged principally as specialized foci on parts of that process, not on relating the parts to other domains. Again the re-emergence of the family physician with his synthesizing functions represents a significant exception, but the main point still holds.

Both pain and behavior have peculiar relationships to that system. Pain cuts across the jurisdictional boundaries. Pain is often specific to a given disease or trauma or to a specific body system, but often it is not. It frequently requires the expertise of several specialties for proper identification and management. There are similarities and differences in relationships to the health care system of pain and behavior.

Behavior, like pain, cuts across specialty boundaries. Like pain, it is a part of all and belongs to none. Furthermore, just as pain often requires specialized expertise to be modified, so also does behavior. A significant part of the spectrum of events that make up a pain problem is behavior.

When behavioral concepts are woven into the evaluation and management of chronic pain, among the most important added dimensions are the need to deal with the patient's current and posttreatment environments and the need to focus on strengthening well behavior as well as reducing sick or pain behavior. When those concepts are added to the treatment planning picture, the ideal treatment plan would try to do what it can to reduce or eliminate the current pain problem, respondent or operant, diminish gaps in well behavior repertoires that threaten the maintenance of treatment gains, work toward a patient-environment relationship that will optimize maintenance of performance, and work with the patient and the family to minimize the future development of operant pain. The constraints of reality will limit how far the system can go in behalf of those objectives. If carried to their ultimate, those objectives would require treatment preparation and resources beyond what is often available. Not all chronic pain patients need that kind of broad-spectrum approach. Many chronic pain patients, particularly those having significant amounts of operant pain, will require just this kind of comprehensive treatment to produce a lasting and overall cost-effective resolution to the problem.

The roster of possible treatment goals requires more precise description in behavioral terms. Before doing that, it should again be noted that these issues are not specific to a particular kind of pain, medically defined. Tic douloureux, the causalgias, the pain of joint inflammation, mechanical low back pain, vascular headaches, and pain arising from cancer, to name but a few, all may have elements in their respective pictures, in regard to a given patient, that make these concepts pertinent. Clinical experience suggests that long-standing low back or abdominal pain of diffuse and spreading character is one of the more common classifications within which to find operant pain.

Viewed in behavioral terms, the roster of target behaviors that a chronic pain management program might and often should be concerned about changing can be summarized as follows:

1. Pain signals or pain behavior
2. Functional impairment behavior (activity or inactivity)
3. Health care utilization behavior (relating to the pain problem)
4. Effective well behavior sufficient to maintain the performance level that was the target of treatment

Each of these four categories of target behaviors has special significance for both patient selection and treatment planning, which requires some elaboration.

Reduction of pain signals or pain behavior

This topic deals directly with the personally experienced subjective discomfort of distress known as pain. Keeping clearly in mind the respondent-operant distinction will help to focus the points that follow.

Respondent pain may be subject to reduction in several ways, apart from that of modifying the source of stimulation. One strategy involves counter-stimulation. Melzack and Wall's gate control theory provides a neurophysiological rationale for how that might work. Counter-stimulation that increases large A fiber input, thereby changing the large-to-small fiber ratio, may inhibit transmission of a pain sensation. Counter-stimulation may be brought about by movement, rubbing, or the like, or it may be produced by exogenous electrical stimulation, as in the percutaneous and transcutaneous stimulators (Loeser, 1973; Shealy and associates, 1970). Counter-stimulation mobilizes central neural mechanisms, which may exercise control or influence over the gate and thereby over the pain experience. Distraction and other pain-inhibitory effects may then occur. These methods do not in themselves emphasize conditioning. However, the program or sequence in which they are arranged or delivered can promote conditioning, or it can fail to do so.

There are several possibilities here, all concerned with respondent pain and all lending themselves to facilitation by operant-based methods.

In the first place, in the face of pain and discomfort when motion occurs, it is often a formidable task to get a patient to engage in the movements that can provide useful activation of inhibitory processes. Treatment involving the systematic programming of rest and attention and perhaps other contingencies may serve to help the patient to get past the initial painful barriers of movement.

One of the more direct examples of this concerns the severely burned patient who must engage in range of motion exercise to avoid disabling contractures and other deleterious side effects. The pain is respondent, and it is severe when a joint is flexed or extended. A simple adjustment in the exercise sequence often will materially reduce suffering and make the treatment process considerably easier for both patient and therapist. The therapist who stretches the painful muscles until it becomes intolerable and then stops has made rest pain-contingent. When, however, he or she works out a quota system with a patient, progress can be expected to become both faster and less stressful. It may, for example, be stipulated that a 30-second pause will automatically follow 10 seconds of stretch at x number of degrees of extension of the limb. The amount of extension and its duration are based on balanced judgment as to how much the patient can handle and how much needs to be done. By engaging the patient in the quota-setting process, the therapist often makes the method yet more effective. As range of motion is restored, pain abates. Furthermore, providing the patient with a mental set to focus on time and on the rest that automatically follows often reduces experienced pain during the process.

If the gate control theory is correct, another possibility emerges. In the first chapter attention was called to the time dimension of the theory. If no conditioning occurred, effective closing of the gate and the inhibition of pain would be temporary and transient. But it should be possible to condition the inhibitory processes. For example, that is probably what happens in part with professional football players. On each of several dozen plays during a game, many of the players experience explosive impact, clearly enough to produce voluminous pain in virtually anyone. But neither the displayed nor the subsequently reported pain seem to approach the level one might expect. Several plausible reasons for this are apparent. One, of course, is that excitement and arousal serve to inhibit pain. However, it seems problematical whether that many players maintain that level of excitement and arousal for so many plays, so many games, and so many seasons. Another set of reasons relates to experience or prior conditioning. Beginning in high school or before, those players underwent systematic reinforcement of stoical and extinction of pain behaviors. Action, movement, and preparation for another impact were behaviors that were targets for special reinforcement. Cues for the imminent occurrence of further impact or action were paired for many years with approval, success, group acceptance, and cheers of the crowd. It is not surprising that those cues now lead to vigorous action rather than pain behaviors. Later, after the game, in the dressing room where modest amounts of pain behaviors are tolerated, the pain is experienced at a greater level of intensity, although still well below what the unconditioned player would probably display.

It will be recalled that one of the principles of conditioning is that stimuli present when reinforcement or punishment are occurring are capable of becoming reinforcers or punishers in their own right. It follows from this that the systematic pairing of pain or of cues indicating that pain is imminent with highly reinforcing consequences may have the effect of letting the pain or its cues become indicators of an imminent positive consequence. These cues may thereby become subjectively pleasant or, at least, significantly less unpleasant, through systematic learning trials. For further illustration of this point, go back to the burn patient undergoing range of motion while immersed in a tank. If the therapist is not handling the situation well and the patient is failing to progress, cues in the treatment process will take on the coloration of the pain. The patient may, for example, begin to display and to report increases in pain when the cart on which he travels to treatment approaches the treatment room or when the therapist approaches to begin the treatment process. That would illustrate spread of initially respondent pain to other cues in the environment. A therapist who has made good use of learning or conditioning principles in laying out the treatment sequence may produce the opposite effect. He or she may make judicious use of rest, as in the quota method, and may optimize the pairing of rest with other reinforcing consequences. The therapist may strive particularly to make rest periods moments in which to make conversation pleasant and stimulating. He or she may use prominently displayed graphs on which to mark progress immediately after range of motion trials. While the patient rests, the therapist also observes the indications of progress displayed by an upward climbing graph reporting degrees of extension. Now the therapist is pairing rest and pleasant attention with cues in the immediate environment that point toward future additional benefits, such as getting better, restored function, end of treatment, and return to more normal activities. In time, the graph with its display of progress can take on increasing reinforcing properties that serve to inhibit further the pain experienced during muscle stretch.

Recent work in biofeedback suggests yet other ways in which respondent pain might be reduced through systematic conditioning (Gannon and Sternbach, 1971; Kamiya, 1969; Melzack and Chapman, 1973; Green and co-workers, 1970; Birk, 1973). One approach has been to train brain wave activity in an effort to dampen or to replace the pain experience with a more pleasant subjective state—and to teach the person how to control that effect so that it may be used as needed. Small electroencephalographic equipment is used to pick up and display for the patient to see or hear the amount of alpha wave activity going on at the moment. Using the visual or audible cues by which to identify immediately the effects of the patient's efforts to increase the amount of alpha, patients can often quickly be brought to a state of considerable facility at controlling alpha wave activity. Early results suggest (Gannon and Sternbach, 1971; Kamiya, 1969) the possibility of significant reduction in experienced pain by enhanced alpha wave activity. Which of a number of possible cortical activities accounts for the pain reduction is not yet clear. Melzack and Chapman (1973) suggest at least distraction from pain to an inner-feeling state, suggestion, relaxation, and development of a sense of control.

The recently emerging and rapidly expanding domain of biofeedback in the modification of pain and other body processes is a whole subject unto itself. A detailed treatment of the subject is beyond the scope of this book. It will be referred to again later in another connection. For the moment, however, the concern is first to illustrate that respondent as well as operant pain may be modified by conditioning techniques. Second, without going into the technical details as to precisely how biofeedback works or how it may be used, one should know that the methods appear most promising. As events move along, more information about them should be sought.

There can be a direct attack on respondent pain in another way. Pain may result from muscle tension. The tension headache or masseter pain resulting from too frequent gritting of the teeth and jaws are common examples. The tense muscle can be taught to relax. Moreover, the relaxation process is itself a skill that can be learned. Patients often can be brought to a level of considerable proficiency in turning off the tension

or turning on the relaxation rapidly and precisely in relation to the target muscles. Relaxation training procedures have existed for many years. More recently, however, the methods for bringing this about have been advanced considerably by the use of biofeedback technology. Using electromyographic pickup of level of muscle activity and visible and audible feedback as to that activity, many patients can learn quickly to exercise effective and continuing control over tension levels. When that is mastered, the cause of the pain is correspondingly reduced (Fowler, 1975).

Another illustration of a conceptually similar process is found in the use of biofeedback methods for migraine or vascular headaches (Green and associates, 1970). The strategy used in this case is to teach the patient to increase peripheral blood flow by using skin temperature feedback. Audible or visible indicators provide precise and continuous information as to the temperature of the finger tip as compared with the forehead. The methods often can produce strikingly effective ability to raise or lower finger temperature and, therefore, peripheral blood flow at will. A significant proportion of long-time migraine victims can come to reduce, eliminate, or abort the headaches.

Thus far in this section the focus has been on methods for reducing respondent pain. The operant or contingency management methods set forth in the preceding chapter can be used to help bring this about, as in the example of the burn patient. Additionally, biofeedback conditioning methods and specialized equipment should always be considered where there is an indication that an underlying body process (for example, alpha waves, muscle tension, or skin temperature) can be modified to reduce either noxious stimulation or the subjective experience of pain.

There is another set of possible treatment objectives here that should not be overlooked. Apart from whether the pain is respondent or operant, there is the question of the effects of the patient's communication about pain on his environment. There often are pragmatic as well as moral virtues to stoicism or prudence in public expression of pain. The very display of pain produces effects in the environment that may work to the patient's disadvantage by setting up systematic reinforcement of the wrong responses or behavior. There are also situations in which getting along in the environment is prejudiced adversely by displays of pain. The patient may become his or her own worst enemy by communicating pain, even when it is respondent in character.

A clinical example will illustrate. The patient was a lady in her 70s who was living with her retired and yet older husband, who was in gradually failing health. She had a long history of abdominal pain problems for which she had received several surgeries, including a subtotal gastrectomy. The medical consensus was that there was indeed systematic respondent pain. One of the ways in which pain was communicated to others was by frequent moaning. After some observation, it became apparent that the moaning, although largely respondent, had operant overtones. Moaning became more audible and more incessant when she was around other people. However, moaning was also present on an intermittent but not infrequent basis through the night.

Treatment focused on a number of issues, but the one of concern for the moment is the moaning. To continue to moan at her rate at the start of treatment would deprive her solicitous husband of vitally needed rest. By history it was evident that her basic style was that of a self-reliant, independent, strong-willed, determined person. Her moans led her husband to try to help or console her. In keeping with her typical manner, she would reject or discourage his ministrations, but the moans would continue, presumably partially respondent and partly operant, reinforced by his attention.

The degree of operant characteristics to her moaning indicated that there was some latitude or leverage by which it might be reduced. Without belaboring with her the point that variations in moaning occurred as a function of whether people were present, the point of helping her husband by reducing moaning was explored. Although skeptical that it could be done, she agreed to try.

The procedure followed was for the nurses to count number of moans on a time sampling basis through the night. Those baseline values were then posted on a graph in the patient's room. Quotas of lowered number of moans were then negotiated with her. The essential reinforcers were praise and encouragement from the staff when progress occurred, and, in her case probably more important, evidence from the graphs that she was indeed lowering the moan rate. Both day and night moaning substantially diminished.

There is always a possibility that the methods by which pain is expressed can be modified or reduced in frequency, even where there is currently a noxious stimulus. Those methods of expressing pain *are* operants. Even though, in the case of a respondent pain problem, they are presently occurring predominantly, or even virtually totally, in response to the noxious stimulus, yet because they are operants, it is always possible that effective contingency management can help the patient to reduce their rate. He or she may develop more socially effective ways of expressing the pain, such as not making it public at all.

The principal treatment theme of this book is the reduction of operant pain. What is reduced for and with a given patient may include both pain behaviors or pain signals in the narrowest use of those terms and the broader associated behaviors listed earlier as possible treatment goals. In a sense, each of the four sets of behaviors listed on p. 105 as potential treatment goals are pain behaviors. They occur in relation to the pain problem. In the interests of precision, a roster of pain behaviors in the narrower use of that term will be restated. Each of these may occur as respondents, stimulated by peripheral noxious stimulation. Each may come to occur as operants, controlled by the consequences to which they lead. Virtually every chronic pain patient will show some of these behaviors. Even where there is a vigorously active organic component to the picture, if the problem has existed for several months or longer, there probably will be some operant features. Perhaps it is true that the longer the problem has existed, the more likely there will have been conditioning for the element of operant pain to have taken over a larger part of the picture. Certainly it is not uncommon to find pain behaviors almost totally operant in character.

Pain behaviors, narrowly defined, include the following:
- Blanching, flushing, alterations in pulse rate, and other such autonomically mediated pain indicators
- Visible and audible, although nonverbal, signals that pain is being experienced (gasps, moans, spasm, compensatory posturing, guarded movement, etc.)
- Verbal reports of pain, including compellingly vivid and precise descriptions of the quality, intensity, and distribution of the pain
- Requests for ministrations or assistance because of the pain (requests for medication, for a heat pad, for a back rub, for relief from a task, or for physician contact and medical assistance)
- Functional limitation or restricted movement reportedly because of the pain (reclining, falling because of a painful and weakened joint or muscle, momentary or enduring interruptions of normal activity)

To the extent that the behaviors listed have come under environmental control by contingent reinforcement, it is possible to reduce their rate, in some cases to zero. If they are occurring on a respondent basis, the extent and duration of reduction in rate by operant methods is likely to be less. However, failure to reduce rate of pain behaviors by operant methods does not establish that the pain behaviors were clearly respondent in character. Such a conclusion may be incorrect because the operant methods themselves were not well carried out; for example, effective reinforcers were not

found, or, if they were found, they were not made contingent.

Conversely, as noted in the preceding section, reduction in the rates of these pain behaviors also does not establish conclusively that they had been occurring on an operant basis. Respondent pain may also be reduced by conditioning, although just how much and in what ways he not yet been clearly demonstrated.

The material presented in the next sections of this chapter deals with the broader definitions of pain behaviors. The lines between the immediately preceding list and what follows are arbitrary and fuzzy, which is a matter of little importance.

Increasing activity level (reduction of functional impairment)

The term *activity level* is used here to summarize the almost endless list of purposeful movements in which people may engage. In the context of chronic pain, the term refers mainly to alterations in the amount and kind of movement a person engages in because of the pain problem. It is a generic term. It may be used to refer to limited and specific motions such as the amount of a given exercise (for example, walking) a person does or to more complex behavioral patterns, as in going to work, performing household chores, or participating in social or recreational activities.

Experience with the operant approach to chronic pain suggests that activity level is a useful measure or yardstick. Measures of pretreatment activity level help to identify those patients who are more or less likely to profit from the operant approach. Measures of activity level during treatment help to identify when things are going well or wrong. Measures of change in activity level provide an index of when the patient is ready to move from one phase of treatment to another. These measures also provide a useful index by which to help the patient and family more precisely to identify change as it is occurring. Finally, activity level can be an index of how well treatment gains are being maintained at followup. The case examples showing uptime graphs illustrate one method for doing this.

Setting treatment goals or objectives in relation to activity level requires, as in any other behavior change process, precision as to what needs to be changed and what is to be changed. The term activity level may be used generically, but in working out the details of a given patient's program, it must also be used precisely to indicate *what* activities need to be increased or decreased.

Removal of the inhibition or limitation on activity by reducing the pain problem does not automatically result in increased activity. A low activity level may persist for any of several reasons. The family may continue to reinforce inactivity or punish activity or both. In addition, if the inactivity has persisted for a lengthy period, sheer disuse may make it difficult for the patient to get going again.

General activity plays a potentially central role in many problems of chronic pain for yet another reason. The posttreatment activities in which the patient is to become involved, and which will serve to help maintain treatment gains, will often not be accessible until the patient has reached a certain generalized activity level.

There is yet one more reason for concern about activity level in treatment planning. It is logically redundant, but it has features worth further attention. For those pain patients whose activity level has diminished markedly with onset of the pain problem, activity is incompatible with many of their pain behaviors. One cannot have it both ways; that is, one cannot be impaired by pain to where much of the day is spent reclining *and* walk a lot. Walking is in part incompatible with reclining. Moreover, one cannot convey to others that pain compels limitation in activity *and* walk a lot or do a significant number of repetitions of one or more vigorous exercises. Increases in activity level, particularly in the form of vigorous motion, are inherently incompatible with major functional limitations because of pain, both to the patient and to those around who have been helping to protect the patient

from too much activity. Exercises such as walking often become one of the most useful mediums in which to develop behaviors incompatible with pain behaviors. The incompatibility, in appropriate cases, helps the patient and, when displayed in the patient's environment, helps that environment to respond in ways more effectively supportive of treatment progress.

The need for precision in the analysis of behavior and the identification of target behaviors to be increased or decreased has been emphasized. That issue is never more clearly seen than in relation to activity level. Some people rest when they hurt, whereas others move around. The former group might be characterized as recliners and the latter as pacers. One obvious and presumably the most important reason for the difference relates to the nature of the respondent pain process. That is, some pain problems are relieved by rest or nonmotion; others are relieved by change of position or movement. Both groups may benefit by avoiding a body position that produces more pain. Pacers are probably also activating more inhibitory or gate-closing mechanisms or producing more distraction or counterstimulation. There are potential social effects to reclining and pacing, which also should not be overlooked. Depending on the people in the patient's environment, reclining or pacing may elicit different social consequences. One may elicit help and support, the other may not. It is enough for the moment to keep in mind that reclining and pacing often have differential effects on a pain patient and on the environment. They receive different consequences, physiological and social. Many chronic pain patients are likely to vary markedly in this regard. They are recliners or they are pacers. They are rarely both. The patient who is a recliner has a lower activity level. Activity level is a set of behaviors to be increased by treatment. Pacers, in contrast, have high activity levels, perhaps too high. Pacers often need a lower activity level. It rarely needs to be increased.

There is another facet to the recliner-pacer distinction that should be noted. In line with the Premack principle and the selection of naturally occurring reinforcers, for recliners rest is almost certainly an effective and potent reinforcer. That is not likely to be true for a pacer. Rest may be aversive to a pacer. Activity and movement are more likely to be reinforcers. The probable differential effects of rest as a potential reinforcer are indicated by pretreatment observations showing whether movement and activity were high- or low-strength behaviors.

Again, some respondent pain problems cannot be modified by treatment, but activity level might be modified to the patient's benefit.

To summarize, activity level is often a convenient index of the functional status of a chronic pain patient, a central treatment objective; activity level is a process that, when changed, may help change the reinforcing characteristics of the patient's natural environment, and it is a guide as to what kinds of reinforcement may help the behavior change process. Precisely which activities need to be increased or decreased will vary from patient to patient.

Reduction of pain-related health care utilization behavior

Health care utilization behaviors may also be considered as one kind of pain behavior. The health care utilization behaviors begin with the onset of the pain problem. That is not precisely the case because the patient will have a repertoire of previously developed ways of relating to the health care system that influence when, under what circumstances, and in what manner he or she seeks medical assistance. However that may be, once a pain problem begins and the patient begins to interface with the health care system, a complex set of behavior-consequence relationships is put into action, which can exert major influence on the course of the pain problem. The influence may be somewhat independent of the effectiveness of the diagnosis and treatment first received for that which for the moment shall be assumed was a respondent pain

problem. There are many reasons for this. They will be considered in this section. They will point to health care utilization behaviors as a set of target behaviors that may need to be modified in their own right. The issue may become a factor even when the health care system does not have a helpful or definitive treatment for the pain problem itself. This issue can be important when dealing with problems of operant or respondent pain.

The major reason for reducing pain-related health care utilization behaviors concerns the risk that the patient may be harmed as well as helped by the health care system.

One source of the difficulty starts with the way pain is conceptualized. As has been noted at several points earlier in this book, as well as in any number of other places, the diagnosis of pain relies in important degree on the visible and audible pain behaviors emanating from the patient. The physician who views those pain behaviors virtually solely from a disease model perspective constantly risks making conceptual and therefore diagnostic errors. Visible and audible displays of pain behavior, including exquisitely detailed and authentic-sounding pain descriptions, do not establish that there is a currently present and active antecedent noxious stimulus. The data from the patient by which diagnosis and treatment are developed may be occurring in small or large part for different reasons. Failure to recognize this point and to take it into account in the diagnostic process can lead to ill-fated and often harmful treatment efforts. Destructive and needless surgeries, excessive and harmful medication regimens, costly treatment programs, and unnecessary restrictions on productive activity are all possibilities.

The risks to the patient of reliance solely on a disease model extend also to some extent to when that model is used to infer that there is psychogenic and therefore mental illness or personality disturbance behind the pain problem. There is ample basis, as noted in Chapters 2 and 3, for expecting that many compelling pain behavior displays relate neither to underlying physical findings nor to underlying emotional or personality problems. Referral for psychotherapy or some similar process is not then likely to lead to a solution. The patient, whether rejecting the referral or failing to gain a solution, is likely to persist in searching the system for a better answer. That search holds potential risks to patient well-being.

It says nothing new to note that when health care begins, the two principal parties, the physician and the patient, are involved in a complicated social and interactional process. The patient, on the one hand, enters the relationship with hopes and expectations for a solution to the problem and related functional impairments. To the patient, the question is not whether health services can solve the problem, but rather, which element of the system will be the most successful. From the patient's perspective, there is only one system. If it fails, there are few if any alternatives, aside from quackery, faith, or acceptance of unending suffering. The patient is therefore virtually beholden to demand and expect a solution. Failing to find it at one door to the system, he or she seeks another door, not another system.

On the other side sits the physician. He or she also recognizes that the patient expects and often insistently demands a solution. The physician further recognizes that his or her diagnostic and treatment efforts, augmented as indicated by specialty consultations and referrals, basically represent the only alternative open to the patient in search for a solution. There is no problem when diagnosis and treatment lead to a successful outcome. But if success does not follow, even after additional specialty resources have made their contributions, there is pressure from both parties to the transaction to do *something*. The physician would be less than human if he or she did not occasionally engage in essentially ineffectual treatment or management procedures, which, however, may yield some relief from incessant patient pressure for action. Perhaps the more common of these endeavors is to try to smother the problem with pain medications: analgesics, narcotics, tranquilizers, or whatever. And so it is that so many chronic pain patients are observed to be addicted or habituated to medications, even when there is little neurophysiological or pharmacological basis for expecting that the protracted medication regimen would move the patient constructively toward a solution to the pain problem.

As noted in Chapter 3, a medication regimen often becomes a problem solely because of the pattern in which it was carried out. Pain-contingent medications promote habituation or addiction. In that sense, too, repeated approaches to the health care system might be said to hold risks for the chronic pain patient, for *prn* regimens may be encountered.

Let it now be supposed that the physician exercises more restraint in response to the patient's continuing requests for help. The physician is satisfied either that it is a respondent pain problem for which the patient is not going to find a further solution or that it is an operant problem that, for one reason or another, is not going to be treated in an aggressive fashion. The regimen that follows might be characterized as one of benign neglect. There may be a placebo or otherwise harmless palliative medication provided in a time-contingent mode. The patient may receive appropriate instruction regarding exercise and activity level. In regard to physician attention, however, things may be left on an essentially "call when needed" basis. Such an arrangement may be reassuring to the patient, but it may also raise some additional social reinforcement risks. A need to go to the doctor often produces potent social reinforcement from several sources. Operant pain tends to gain a kind of social confirmation and therefore additional social reinforcement when it is further legitimated by physician visits. The family may be expected in light of this legitimating to maintain protective and solicitous behaviors that have been supporting the operant pain behavior in the recent past. They may even increase the intensity of their overprotective efforts. Similarly, broader social consequences such as the maintenance of wage replacement funding (compensation) may result from the frequent physician contacts. Even more directly, physician attention occurring on a pain-contingent basis has the potential to develop or maintain operant pain. That attention is usually a potent reinforcer.

Those are some reasons why it may prove desirable to reduce in a selective fashion some of a patient's health care utilization behaviors.

There are additional considerations in this context. When a patient expects a solution and does not get one, anger often follows. That anger can in turn interfere with compliance with physician-specified regimens, in relation either to the pain problem or to other unrelated illness events. The patient may become less cooperative and prudent.

The patient who continues to expect success and finds no end to the pain problem also may seek quacks or marginally adequate sources of help. Those sources may prove harmful. They also may prove costly. They are not likely to be helpful.

The hazards involved in dealing with the health care system become a particular issue with chronic pain because of the personal and social pressures on both sides to take action. It might be reasoned that the solution lies in adequately informing the patient and the family as to the realities of the situation. Explain that it is a pain problem for which there is no further solution and that continued efforts to seek help from other doors to the health care system or from other systems (such as quackery) may be risky. Such an approach is fine if it works. It represents an effort to change behavior by dispensing information and perhaps exhortation. Such a simple procedure always deserves a chance. The problem arises if it does not succeed. The patient may perceive the information and advice as a rationalizing of failure or as a rejection. He or she may persist in a resolve to knock on doors until answers are found. That often happens,

and when it does, more systematic efforts to help the patient and family to alter their utilization behaviors are desirable.

Treatment methods set forth in later chapters will deal directly with some of the ways to work toward these ends. In addition, however, it should be recognized that one set of treatment goals to consider in regard to chronic pain is legitimating the chronic but essentially stable level of the problems. The legitimating process may be brought about by such arrangements as prudent levels of time-contingent medication coupled with fixed-interval physician attention. There can be scheduled office visits, not as needed, spaced to the longest possible interval that nonetheless helps dissuade the patient from engaging in further doctor shopping in fruitless search of a final solution. Further strength to the program can be gained from scheduled exercise regimens, basically on a maintenance level. Finally, active participation of the family by helping to monitor exercise performance and continuing recording of activity level can serve to forestall family pressures to seek additional help. These procedures, which are essentially maintenance in character, may also legitimate the illness in the eyes of friends and associates and thereby reduce that source of social pressure to seek help elsewhere.

The matter of legitimating retirement arises in the context of chronic pain for yet another set of reasons. A pain patient who has been on the sidelines for long periods of time, even when treated to bring pain behavior down and activity level up, may find limited opportunities for normal performance in the environment. There may be, for example, too many skill deficits to make it a practical and cost-effective matter to prepare the patient for employment. The prototype of this kind of problem is the laborer who is now in his late 40s, has limited intellectual and other vocational retraining potentials, and has enough of a residual back pain problem to preclude return to heavy labor. There are many other possible examples. Any wage earner who has been on the sidelines for several years because of a pain problem is not likely to find an employment opportunity, however resoundingly encouraging are physician statements about the patient's ability to work effectively from a health standpoint. Finally, medical liability insurance programs carried by employers often specifically forbid the hiring of chronic pain patients because they are perceived as high-risk cases for future costly medical liability. Thus, no matter how effective treatment and preparation for employment might be, the patient often does not have employment as a viable option. When that happens, the patient is in a most difficult social bind. His or her rationale to the rest of society for not working is not likely to rest comfortably on the grounds that "no one will hire me!" A much more socially reinforcing definition to the patient is that "my pain is too severe to permit work." For these reasons, as well as those set forth earlier in this section, the patient may engage in the fruitless pursuit of additional medical treatment partly to continue to reaffirm to others that he has a medical problem. It behooves the health care system at that point to legitimate retirement to protect the patient from risks inherent in endless seeking of further treatment. These are positive treatment goals or objectives. They often require aggressive management. Any process that can have such far-reaching benefits to the patient can hardly be considered a treatment failure.

Cost factors have, to this point, barely been touched on. In certain respects they are important. Treatment in depth of this issue would go too far afield because cost issues relate to so many other factors. Those other factors can perhaps be consolidated into one: whose money is being spent? Out-of-pocket cost is simple and direct. Costs deriving from third-party carriers are much more complex. Costs subsidized all or in part by governmental sources represent another and further removed kind of third-party source. It is difficult to separate who pays and to whom it costs when treatment succeeds or fails. The problem is further complicated in a chronic illness such as chronic pain. The duration of the problem and the spread of its effects to interference in work and wage earning brings in additional cost factors and even more indirect cost burdens. Those issues cannot be dealt with in meaningful detail here except for the recognition that chronic pain and its associated functional impairments cost *somebody* when they entail either health care services or interference in generation of income. The allocation of those costs is a concern of others.

Most of the cost issues relating to chronic pain appear to be self-evident and do not require further explication here. Early and effective treatment pays off financially as well as in other ways. Misdiagnoses, treatment failures, and problems for which helpful treatment is not available, all may lead to long-term disability and expensive wage replacement or governmentally subsidized family maintenance costs. These costs can mount into the hundreds of thousands for a single patient.

There are two points relating to the cost factor that need further comment here. One is that when the pain problem is weighed in the context of deciding which treatment or management paths to embark on, one needs to give special attention to the probable spreading costs of chronic pain. It is not only that the patient may be disabled and unable to work or that he or she may require wage replacement or family maintenance funding. There is additional likelihood that a narrow approach to treatment that fails to consider the learning or behavioral model perspective all too often is followed by increasing medical costs as well. Conditioning can maintain pain, with or without effective medical care. When it does, office calls, medications, hospitalizations, and surgeries can and do needlessly occur. Across time, these costs tend to rise, not fall, for each patient. The costs spread medically, as well as in other ways.

The second point about the cost factor is essentially a restatement of the first, but now in terms of treatment objectives. The *effective* maintenance of the medical status quo in regard to a given pain problem is often both cost-important and cost-effective. The reduction or the avoidance of future increases in health care utilization behaviors in relation to the patient's pain problem is important for cost reasons. It is also important because it helps the patient to keep out of the other kinds of trouble described in the immediately preceding pages. Somebody pays.

The question is sometimes raised as to whether training a patient toward less frequent health care utilization behaviors might not entail risks for the patient. For example, could a patient be brought to the point where new and medically significant pain experiences would not be experienced or would not lead to consulting his or her physician? Conceptually, the problem is real. In the practical case, it hardly seems real for several reasons.

In the first place, a learning or conditioning program that effectively influences patient responses to cues previously identified as painful and requiring some kind of protective action is mainly a discrimination learning process. It is not that the patient comes not to experience the pain cue or stimulus. Rather, what happens is that the patient better discriminates it and makes a different response to it. Perhaps a return to the example of the professional football player will provide a useful illustration. By the time he is a professional, he has long since learned different ways of responding when he smashes into another player or is smashed into in return. At age 10, with or without protective padding, under proportional levels of impact he probably would have collapsed, would have experienced severe subjective distress identified as pain, would have been rendered at least temporarily nonfunctional, and probably would have freely communicated to those around him that pain was severe. Now, some 15 years and innumerable learning trials later, the response is different. The player does not lose the ability to detect that he has been hit. What changes is the manner in which he (and his body) responds. He does not collapse, nor is he rendered nonfunctional. Public displays of pain are minimal or missing altogether. Subjectively, he also feels much less distress. As more than one professional athlete has been quoted as saying, "It's only pain."

That same professional player has not lost the ability to detect the occurrence of special and significant forms of body damage beyond the routine wear and tear of a football game. A sprain, a spasm, a muscle tear, or a bone fracture are rapidly detected except under the most unusual of circumstances. The player has learned to discriminate between routine impact pain, if it can be called that, and other kinds of pain signals. Moreover, apart from what he immediately experiences, his body has not lost the ability to take reflexive protective action, as in spasm.

The discrimination learning just described tends to be precise and specific. To continue with the example of the football player, there is no basis whatever for expecting that that player would be less competent at detecting a state of unwellness on awakening in the morning with a bout of influenza or of cardiac-related pain. Impact pain about which learning has occurred is easily and consistently discriminated from other forms of body distress.

The contingency management methods outlined in this book modify behavior or actions or responses. They do not modify signal information except in the special instance of reducing signal intensity of respondent pain by promoting partial gate closure. They may modify how a person responds to a particular signal, but those behavior changes are specific to the signals—and not to just any signal. A treatment program that seeks to modify a patient's health care utilization behaviors must of course exercise prudence. The patient is not expected to learn to ignore pain. He or she is not to fail to consult a physician when significant pain events (or other illness events) appear to be occurring. The targets for behavior change are the pain behaviors and excessive health care utilization behaviors relating to *that* pain sensation from *that* source, which occurs under *those* conditions. The discrimination learning process appears to be both simple and virtually automatic. The issue now under consideration will receive further attention in Chapters 9 and 10 in relation to dealing with other illness events during the course of treatment pain.

There is one final issue to be considered in regard to adding health care utilization behaviors to the list of potential treatment objectives. As with any other set of behaviors to be changed, the change process must consider the sources of reinforcement that presently help to maintain the target behaviors. Health care utilization behaviors have, to say the least, some reinforcing qualities for the physician as well as the patient. The physician's professional life is tied closely to maintaining a caseload. Physician reinforcement for these efforts comes in many forms. A few of the more apparent include professional recognition, which is a form of social approval, the positive and approving regard of the patient, money, and sense of accomplishment. Were the physician solely or collaboratively with others to work to reduce a particular subset of utilization behaviors in a given patient and to do it well, money is about the only one of that roster of reinforcers that might be diminished. Even the prospect of loss of income may be more apparent than real. It is to be hoped that effective management increases the likelihood that the patient will continue to consult with that physician in regard to other illness-related events. In addition, the number of chronic pain patients actively seeking effective management appears to be considerable, and more referrals may follow.

In viewing this issue in relation to chronic pain, the blade cuts both ways. That is, it is to be presumed that one of the factors that maintains ineffective physician management of pain problems is the continued health care utilization behaviors and their attendant attentional and monetary consequences. Failure to end the problem

may under certain circumstances keep the patient returning for more attempts. That is unfortunate if true, but it is also a side issue that will be left where it is except to note that the physician also needs to assess his or her reinforcers.

The increasing movement in health care delivery systems toward health-contingent rather than illness-contingent monetary payoffs should make even the monetary reinforcer matter an issue of lessening concern. The rapidly expanding health maintenance organization concept, for example, provides monetary reinforcers for the kinds of effective and selective utilization behavior reductions under consideration here.

Apart from economic matters, the physician who would work to reduce selected utilization behaviors faces another problem as well. The patient who is insistent on immediate, aggressive, definitive help is not easily going to lessen health care system contacts for the continuing pain problem, even when the absolute level of discomfort has diminished. It will sometimes be difficult for the patient to distinguish prudent maintenance of the medical status quo from rejection and inadequate performance by the physician. If the patient does not receive the expected amount of help or attention in one place, he may seek it in another. Conversely, a physician will often find it difficult to proceed with these matters for fear that the patient will feel rejection or will pursue efforts for help elsewhere. Elsewhere, of course, may mean other physicians, or it may mean quackery.

Those are reality issues for which there are no simple answers. Until the health care delivery system and consumer expectations become more aware of the implications of conditioning factors on chronic pain, it will often be difficult to develop truly effective approaches to help a given patient and his family to maintain a prudent course. Conceptually, the desired strategy is to do all that is possible to maximize the reinforcing characteristics of patient well behaviors.

Help the patient and his family to find effective and reinforcing activities that are alternatives to sick or pain behaviors. This brings us to the fourth and final category of target behaviors in a contingency management approach to the treatment of chronic pain: effective well behavior.

Promotion and maintenance of effective well behavior

Any effort to provide a detailed account of what well behavior is and of how to bring it about could quickly bog down into a treatise on mental hygiene, mental health, or how to achieve happiness. That endless task shall be foregone. For the purposes of this book, well behavior consists of behaviors that keep the person out of trouble medically, legally, financially, socially, and ethically, and that gain access to effective reinforcement. They receive what is for that person positive reinforcement, and they do not lead to aversive consequences. So much for the definition.

The basic reasons for concern with well behavior have been set forth in preceding parts of this book. At this point the major elements of the issue need to be restated only briefly to complete the treatment goal setting picture.

There are three kinds of situations in which the promotion of well behavior is likely to be a significant concern to the patient's program. The first situation was one of the concerns of the immediately preceding section. It is where the nature of the pain problem, the debilitating effects of surgeries or other prior treatments for it, or a low probability that the patient will be able to return to work, for whatever reason, indicate that posttreatment target behaviors must be some variant of retirement. The matter of legitimating retirement to help keep the patient out of medical trouble has already been considered. That really is not enough in some cases. Some patients (and a lot of other people) do not know how to retire effectively. To tell a chronic back pain patient to take it easy for the rest of his or her days often sounds pleasant. It often does not prove to be pleasant. The patient who was an active

person before onset of the disabling condition was gaining reinforcement from activities no longer available because of the pain problem and related functional limitations. How are these or other reinforcements now to be gained? Finding effective alternative sources of reinforcement is not an automatic process. One only need observe the high rate of depression among elderly retired people to confirm that point. They are suffering a deprivation of reinforcers. Another illustration comes from the number of patients in virtually every physician's caseload who, as noted in earlier chapters, come with synthetic complaints because these complaints provide access to the reinforcing consequence of physician attention. The people who do that are, by definition, living a style of life that provides deficient reinforcement.

It is not suggested here that the health care system can be expected to deal with all of these problems. It is proposed, however, that each patient's future course is likely to be influenced significantly by these matters. Somebody will pay if they are not attended to. Some efforts need to be made to help. The more the patient is helped to become effectively involved in alternative behaviors, the less likely that patient will resume increased suffering behaviors or the hazardous and costly pursuit of additional health care.

The need to strengthen well behavior also arises with a patient who is having difficulty gaining access to or performing the mutually agreed on posttreatment target behaviors. A patient who has an employment objective may need additional job skill or assistance in finding a job. It may be necessary or desirable to change vocation. Vocational counseling resources should be called on to provide some of the needed assistance. However, the process of vocational re-engagement should be woven into the fabric of treatment and not tacked on at the end as an afterthought. For example, prescribed exercise and activity should begin in later phases of treatment to involve increasing proportions of job-related and job-seeking behaviors. This is an aspect of generalization to be dealt with in Chapter 13. The issue needs mention at this point because of the importance of incorporating into overall treatment planning a detailed consideration of what the posttreatment behaviors are likely to be and need to be.

Treatment planning sometimes moves ahead on too narrow a base. The assumption is made that the reinforcers relating to work (money, companionship, peer recognition, sense of accomplishment, and career advancement) are sufficient to maintain a host of well behaviors, including the appropriate levels of activity and exercise essential for the maintenance of treatment gains. Effective job placement can indeed help a patient into a richly reinforcing environment. Those reinforcers may then maintain a spectrum of behaviors from exercise and job-related activity to staying away from excessive health service demands and pain-contingent attention. It is also true, however, that many people find much of their sustaining reinforcement for daily effort in avocational or leisure time pursuits. Any number of people are content to put up with a dissatisfying or uncomfortable job because of the fun they have in the evenings or on weekends. Conversely, effective job placement, if it is not associated with at least a modicum of pleasant leisure time, may be inadequate to maintain performance. Sometimes a little effort at helping a patient to develop more skill at leisure time activity, or to gain better access to attractive (for him or her) leisure time outlets, can go a long way. People will often do a lot of otherwise uncomfortable or less-than-attractive things if pleasant leisure awaits them at the end of the day.

Work and play are considered here as both skills and potential sources of reinforcement. The latter concerns us because of the desirability of doing as much as one can to optimize the maintenance of treatment gains. The skill issue is of special interest because chronic pain patients so often have major skill deficits. The skill deficits may have antedated the pain problem, or they may

have arisen because of the long interval of relative inactivity associated with the problem itself. In either case, treatment planning and goal setting need to assess carefully what help is needed to reestablish the patient in the community.

One additional need for concern about promoting effective well behavior is probably the most commonly encountered. One of the major sources of reinforcement for operant pain is the time out it buys from aversive events, which was dealt with in Chapter 3. The issue reappears here because of the importance of reducing or eliminating that source of reinforcement for pain behaviors—as well as reducing the pain behaviors themselves.

Treatment goals must be concerned with solving or working around the problem or aversive consequences that pain behaviors were developed to avoid. Treatment gains soon disappear if the problem underlying avoidance learning is ignored or overlooked. The wage earner whose pain buys time out from repeated job failures needs job skill assistance. The housewife whose pain behaviors keep her otherwise neglectful husband closer by and more attentive has a pain problem that earns time out from loneliness or neglect. That marital pair needs help; perhaps only in how better to relate with each other or perhaps to find more stimulating shared recreation. Either the impotent husband or the frigid wife may find that pain buys time out from aversive intercourse. Referral to a sexual dysfunction clinic may be an essential adjunctive treatment. The list of possibilities is endless. The point is simply that well behavior leading to aversive consequences will not long endure.

The preceding discussion of treatment goals and patient target behaviors boils down to a need to recognize that treatment of chronic pain cannot be an enterprise solely in reduction of illness or disease. Treatment-effective and cost-effective issues both require that goal setting be broadened. On the conservative or pessimistic end of the spectrum, there are many important positive and highly beneficial consequences that accrue to a patient's program that strives only to establish and maintain a medical status quo. The pain or illness factor may not be capable of reduction, but the patient and family can be helped not to engage in further hazardous and costly treatment-seeking efforts. In another case, pain and functional impairment may have been reduced and perhaps even eliminated, but legal or economic factors prevent a return to competitive employment. The patient and family then may be helped to legitimate retirement, however that is labeled. When helped to enjoy retirement they are better able to maintain a medical status quo. Objectives of that conservative or, by some standards, pessimistic level, may neverthe-less provide both treatment-effective and cost-effective benefits.

On the more optimistic or ambitious side, where treatment is expected to lead to a broad expansion in activity level, including perhaps competitive employment or full resumption of housekeeping or parenting roles, treatment goals must be concerned with ensuring that those posttreatment activities are accessible. There must be concern that they are effectively reinforcing and that the patient has the skills and resources to gain access to them. The reduction of illness does not mean an increase in health. The increase in and maintenance of health or well behavior is a central issue in chronic pain.

6 The behavioral analysis of pain

The objectives of this chapter are to prepare interviewer set and to outline an interview or behavioral analysis guide for chronic pain.

When is a behavioral analysis called for? The first diagnostic or evaluative line of approach should be based on a disease model. There should be a thorough exploration of possible physical findings that account for the reported or displayed pain or that play a significant role in it. The medical evaluation or diagnosis of pain is a topic for which I have no professional competence. There are innumerable references from which additional information about the medical diagnosis of pain can be obtained. One that seems particularly to warrant mention is The Management of Pain (Bonica, 1975). The contributors to that book share a particular interest in and experience with pain in its various forms.

It is simply a matter of prudence to explore first in disease model terms. Conceptually, the indications for proceeding with a behavioral analysis after a disease model study of the problem can be depicted as shown in Fig. 16. Resorting for the moment to an S-R or stimulus-response descriptive mode, one looks for situations in which there is little or no stimulus (organic or physical findings) to account for the pain behaviors, where the magnitude of pain displayed seems disproportionately great relative to the kind or amount of body damage identified, or where the conclusions about body damage or the organic factor are themselves speculative or questionable.

It is easier to allocate to physicians and the medical diagnostic process the responsibility for making those determinations than it is for them to do it. Afferent impulses are not observed. Their presence and periodic activity are inferred. The inferences are based on some mixture of observations about body damage and of the patient's pain behaviors in all the forms those behaviors may take. Still, precision, experience, and sophistication of procedures and equipment all help. However good those resources are, at least two sources of error or misperception remain. One is that the patient's pain behaviors, however consistent and persuasive, are forever vulnerable to learning or conditioning effects. What the diagnostician sees or hears from the patient because of conditioning effects may not mean now what it meant earlier in the history of the problem. Second, observations of physical findings and correlated—even highly correlated—pain behaviors do not establish a causal relationship. This point may possibly be illustrated by patients who have received multiple surgeries at a given site (for pain relief or for other reasons) and who continue to report pain or who resume reporting pain after several weeks of postoperative relief.

The pain is sometimes explained as resulting from scar tissue or some such other by-product of the surgical process. The presence of scar tissue does not in itself establish that such scar tissue causes the reported pain. It only establishes a plausible explanation. Presumably, the greater the correlation between type and quality of pain behavior and information about the location and amount of scare tissue, the higher the plausibility. But the medical diagnosis of chronic pain, based on a disease model perspective, is fraught with difficulties. Diagnostic conclusions must be recognized as probability statements. To expect more from the diagnostician is unfair.

It is also difficult medically to assess how much pain or functional limitation can rea-

Stimulus	Response
O'	R
s^2	R
"S"^{3}	R

O' = No physical findings
s^2 = Physical findings present but insufficient to account for pain behavior
"S"^{3} = Physical findings hypothesized but with doubts

Fig. 16. *Schematic criteria for patient selection.*

sonably be expected from a given type or amount of physical findings. Conclusions about that issue usually represent a weighing of judgments about physical findings and assessments of the patient's age, general health, pain tolerance, and extent of hypochondriacal tendencies—from none to many. The last two, as noted previously, seem more prudently viewed as pain behaviors and not as personality traits. Judgments about them will not be drawn reliably from observations about a kind, location, and amount of tissue damage. Judgments about them based on knowledge of and observations about the patient as a person are helpful. But if those data take one back into the motivational model perspective, they are fraught with imprecision. Predictions as to what a person will do (including how much activity is to be expected in the presence of a given amount of physical findings) based on judgments about what the person *has* (personality traits) are simply less precise than those based on careful observations of what the person *does,* that is, behavior consequence relationships. It is therefore sometimes desirable to round out a disease model analysis of a pain problem with an additional behavioral analysis. When there is doubt as to whether functional limitations are appropriate to the physical findings, a behavioral analysis may help by providing negative evidence; that is, the amount of limitation observed seems not to be accounted for in operant terms and may therefore more certainly relate to the body damage factor. This negative evidence may encourage additional disease model evaluative studies. Alternatively, the amount of functional limitation may bear systematic relationships to environmental consequences. The evidence would then suggest that significant degrees of the limitations relate to nonorganic factors. They are largely or partially operant in character.

If a disease model evaluation identifies the problem as predominantly one of respondent pain and points clearly to a course of action, there is rarely any need to proceed with a behavioral analysis.

The next point to be made about when to do a behavioral analysis is that the behavioral analysis has nothing whatever to say about whether there is respondent pain. This is a point of fundamental importance. Establishing what appear to be tight relationships between the occurrence of pain behaviors and what appear to be reinforcing environmental consequences does *not* by itself indicate that there are not physical findings to be found to account for the pain. A behavioral analysis is not a substitute for a disease model analysis. A behavioral analysis can only indicate the viability of learning factors as an alternative explanation for the pain problem. Even in situations in which pain behavior–reinforcing consequence relationships are close and persuasive, all or part of the pain problem may in fact be a result of some organically-based factor. Behavioral analysis is neither a diagnostic nor a treatment panacea. It should follow, not precede, a disease model analysis.

Situations fitting one of the categories set forth in Fig. 16 indicate the potential utility of a behavioral analysis. This assumes that the pain problem has existed for several months or longer or is the reappearance of a previously long-standing pain problem or that the patient has previously displayed lengthy episodes of pain of a roughly similar nature, although perhaps at different body sites. Conditioning requires opportunity for practice. If there has been inadequate opportunity for learning to occur, there is no point in looking for conditioning effects.

Interviewer set

The experienced chronic pain patient has undergone many diagnostic evaluations. Understandably, the patient has a set of expectations as to the kinds of questions that will be asked as well as the kinds of non-interview types of examinations that are to be expected. Alterations in the diagnostic process, particularly the introduction of different lines of questioning, may produce or increase patient apprehensiveness or even suspicions. This can raise serious difficulties in the interview process. The scope and nature of this problem needs to be fully understood.

The chronic pain patient is, by definition, a loser in the health care process. If that process had been successful, the pain would not have persisted to its present chronic state. It follows that the patient enters these later or chronic stage evaluations with some mixture of fear, anger, resentment, suspicion, and sheer resignation. The problem is really more severe. As was noted earlier, pain often occurs in relation to causes that are invisible to the eyes of observers. For one to state that he or she cannot perform a task because "my back hurts" may raise few problems in the minds of those around the patient the first time or two. However, if the problem persists and endures beyond prescribed treatment programs, there is increasing probability of growing doubt or skepticism by observers. Sometimes it is only that the patient may fear that others doubt the reality of the pain. In either case, patients often develop concern or suspicion that others question the authenticity and severity of the pain and associated impairment. It is in that context of suspicion and resentment that diagnostic interviews often are perceived by the patient.

The problem is sometimes even more pointed. It was noted earlier that a disease model view of pain encourages the idea that there are essentially two kinds of pain, organic and nonorganic. The former is often accompanied explicitly or implicitly by such qualifiers as "real" and "physical." The nonorganic type, more often called psychogenic,

usually carries such explicitly or implicitly stated qualifiers as "imaginary," "unreal," "all in the head," "hysterical," or "hypochondriacal." These two characterizations of pain have accrued a good deal of currency, both by physicians and lay people. Most chronic pain patients who have undergone a number of diagnostic examinations and treatment programs report having received allusions or direct statements from physicians that all or part of the pain problems was psychogenic with all of its socially unattractive connotations. This may truly be the case, or it may be only that patients think it is. The frequency of this feeling in patients is easily confirmed. One may comment to the patient at the outset, "I suppose by now one or more people have said or implied to you that some or all of your pain is imaginary or all in your head." Such a statement leads virtually without exception to a vividly affirmative comment by the patient.

Another factor influencing how patients view the diagnostic interviewer is that the patient with much operant pain is often a chronic loser in life. Sternbach and associates (1973, p. 136) have described a type of pain patient often encountered who "Because he has little likelihood of future gainful employment . . . seems to be a loser in the game of life." Whether the patient's difficulties focus on employment or on other matters for which avoidance learning helps to maintain pain behaviors, he or she is likely to have had many unsuccessful life ventures and to be apprehensive, suspicious, and excessively guarded in relating interview information. Among other discomforts they may face, there is the threat of loss of the relative haven of illness, with no tenable alternatives yet in sight. If those among this group for whom it is appropriate knew that legitimate retirement was a viable potential alternative, they might feel differently.

The search for valid information from which to judge the nature of chronic pain problems and what to do about them is burdened with these special difficulties. It follows that the gatekeeper to the evaluation process needs to be skillful to cope with the communication problems surely to be encountered.

A behavioral analysis of a pain problem explores alternatives to a disease explanation. The patient may assume that this analysis represents a challenge to the reality or authenticity of the pain. That is unfortunate, as well as untrue. The issue should be met squarely. That proves surprisingly easy to do.

If there are indications in the situation that the patient does have these concerns, as a preliminary to the anlysis, it is worthwhile to take the time to point out one's entering premises to the patient. There are four major points that experience suggests deserve attention. These can be summarized as follows:

1. The idea that there are two kinds of pain, (1) organic, physical, or real and (2) nonorganic, psychogenic, or imaginary, is nonsense. Pain is what one feels when one hurts. Of course it is real. The proper question is not, Is it real? The proper question is, What are the factors that influence or control the pain?

2. Pain, like virtually every other body process, is subject to the influence of learning or conditioning. A pain problem does not begin because of learning, but it may come to be maintained or controlled by learning factors. When that happens, it still feels the same, but it is now controlled by different factors.

3. Learning or conditioning is automatic. If conditions are favorable for learning to occur, it will occur, whether we want it to or not. Learning can neither be turned off nor on. We can only help ourselves to get into or out of situations where learning can occur.

4. If what you, the patient, now have is a significant amount of learned or conditioned pain, you are suffering more than you need to. There is something that can be done about it.

If learning has occurred, unlearning can also occur.

Those points and some suggested ways of describing and illustrating them are provided in more detail in Chapter 8. A few moments devoted to these issues at the outset of evaluation of a chronic pain patient are a good investment toward patient cooperation and understanding and toward greater precision of information exchanged.

Much of the diagnostic information needed must come in part from the patient and in part from a key family member, usually the spouse. Additional useful and often critically important information will come from measures of patient activity level. The simplest and most direct way to obtain that information is to have the patient complete daily diary records (see Appendix A) before the workup. If diary recording cannot begin until the time of the behavioral analysis, the final conclusions will often need to be delayed until completed diaries have been examined.

Diaries provide an additional advantage. Patients should record directly on the diary forms the kinds, amounts, and times of pain medication intake.

The importance of the spouse accompanying the patient to the workup and of diary data being completed before diagnostic and treatment recommendations can be made should be spelled out to the patient at the first consideration of a behavioral analysis of the pain problem. Experience with a pain clinic (Bonica, 1973) and with operant treatment methods go beyond that. Experience suggests that virtually all chronic pain evaluations would be bolstered and facilitated by the requirement that the spouse be available during the workup process and that 1 to 2 weeks of diary data be completed and returned by the time of first workup. When such a policy is adopted, it is wise to be sure the point is clear to the patient. Patients are not accustomed to having family members participate in the workup. As a consequence, patients are not infrequently casual about arranging for the spouse to come along or to come at another time. The same casualness is sometimes applied to diary recording.

The patient and the spouse should be interviewed separately. A few moments should be taken with the two of them before proceeding to point out that the separate interviews are not a matter of questioning the accuracy or honesty of one against the other. Instead, with a problem as complex and long-standing as chronic pain, it simply makes sense to expect that each of them will be able to see things about the problem that the other has not recognized. They are both so caught up in the problem that there are bound to be some differences in their perspectives and their observations. Evaluation is too important to ignore that and to pass up the opportunity to develop all the information that can be developed to determine how help can be provided.

The issue as to which questions to direct to the patient and which to the spouse is one for which little firm guidance can be provided. It is largely a matter of judgment as to the adequacy, depth, and precision of the information that has been obtained. When in doubt, ask the spouse as well as the patient. One certainly would ask both about the time patterns of the pain, how pain is displayed or communicated, what activities and events systematically do and do not occur (that is, time out), when pain occurs, and what actions are taken to ease or relieve pain. In addition, if an operant treatment program is being considered, both patient and spouse need to be queried about probable and feasible posttreatment activities.

Patient evaluation may in a given case be concerned only with the narrower issue of defining the problem. Alternatively, the evaluation mission also may be to identify possible treatment methods. These two workup missions will be linked here to avoid needless repetition. The evaluator whose charge is only to determine whether the patient's pain problem could be accounted for in behavioral terms can omit elements of the interview guide, although the two missions'

diagnosis and treatment are not entirely separable. The concern about the interplay between patient and his or her environment inevitably leads one into some of the more treatment-oriented questions and topics. They will, however, be separated as much as seems practical in the behavior analysis guide.

The issues to be determined by a behavioral analysis of a pain problem can be formulated as follows:

A. The search for evidence indicating or contraindicating operant pain, that is, systematic and effective
   1. direct positive reinforcement of pain behavior
   2. indirect positive reinforcement of pain behavior by avoidance learning
   3. punishment of or failure to reinforce patient well behavior
B. The search for reinforcers holding promise of effectiveness in treatment
C. Identification of feasible and accessible posttreatment target behaviors
D. Determination of the readiness of family and the patient's environment to support change by
   1. reduction in reinforcement of pain behavior
   2. effective reinforcement of well behavior

The key element in searching for operant pain is *systematic* pain behavior–environmental consequence sequences (that is, repeated consistently and with time and consequence relationships capable of yielding effective reinforcement).

The next step is an interview guide. The procedure will be to present the key issues or questions, accompanied by explanations designed to relate them to material presented earlier in the book about the development of operant pain (Chapter 3), operant rudiments or behavior change technology (Chapter 4), or identification of treatment goals (Chapter 5).

The items presented are intended as guidelines. There are innumerable ways by which one might explore by interview for given bits of information. Furthermore, the special circumstances of the patient, of the context in which the interview occurs, and information developed within the interview all may lead one to abandon or to expand a given area.

Before commencing the step-wise assessment of issues set forth in the interview guide, it is usually a helpful shortcut to ask the patient to describe a typical day. ("When do you awaken? Do you get up? What happens during the morning and the afternoon? How ordinarily do you spend your evenings? When do you usually go to bed?") For the patient who stays home and is relatively inactive because of pain, determine also whether he or she dresses, how much time is spent reading or watching TV, and how often he or she goes out of the house.

The foregoing information should permit one to estimate roughly how many hours of each 24 is spent reclining, sitting, or moving about. That information, coupled with the diary data, will provide a useful check point against later items as well as being a convenient shortcut to several questions.

A. *Time pattern* (core issue: What is going on around the patient, or what activities preceded pain behaviors?).

1. *Episodic pain* (example: When do you have pain? Are there periods of several days or weeks free of pain, followed by episodes in which pain occurs almost around the clock?). Some patients will report episodes in which pain is virtually unremitting for several days or longer, followed by intervals of almost total relief. That kind of time pattern rarely bears systematic relationship to the environment unless it can be shown that pain episodes consistently follow certain patient activities or certain environmental events. The housewife who scrubs her floor once a month and then has 4 days of pain is illustrative. If pain seems to occur only when those kinds of physical demands occur, the episodic character of the time pattern is incidental.

Occasionally pain episodes coincide with the activities of others in the environment. Pain-free intervals may coincide with the spouse being away, as with the husband who travels or the wife who visits relatives.

Periods of around-the-clock freedom from pain when activity and circumstances in the environment are essentially normal are likely to be indicative of respondent and not operant pain. Systematic pain behavior–environmental consequence relationships are missing.

Consistent relationships between pain episodes and certain activities or environmental arrangements indicate that operant pain should be considered. More detail will be needed as to what these relationships may be.

2. *Nocturnal time patterns* (example: Is there any particular or consistent time of night when the pain is better or worse? What happens with the pain when you go to bed at night, turn out the lights, and begin to go to sleep?).

The patient who reports that the reduction in sensory stimulation accompanying lights out leads to increased pain is more likely to have respondent pain because reduced distraction opens the gate to peripheral noxious stimuli or because the reclining body position is specifically productive of pain.

One exception that occurs occasionally is the long-time pain patient who has evolved a pattern of sleeping or resting all day while the spouse is at work or is quietly supporting the apparent need for full-time rest. Nighttime may, for that patient, be boredom time, an antidote for which is the movement and attention generated by displays of pain. Patients *will* sleep sooner or later. It is common for pain patients to report that each night is marred by pain to the point where but a few moments or a handful of hours of restless sleep were gained. More detailed exploration with the patient or the spouse often indicates that the amount of nighttime sleeping is underestimated or that it is compensated for by ample daytime sleep.

If those alternative rest patterns cannot be identified, it is more likely to be respondent pain.

Nocturnal awakening (example: How often do you awaken at night because of the pain? How many times do you awaken each night in an average night? How many nights each week are you likely to awaken because of the pain?—each month?).

The overlapping questions are essential because of the frequency with which the first response is vague or off-hand: "Oh, several times every night." It often comes out that awakening is much less or more frequent than initially implied. Assuming that the patient's or spouse's reports indicate frequent or consistent awakening during the night, find out what happens when the patient awakens. Precision is needed here, as in all behavioral analyses. General or vague responses such as, "Oh, I get up and have a smoke," "I sit up for a few minutes," "I toss and turn for awhile before going back to sleep," often omit key systematically occurring events. If one is not satisfied that the question is receiving the kind of detailed thought it deserves, an often helpful remedy is to pose it this way: "If I were there when you awakened, what would I see and hear?"

There are several things to watch for. The patient who, on awakening, takes private action to relieve the pain (aside from medication, which will be considered in a moment) or to seek distraction from it is more likely to have respondent pain. The patient may quietly steal from the bed and go to another room to read, pace, sit up, or whatever. This arrangement is to be contrasted with the patient whose awakening activities also awaken the spouse, whether deliberately or ostensibly accidentally, and then lead to systematic spouse action. It would be a mistake to assume that spouse action must be obviously beneficial. It may be obvious as in providing a back rub, bringing the heat pad, bringing medications, or simply providing reassurance or expressions of concern. In some situations, the sheer act of awakening and disturbing the spouse has more subtle reinforcing effects for the pa-

tient. To awaken the spouse may, for example, serve to reassure the patient that the spouse continues to be aware of the extent and duration of the patient's suffering. There may even be sadistic pleasure at harassing or disturbing the spouse, particularly if the patient is resentful at being impaired when the spouse sails through life unburdened by chronic pain. The key thing is systematic spouse action, whatever its form. When there is systematic spouse action, there is always the possibility that it represents pain-contingent social reinforcement as well as perhaps direct palliative relief.

Frequent nocturnal awakening may only mean that something else awakened the patient and, in retrospect, the patient incorrectly attributes awakening to pain. The interestingly frequent illustration of this is the patient who, on awakening "from pain," always goes to the bathroom to empty his or her bladder. When, under further inquiry, it becomes evident there is consistent and reasonably frequent bladder urgency, day or night, the alleged nocturnal pain is sometimes an innocent mislabeling. Perhaps it was only that, having awakened because of bladder urgency, the patient was then reminded of and experienced the pain. Under those circumstances, that part of the pain pattern may be said to have come under control of other factors. Nocturnal awakening by itself does not support the inference of respondent pain.

Nocturnal medications. Another issue to explore in regard to consistent nocturnal awakening is pain medications. A two-step approach to this issue seems to work better. First determine the frequency and time-spacing of the awakening (example: How soon after going to asleep do you awaken? How long is it until the next time you awaken? Are there fairly consistent times at which you awaken or are likely to be awake, such as 1 AM or 4 AM?). Once it has been established that the patient is often awake at certain approximate times, ask if medications are taken at those times. Sensitivity must be exercised here, for the patient may be apprehensive or guilty about the amount of medication being consumed. The responses one gets are potentially burdened with patient concerns about how the interviewer will react. This is also one of the topics about which spouse observations may prove particularly helpful. If it can be shown that the patient takes medications in a consistent time pattern (for example, every 3 to 4 hours), addiction or habituation must certainly be considered. But more than that, the nocturnal awakening from pain may not be that at all. It may be that the systematic consequence to awakening is the reinforcing effects of medication. Under those conditions, the pain behavior of awakening and taking medication may be substantially or even totally under control of addiction or habit. There will be more about that later.

3. *Diurnal time patterns* (example: Is there any particular time of day when pain is likely to be better or worse? What is the pain like when you first awaken in the morning and get out of bed? What is the trend of that across the day? Does pain tend to get better or worse as the day goes along?).

Pain that is specific to activity or movement can often be expected to occur or increase in daytime and diminish or disappear at bedtime. It follows that a pattern of pain only in the daytime is not necessarily operant.

Daytime pain time patterns do not often have significance except when they point to specific pain-activity or pain–social reinforcement relationships. Those relationships will be explored more directly further along. Examination of the trend of the pain across daytime hours usually quickly indicates whether it is activity related. Unremitting pain or lack of variation when the day's activities vary suggests respondent pain. A trend toward lessening pain as the day wears on also argues against rest or time out from activities as sustaining operant pain.

Systematic time periodicity to increases of pain should be checked. If, at the time of the increases, the patient takes medication, the problem may be addiction or habituation, which, in turn, may indicate operant pain and a minimal respondent component.

To sum up the time issue, without systematic pain behavior–environmental consequence relationships, there can be no operant pain. Time patterns, that indicate such relationships may reflect operant pain, respondent pain, or a mixture of the two.

B. *Pain behavior* (core issue: How do those around the patient know when pain is experienced or is severe?). If the patient's pain and associated functional limitations remain a totally private matter, systematic social reinforcement cannot occur. Although it seems a straightforward matter, it is often difficult to obtain precise information from the patient about this point (example: How do people around you know when you are having pain? How do they know when the pain is severe? How do people know what activities you cannot do or must limit because of your pain?).

Perhaps the most common initial response to this topic is, "I don't let people know I am hurting!" or "I don't say a word. I keep it to myself." Such a response is of course more attractive because of its higher social desirability. In addition, however, people who have long been experiencing pain often will have developed ways that may seem to mask the occurrence of pain but in fact signal to others that it is being felt. These signals are often subtle. Even the spouse may no longer be aware that they are occurring or that they successfully elicit systematic spouse responses. This issue becomes of major import in the matter of spouse retraining, a topic of Chapter 12. It is also essential now to pinpoint whether there is ample opportunity for people in the patient's environment to make systematic responses. They must receive cues to do so. It is often helpful to ask, "If I were in your living room when you were present and were experiencing pain (or severe pain), what would I see you do and hear you say?" The pain behavior may be nothing more than not doing something else. For example, the patient may recline on the sofa when, were there no pain problem, some other activity would be underway at that time. The key element is that those around the patient can reliably discriminate pain-free states from those in which pain is experienced or anticipated.

Pinpointing pain behaviors does not bear directly on the question of how much is respondent and how much is operant. The information helps to identify the consequences, social and otherwise, to those pain displays, as will be explored next. Whether those consequences are systematic *and* reinforcing remains to be determined.

C. *Environmental responses* (core issue: How do those around the patient respond when pain is signaled?).

1. *Direct reinforcement of pain behavior.* Patients commonly interpret this question to be, "Do others help 'baby' or protect me?" Occasionally the question is interpreted as aimed at determining whether the spouse is loyal in the face of adversity or is fed up with the pain problem. The task is made easier by clarifying that the information being sought is description and not judgment (example: What I'm after here is not whether what others do is good or bad, helpful or harmful, or anything like that. It is just that when a patient problem has lasted a long time, people often develop ways of behaving or responding to the pain of which they no longer are aware. Sometimes knowing what those are can help—can make a difference.).

The most common first response is, "They don't do anything." Taken literally, people cannot do nothing. The point should be pursued further (example: If I were there when your husband/wife came into the room and could see that the pain was bad, what would happen? What would I see and hear him/her do? What would you do next?).

The major thing to watch for here is consistency. The content or quality of the spouse behavior when pain is signaled is a second-order question. Data from the patient and, separately, from the spouse indicating much variability or almost random behavior precludes effective social reinforcement for pain behavior or punishment of efforts toward activity or well behavior. On the other hand, consistency of spouse response to pain behavior increases the possibility of social reinforcement as a significant factor.

It can hardly be overemphasized that the content or quality of the spouse response may have systematic effects on the patient, regardless of whether the interviewer thinks that spouse behavior is reinforcing, aversive, or whatever.

There are some obvious and direct things to watch for. The spouse may be immediately solicitous or helpful; he or she may reassure or console, offer medications, or step in to take over a pain-producing task. The reinforcement may be more subtle. The spouse may consistently change the subject ("I am trying to divert his/her attention—get his/her mind on other things"), may turn toward (or away from) the patient, without saying anything, or may become angry or disgusted and express that feeling openly. All but the last named clearly can have positive reinforcing value. Negatively toned spouse affect in response to pain displays is also capable in several ways of being reinforcing. The negative affect may be followed consistently by helpful behaviors. The angry response may reassure the patient that the spouse is still aware of the pain problem. The patient may delight in bedeviling the spouse. The possibilities of the subtleties are endless.

2. *Discouraging activity (punishing of well behavior).* After direct reinforcement of pain behavior, the punishment of well behavior must next be considered (example: When you try to do things and your husband/wife knows you are having pain or expects that you will have pain if you continue with what you are doing, what does he/she say and do?).

Discouragement of activity may await a cue from the patient that pain is present and thus be a response to pain behavior. Matters may have progressed to the point where the spouse asserts protective action in anticipation of pain. Seeing the patient begin some action, or even simply signaling that action is being considered, may be enough to elicit spouse response or intervention. That response may be to step in to take over the contemplated task or in some other fashion to discourage the patient from proceeding. Routine assumption of tasks by the spouse, without a pain behavior display as a cue or reminder, will be dealt with later. At the moment, the concern is with direct responses to pain behavior.

The content or emotional tone of spouse response is of secondary importance. If it is systematic, it may be an effective punisher or inhibitor of activity, whether presented solicitously or with bitter overtones.

Discrepancies between patient and spouse are common in response to those areas. That is to be expected. Interchanges between them about pain have been going on long enough to lead inevitably to some routinized responses about which one or both parties may have become unaware. Conflicting accounts must be weighed. It becomes a matter of clinical judgment as to where the greater accuracy rests.

In this section the spouse has been the target and not other people around the patient. One occasionally finds situations in which others in addition to, or instead of, the spouse play key roles. That is uncommon. The exceptions are mainly to be found relating to adolescent children in the household or to parents of the patient. There are always potential exceptions. But experience indicates that neighbors, co-workers, and relatives or immediate family members living outside the household almost always play, at most, secondary and noncrucial roles. Contact is too infrequent for them to be sources of effective social reinforcement for

pain behavior or for discouragement of activity and well behavior. They may play a role, but it is rarely enough to sustain the pain problem if the spouse is not also contributing.

The single patient is, of course, another exception. It is usually a simple matter to judge whether there is someone in the picture with whom the patient has sufficient contact to derive sustaining social reinforcement for operant pain. When such a person emerges in the picture, he or she should be called in for an interview in the same fashion as is done routinely in the case of a spouse.

D. *Pain activators* (core issue: What increases pain or causes it to occur? There is a closely related issue: What is the reinforcement value or importance to the patient of the activities that bring on or aggravate pain?).

At this point the concern is with kinds of movement or physical demands that may increase pain. Later these will be studied again in larger units that combine these activators. "Taking care of the housework" or "going to work," for example, represent clusters of bending, lifting, and walking. The issues here have complex interrelationships. One way of posing the central question is to explore the relative costs of pain versus activities. If onset or increase in experienced pain results in termination of a high-value, high-strength activity for the patient, it might be said that the cost of pain is high. *Cost* here is used in a psychological sense, although it might be economic as well. The patient must, because of pain, limit or forego reinforcers that ordinarily accrue to the relinquished activity. His or her pain costs that much. Furthermore, continuing to engage in the activity for a distinctive period of time or to a significant amount, after onset or increase of pain, supports the idea that the pain costs a great deal. The patient is willing to suffer to gain the reinforcers relating to the activity. The cost-benefit ratio of pain to activity is high. Stated another way, the payoff or reinforcement for pain behavior is low.

A quick termination or militant avoidance of the activity when pain begins or increases suggests that pain behavior (in this instance, stopping to rest or avoiding a particular activity) is relatively more reinforcing. Logically, there are two possibilities here. One is that the pain is so severe or uncomfortable that the patient is willing to undergo the reinforcement deprivation resulting from limited or avoided activity to gain relief from the pain. The second is that the amount of reinforcement from the activities is not great. In the latter case, rest and time out readily yield equal or greater reinforcement than do the activities. The pain-activity cose-benefit ratio may be said to be low.

One must determine what activities increase or aggravate pain. The relationships between amount performed and stopping or limiting one's effort must also be determined to judge whether contingent reinforcement relationships exist. Finally, one needs to determine the potential reinforcing value (high or low, positive or aversive) of the activities.

1. *Roster of activators* (example: What are the things that produce or increase pain? What makes your pain worse?).

    Care again should be exercised to gain accurate detail. General comments ("Any kind of movement," "Any kind of bending or lifting") should be elaborated. The housewife can be asked to indicate a typical list of household chores that produce or increase her pain. The wage earner can develop a similar set of details. The list need not be exhaustive. It should be broad enough to help later in pinning down what activities are indeed avoided.

    Patients occasionally will report that the pain keeps them from doing so many things that they no longer know what aggravates the pain. They can be asked to recall which activities previously engaged in brought on the pain. At the other extreme is the patient who steadfastly claims that all activities increase pain. He or she should be asked to discriminate a few that produce greater amounts of pain or more rapidly or consistently aggravate pain.

    Patients often fail to distinguish among pain, weakness, and fatigue. An activity, limited in relation to the pain problem, may now be curtailed because of weakness or fatigue resulting from infrequent or insufficient exercise. Or perhaps it is limited as a by-product of heavy medication intake and associated lethargy or discoordination. The error works both ways. The patient may state that an activity is curtailed because to continue with it is to produce an increase in pain, when in fact it is weakness and fatigue that now are experienced. Alternatively, the patient may have limited an activity for a lengthy period because to do otherwise would have resulted in significant aggravation of pain. Long periods of disuse lead to ease of fatigue. Subsequently, when the activity is attempted, fatigue or weakness are experienced and reported by the patient, and he or she must stop. For the purposes of behavioral analysis, the distinction between pain, on the one hand, and weakness or fatigue, on the other, are usually unimportant. It is the systematic relationship between doing or not doing (behavior) and rest or other consequences (contingent reinforcement) that matters. It follows that questions about activity or nonactivity can be posed such that pain, weakness, and fatigue are essential equivalents.

    Once a representative roster of pain activators has been identified, these should be sampled to learn how soon pain follows. Determine how much is done before pain begins or before the patient stops or modifies the activity because of pain, weakness, or fatigue.

2. *Activity-pain time interval* (example: When you do an activity leading to pain, how long is it from when you begin until the pain begins? When do you stop—when the pain begins? before it begins? If you stop before the pain begins but the pain comes later, how long is it after you stop before the pain begins?).

    Pain that begins many minutes or even many hours after an activity has terminated is not likely to be reinforced by rest, by time out from the activity, or by contingent social consequences. Rest and attention both occur too late to be considered effective reinforcers. The patient who no longer engages in an activity reportedly because of pain it produces, although delayed by several minutes or hours, may have time out or avoidance learning sustaining pain behavior. Always assuming that medical evaluation has raised doubt about whether physical findings account for the functional limitations reported, the question of whether this represents avoidance learning can best be judged by assessing the reinforcing value of the activity itself, apart from the issue of pain.

If the patient persists in engaging in the activity, when to do so surely produces delayed pain, it is almost certainly respondent pain. There is no time-out reinforcement.

Enquire about how much of each of a sample of the pain activators ordinarily is attempted before halting, resting briefly, or significantly restricting how the task is performed. One can then weigh the relative costs of pain behavior versus rest or time out. If little is attempted and it is reported that pain, weakness, or fatigue quickly lead to termination, the distress is highly aversive, the activity is not reinforcing, or both. The patient who imposes pervasive functional limitations on himself or herself such that only limited amounts of activity are attempted, providing a clear basis for this from the preceding medical evaluation, may well have much operant pain. The prime exception to this is the patient for whom this much inactivity is a striking contrast to premorbid behavior. Such a patient as that shows by history that activity is highly reinforcing.

Particular attention is needed here in regard to patient–spouse and patient verbal report–diary data discrepancies. The spouse may not observe how much the patient does but may only infer it. Patients and spouses sometimes form word habits describing much or little activity when in truth what they are describing is what used to be the case but is no longer true.

To this point, in regard to pain activators, information has been developed on what they are, on the time relationships between activity and reported pain, and on amounts of the activity leading to significant pain or functional impairment. The matter of the reinforcement value (high or low) of those activators remains and will be explored later.

E. *Pain diminishers* (core issue: What actions or events, in addition to responses of others, are pain contingent?).

The objectives here are specific. The responses of others to pain behaviors have been explored. How much they reinforce pain behaviors or discourage well behaviors should be clear. If not, that matter can be reopened here. In addition, however, it is important to determine whether rest is a reinforcer and is pain contingent (example: When the pain becomes bad, what can you do to ease or relieve it? What helps?).

1. *Rest as a pain diminisher.* If the response indicates rest (reclining, sitting, some form of taking it easy) helps, the time relationships should be identified. This was accomplished in part in the immediately preceding section (D.2) when it was determined how soon rest begins after the start or increase of pain. The information to be added now is the length of time it takes for rest to have a beneficial effect. Rest taking many hours to be felt as significantly easing the distress is less likely to maintain operant pain. Furthermore, if the patient arises after a period of rest and resumes the activity that led to pain, the cost of rest must be nearly as high as the cost of pain. Rest in that pattern is not likely to sustain operant pain, although it still might relieve respondent pain. Finally, rest used only episodically, to help control pain, is not a systematic reinforcer.

2. *Medication as a pain diminisher* (example: How many times each day do you take pain medication? About how many hours between doses? What do you take? How much difference is there between amounts of daytime and nighttime medication?).

It is often difficult to gain sound data about pain medication intake from chronic pain patients. Errors come from many sources. Some patients understate what is taken out of concern that they will be criticized or to disguise secret or secondary sources of medications that, if revealed, would risk being lost. Other patients err by overstating what they consume. This phenomenon seems like the heavy smoker who always carries a spare pack "just in case." Some patients taking much medication overstate current consumption in an effort to provide a safety factor by seeking prescription of an ample supply. Other patients are toxic or sedated to the point that they are incapable of accurate recall. Yet others routinely substitute large amounts of ethanol (alcohol) as a supplemental source of sedation and so, although honestly reporting medication intake, seriously underestimate the amount of sedation they consume. In regard to interview sources, clinical judgment from close questioning of patient and spouse and cross comparisons with diary data and medical records of prescriptions are about all that can be done. As will be noted in the section on treatment, direct inpatient observation is sometimes necessary.

The major issue here concerns habituation or addiction or systematic, pain-contingent sedation. Medications taken in a consistent time pattern (for example, each 3 to 4 hours), day and night, make habituation or addiction a strong possibility. That in turn is a strong indication that pain behaviors may be under control of the medication habit rather than physical causes.

Other sources of relief encountered with some frequency, such as heat pads, massage, a vibrator, or hot baths do not often maintain operant pain except as they also entail selective and pain-contingent attention or time out from aversive activities. The visible use of these other sources of pain reduction may better be thought of as pain behaviors in their own right. They serve as cues from the patient to others that there is a pain problem for which special help or protection may be needed. The persistent use of a cane, long after it no longer has ample respondent basis, illustrates the point.

F. *Tension-relaxation* (core issue: Does tension increase and relaxation decrease pain, or does the opposite occur?).

This subject is better dealt with separately. There are many reasons why tension and emotional distress might increase pain and why relaxation or escape from tension might decrease it. An opposite picture occasionally emerges: tension decreases and relaxation increases pain. Increased pain associated with emotional or muscle tension can be a purely respondent phenomenon. However, if rest eases the pain and permits the patient to avoid the source of emotional distress, the conditions for avoidance learning exist. The pain behaviors may yield time out from situational or emotional problems because they require the patient to rest to gain relief.

The restless, driven, life-is-a-racing-treadmill patient with chronic pain may yield the opposite picture. For such a person, rest and idleness may be threatening. Activity is a critically important source of reinforcement. When a pain problem occurs and a lightening of the workload appears desirable, the patient may work against himself or herself. Prescribed rest creates distress, and so the patient prematurely or excessively resumes activity, thereby worsening the pain problem. This is what might be called operant abuse of a respondent pain problem. The central behavioral problem now is to help the patient to reduce activity, not increase it.

If relaxation, like rest, fails to ease pain, there is less likelihood that it is an operant pain problem. If relaxation does ease pain, it may still be a respondent pain problem. In this case, relaxation training, for example, biofeedback, training in relaxation or self-hypnosis, may prove helpful. Alternatively, relaxation that eases pain should also be considered as a potential form of rest or time out and judged in that light.

The behavioral analysis has now completed exploring whether pain behavior receives direct positive reinforcement from attention, rest, or medication. The question of whether functional impairment was a direct result of zealous compliance with physician prescription will also have been clarified. The question of the direct punishment or discouragement of activity or daily chores (well behavior) has also been explored. The groundwork has been laid for exploring the third possibility, indirect positive reinforcement of pain behavior through time out or avoidance learning. The roster of pain activators and pain diminishers serves as a foundation for exploring what activities the patient no longer engages in and their positive or negative reinforcing properties.

There are other problems the patient may have alone, in marriage, or in other vocational or social ways. Everyone has problems. Establishing that the patient has problems or displays what some may characterize as a neurosis, deviant personality, interpersonal difficulties, or whatever, is not enough. For these problems to influence the pain problem or have functional relations to it, it must be shown that there are contingent relationships. Pain behavior must lead to time out from or to reduction of the other problems. If those pain-contingent relationships do not exist, the other problems are unlikely to be relevant to the pain problem.

There are many forms in which the time-out or indirect reinforcement effect may exist. They usually can ultimately be reduced to some combination of these: the patient now does something because of the pain problem that was not done before, quits doing something previously done, the spouse now does something not done before, or the spouse quits doing something previously done. In each of the four possibilities there is a pain-contingent relationship. *What* is (or is not) done might be anything from taking tranquilizers to changing jobs or recreational pursuits.

The material covered to this point also tells the extent to which rest, attention, and medication, the three naturally occurring and fairly readily programmed consequences in treatment settings, are likely to be effective reinforcers, should a treatment program begin. Any of them which has been sustaining a patient's operant pain is, by definition, a high-strength behavior. As such, it can, if properly reprogrammed, serve to strengthen well behavior.

G. *Changes in activity as a result of pain* (core issue: What changes in the patient's and spouse's ways of life have occurred, and are those changes costly or reinforcing?).

Distinguish vocational from leisure pursuits and explore them separately. They often show different amounts of change and may have widely different reinforcement characteristics. Leisure pursuits tend to reflect what a person likes or wants to do. That is another way of stating that leisure is reinforcing or provides access to yet other effective reinforcement. Vocational pursuits provide access to reinforcers, but sometimes the reinforcement is only that it makes possible desired leisure time pursuits. For these reasons information about a person's leisure time activities tends to shed more precise light on what is reinforcing for that patient. It is important also to determine the premorbid frequency or baseline of the activities so that change can better be assessed. Patients sometimes report they no longer do something because of the pain that they had not done for years anyway.

The question of how much of an activity was done before onset of the pain problem or before reduction of the activity because of pain has an even more important implication. Behavior that has been occurring at a high rate has, by definition, been receiving *some* form of effective reinforcement. Once one knows what behaviors have been reduced in rate, it becomes possible to assess the cost in reinforcement deprivation from the pain problem for the patient and the spouse. Loss of an activity usually also means loss of the reinforcers that sustained it. That is the case, of course, unless it is also shown that the reinforcers previously sustaining premorbid behaviors continue to be available. In that event there is little or no deprivation of reinforcers.

The sustaining reinforcement for leisure

activities usually will become evident from the nature of the activities. Leisure activities tend to be reinforcing in their own right or because the spouse or other family members richly reinforce them. It is, for example, usually easy to determine what the reinforcers are for a housewife who reports that she used to do much gardening before her back pain. She may have been reinforced by the exercise and sunshine, the pride or esthetic values of a pretty garden, either in her own eyes or those of family and neighbors, or by the access that gardening provided to a garden club in which she could socialize with others.

The key reinforcers sustaining vocational efforts are not always so apparent. It is well recognized that what it is about a job that provides the payoff to the worker is often a complex mixture of many factors. To name a few—money, career enhancement, status, exercise, sense of accomplishment, opportunity to interact with (or to not have to interact with) people, opportunity to be indoors out of the cold or outdoors in the fresh air—all play a role. Some sense of what these reinforcers have been should be developed to determine how much of a deprivation now exists. There should also be exploration of whether significant changes in the reinforcing characteristics of the job occurred at or shortly before onset of the pain problem. Work or leisure that has become less reinforcing or less accessible may change from attractive to aversive, and avoidance learning may follow.

The issue here benefits from being approached in two different ways. One is to enquire about what was done but now occurs on a reduced and perhaps zero frequency. The second is to enquire what would be done in the future if there were no significant limitation because of pain. Contrasts between the two approaches are common. Those discrepancies help to identify what the patient and spouse expect and want and what they will reinforce, which are vital issues in setting treatment goals and posttreatment target behaviors. The slightly different approach reflected in asking what one would do in the future sometimes leads patients to describe lucidly and spontaneously what is reinforcing and

what is not. The wage earner or the housewife often will respond to this question by elaborating many pleasant activities but make no mention of work or housework. These omissions often are made after earlier assertions about the pleasures of work. They sometimes reveal more about what is truly reinforcing than the patient expects.

1. *Patient activity modifications* (example: What are the things you no longer do because of the pain? About how many times a day, week, month—as indicated—did you do those things?).

The patient who reports that he or she is continuing to go to work or to do the expected daily chores should also be queried as to whether there is any change in what is done on the job and whether others have taken over parts of the load. This latter point also may lead to further description of how others respond to displays of pain behavior.

Next, explore what the reinforcers were for the job (example: Did you enjoy the job? What was it about the work that kept you at it?). When all the data are in, it is usually a simple process to judge how much those reinforcers continue to be available in spite of the pain. If they are, there is no deprivation, no cost, and no avoidance of aversive conditions through pain behavior. Operant pain is then not being supported in this fashion.

Next, be sure there has not been a significant change in the work or leisure situation, independently of the pain problem. Several wives who were pain patients have described situations in which social and leisure pursuits were markedly disrupted by husband transfers to other cities. Old friends (and social reinforcers) were no longer available. The patient who had limited skill at forming new friendships then suffered a major deprivation. In similar vein, it is not uncommon for wage earners to report significant job changes at about the time of or before the onset of pain. A job that previously was reinforcing became less so and perhaps even aversive.

If there has been no significant

change in vocational or leisure activities because of the pain, there is no opportunity for time-out effects. The likelihood of operant pain being supported in that fashion is accordingly diminished.

Where changes in activities have occurred, the challenge is to judge their net cost in reinforcement to the patient. This task is usually not difficult so long as it is kept in mind that reinforcers are much more than money and that leisure activities are an easier way to determine the effective reinforcers for a person. Pain that significantly changes leisure pursuits is indeed almost always costly to the patient unless it can be shown there continues to be effective reinforcement from the altered leisure pursuits.

2. *Pain-free activity plans* (example: If you had no significant pain problem, what would you do that you do not now do?).

This point usually can be covered briefly because of the great overlap with the preceding item. The additional information developed here, if there is any, sometimes reveals that the patient or spouse is content with the status quo. No activity change is anticipated or desired. If that is the case, spouse responses have limited relevance to the pain problem. Alternatively, the pain problem provides one or both of them with considerable reinforcement.

Responses to these items should be checked to determine whether they reflect realistic assessments of the future. It is sometimes easy to confuse what one would like to do with what one is likely to do. The central point of the activity modification items is to determine what has been given up or reduced because of pain *and* would be resumed were the pain problem eased.

3. *Spouse activity modifications* (to the patient: "What are the things your husband/wife used to do but no longer does because of your pain problem? About how many times a day/week/ month were they done?" The same question is then asked of the spouse,

both about the patient and about the spouse.).

The issues here are as in G.2: What are the costs in reinforcement to the patient for pain behavior? These items amplify data obtained directly from the patient. More importantly, however, they also explore that vital source of reinforcement and punishment or nonreinforcement for a patient, the spouse.

No significant change in spouse activity because of the patient's pain problem usually means that the spouse is not indirectly reinforcing pain behavior or indirectly discouraging well behavior—direct reinforcement, perhaps, as explored in item C, but not indirect. The spouse is not gaining time out from some aversive activity because of the patient's functional impairments. The spouse is also not undergoing a deprivation of reinforcement from loss of access to a previously reinforcing activity.

The importance of this issue should not be overlooked. Clinically, one finds repeated examples of a spouse systematically reinforcing pain behavior or discouraging well behavior because the pain problem has produced reinforcing activity changes for the spouse. An earlier example described a husband with secondary impotence who reinforced his wife's pain behaviors with enormous effectiveness. Maintaining her pain problem yielded him time out from the now threatening activity of intercourse. He was apparently unaware of what he was doing, but that is beside the point. One need not be aware of a contingent reinforcement relationship for it to be effective, and awareness does not by itself reduce effectiveness.

In another case, the solicitous and now lonely mother of a 19-year-old son actively reinforced his pain behaviors and sabotaged treatment programs that threatened her with his emancipation. In both illustrations, patient pain behavior led to the successful avoidance of aversive events in and for another person, not the patient.

Evidence that a spouse gains indirect reinforcement from pain behavior increases the likelihood of operant pain. It also means that changes in that situation will be essential for treatment to succeed.

Evidence that a spouse suffers a loss of reinforcement as a consequence of the pain problem argues against the spouse contributing to operant pain. That evidence also indicates that the spouse is more likely to be an effective reinforcer of increased patient activity level although he or she may need help in learning how to do that. Treatment is likely to move ahead more easily.

4. *Spouse pain-free activity plans.* This item should require no further elaboration. It is the twin to G.2, the patient's pain-free plans.

5. *Sexual intercourse* (example: What changes in your sexual life have been caused by the pain problem? How often each week do you have intercourse? How often did you before the pain problem began?).

Sexual problems occur with sufficient frequency in relationship to chronic pain to warrant separate treatment.

The central issue here is to determine indirect reinforcement of pain behavior or indirect punishment of well behavior. Changes in frequency or quality of sexual activity in a marriage probably—although not certainly—have major reinforcing properties. Therefore, when changes in sexual activity result from a pain problem, whom does it cost and whom does it reinforce? Time out from intercourse is not likely to be a reinforcer helping to maintain operant pain if both patient and spouse experience sexual deprivation. But if one of the marital pair experiences intercourse as aversive, the opportunity for strong reinforcement exists, and the matter should be explored.

Sex-related questions presented as but one of a series of enquiries regarding activities potentially influenced by pain do not often raise interview problems. Information about the frequency of intercourse, before the pain problem and presently, should be elicited from patient and from the spouse.

Questions about frequency of intercourse can be followed with an enquiry regarding the quality of the relationship. ("How would you describe the sexual adjustment in your marriage?" "Is there much difference between you and your husband/wife in how often intercourse is desired and in how much it is enjoyed?") This brief enquiry, when directed to both the patient and the spouse, appears sufficient in most cases to provide a judgment as to how likely intercourse is either aversive or reinforcing to one or both members of the marriage.

When major problems emerge in regard to sexual functioning, there remains the question of what to do about them. Clearly, when sexual dysfunction appears to help maintain a pain problem, the sexual problems need to be dealt with if treatment gains are to be maintained. Reduced sexual activity is sometimes related to side effects of pain medications. Reducing medication intake usually handles that problem. Other sexual problems may not be so straightforward. They may represent gaps in effective well behavior for which no solutions are in sight. If that is the case, they may prejudice treatment success. Severe impotence, frigidity, or disabling problems of sex-role identity may be examples.

Earlier in this chapter, four potential objectives of the behavioral analysis were noted: evidence for or against operant pain, the search for reinforcers helpful in treatment, identification of posttreatment target behaviors, and determination of family readiness to support treatment and behavior change. The data obtained from this kind of interview, often supplemented by such additional explorations as will be set forth immediately following, provide the basis for judging the extent to which learning or conditioning can account for the pain behaviors and associated functional impairments. The data also provide much, although not all, of the essential information for the other three objectives. Those, too, will be spelled out in more detail in the following sections of this chapter.

Supplemental "behavioral" data

It will be evident that parts of the interview guide presented above are also found in social history or psychiatric diagnostic interviews. Data from those sources should be drawn on when available. They are not, however, adequate substitutes for a behavioral analysis in most cases because of differences in focus and because they do not explore certain key areas. There are additional behavioral samples that can prove useful in assessing the probable reinforcing or nonreinforcing characteristics of pain or functional impairment to the patient. These will be dealt with briefly.

Diagnostic evaluation of diary data

Diary data are simple, inexpensive, and useful. It is a tactical error not to make routine use of diary data in the evaluation of chronic pain. Analysis of the diary data is easy.

The patient is instructed to record medication intake on the diary form: what, when, and how much. That information may not be precise nor complete and so should be viewed cautiously. A quick scanning of one or two weeks of diary forms should suggest the approximate frequency of medication intake and the rough average of hours between doses. Consistent time spacing, unless on a prescribed basis, suggests addiction or habituation and warrants more careful examination. Random and infrequent intake may reflect lack of a medication problem or lack of judicious recording.

The patient will also have been instructed to record (see Appendix A) how much of each day is spent sitting, standing or walking, and reclining and when during the day each of those occurs. At the bottom of each daily sheet is space for totaling the hours in each of the three categories. The combination of sitting and standing, known as uptime, and rest provides a quick index of activity level. A weekly total uptime normally is approximately 112 hours (7 days × 16 hours). A quick totaling of uptime for a 1- or 2-week diary sample should be made. Weekly uptime totals of less than approximately 80 hours indicate that the patient has considerable functional impairment, finding rest or time out effective reinforcers. Patients with more than approximately 80 hours of uptime per week are much less likely to find rest reinforcing.

Occasionally uptime figures are distorted because the patient spends many hours sitting. That can be checked by noting the sitting and standing or walking totals or, even more easily, simply by scanning morning and afternoon hours to see how much is entered in the sitting column. Patients who sit much of each morning or afternoon without compensatory pacing at night are also likely to find rest reinforcing and to experience time-out benefit from pain behavior.

Psychological tests

Some but not all psychological tests have the advantage that information may be obtained in minimal professional time. Moreover, some of these tests have yielded considerable empirical data bearing on issues pertinent to the behavioral analysis of chronic pain. It is too much to expect that there be a comprehensive review here of all of those data. In Chapter 2 reference was made to the MMPI and to data drawn from it in describing a variety of patient groups. That test is the most commonly used instrument in the context of pain and so deserves some attention here (Butcher, 1969; Dahlstrom and co-workers, 1972; Mischel, 1968; Welsh and Dahlstrom, 1956). It will be the only so-called personality test discussed.

The MMPI can be used with English-reading, American-educated people who are age 16 or over and above mental retardation levels of intellectual functioning. The test requires but a few moments to explain to the one who is to take it. That explanation can be done satisfactorily by an appropriately oriented clerical person, office nurse, or other health care professional. The test can be scored by a clerical person (with practice in 20 to 30 minutes), or it can be mailed to scoring services for processing for a fee. It yields scores on a series of scales. The most commonly used scales (three validity and ten clinical) are reported on a graph or test profile. The MMPI processing services to which answer sheets may be sent also usually report a narrative test commentary, which is a printout from computer-based experience data. Those printouts vary in their relevance to questions about chronic pain.

The relationship of personality and personality tests to behavioral perspectives needs a brief consideration. The distinction has been drawn repeatedly in this book between what a person *has* (his or her personality) and what he or she *does* (behavior). Most personality tests, including the MMPI, originated in the context of motivational or personality conceptual schema. The MMPI scales, for example, although constructed empirically, soon came to be described and thought about as states of the person or as personality traits. The descriptions of a person derived from the MMPI and other personality tests aim principally at characterizing what he or she *has*. It is assumed that knowing what a person *has* permits one to predict and understand what that person *does*. The long history of studies of how well, in fact, personality tests predict behavior indicates only modest effectiveness (Butcher, 1969; Dahlstrom and associates, 1972; Mischel, 1968; Welsh and Dahlstrom, 1956). Aggregates of subjects meeting predetermined selection criteria often yield statistically reliable trends in behavioral prediction. However, those trends often prove to be clinically trivial in the individual case. Knowing, for example, that 586 of 1000 subjects scored high on a given test scale and displayed more signs of depression, excitability, right parietal headaches, or whatever was the subject for study and that the other 414 subjects had lower scores on the scale and less often displayed the criterion be-

havior does not permit one to judge wisely whether a particular patient belongs in one criterion group and not the other. For example, the studies reported in Chapter 2, which compared various pain-related criterion groups on personality tests, indicated trends or tendencies of the target populations. Not all subjects had high scores on a given scale. Inferences drawn from those studies were based mainly on mean test scores of criterion groups.

An alternative way of viewing MMPI data is to consider patterns of responses as reflected in test profiles and the configuration of high and low scale scores. These may be seen as indicating high-frequency or low-frequency behaviors. That is, a person with a particular score configuration may display a higher rate of some class of behaviors than a person having a different score configuration.

The point is illustrated by an MMPI issue highly central to chronic pain. Scales 1, 2, and 3 (Hypochondriasis, Depression, and Hysteria, respectively) are usually involved in studies of pain. This was true of studies cited in Chapter 2 (Fordyce and associates, 1975; Janis, 1958; Pilling, 1967; Sternbach and co-workers, 1974). A high score on scale 1 might, to the personologist, indicate the person *has* hypochondriasis and a low score that he or she does not *have* it. Behaviorally, the person with the high scale 1 score might be expected to complain readily about bodily distress. That is what is *done*—the behavior. To this point the personologists and the behaviorist are saying essentially the same thing. Where they may part company is that the behaviorist views those high-frequency behaviors as somewhat more related to reinforcement patterns of the immediate environment. Were the environment to begin to honor different contingency relationships to patient behavior, the behavior would be expected to change. What he or she *does* changes. The personologist may still see the person as *having* hypochondriasis, since alleged underlying personality characteristics were not changed.

This is not simply an intellectualized conceptual debate having minimal pertinence to the subject at hand. The part about this issue that makes a difference in using instruments such as the MMPI relates to the extent to which the patient's pain behaviors are operant or respondent and, whichever is the case, what might be done about it. Those are the questions one asks of test data. The central questions from the MMPI, as they relate to the evaluation of chronic pain, might be posed in this fashion:

1. *How ready is the person to signal pain?*

If scale 1 is high, those around the patient are more likely to receive repeated cues that pain is being experienced. They may or may not reinforce such behavior. The behavior may or may not be a direct consequence of physical findings.

2. *How much does pain behavior cost the person?*

Indications of emotional distress (elevations on F scale and scale 2) suggest that pain has a high emotional cost for the patient *or* that pain is occurring in someone already having significant emotional distress. In the latter case, pain, instead of costing, may yield time out from sources of distress and therefore be reinforcing.

Indications that the person has been restless and energetic (elevations on scales 4 or 9 or both) or persistent and self-demanding (elevations on K plus scales 2 and 7) suggest that inactivity from pain (if that is the effect of the pain) probably has a high personal cost. Inactivity is not likely to be reinforcing to that person.

This second question relates only indirectly to whether the pain is respondent or operant. The question explores reinforcing or nonreinforcing characteristics to impairment from pain.

3. *Are there other problems for which pain behavior may yield reinforcing time out?*

Indications of marked anxiety (elevations on F, 2, and 7) or of depression (elevations on F and 2, low score on 9) may point to long-standing emotional or interpersonal problems, or the distress may be a product of the pain and related problems.

Indications of severe disorganization (for example, psychotic states, delusional thinking, or deficient reality testing) (there are a number of possible test profile configurations that may occur here, but perhaps the most common are elevations on F, 2, and 8—perhaps also 6, with a low K and with 7 lower than 8) immediately raise the possibility that inactivity or functional restrictions from pain may yield rich reinforcement in the form of time out from emotional threats. That would not refute the presence of respondent pain. It would indicate that operant pain may be present.

4. *How probable are addiction or habituation to medications?*

Indications of tending toward addiction or habituation (a configuration of scale 1 elevated and higher than 2, which is higher than 3. If scale 4 is also elevated, whatever its height relative to the others, further confidence in the inference is added) help to assess adequacy of patient information about medication intake. It also raises the possibility that it is addiction that now maintains pain behaviors and encourages the precautionary use of time contingent pain medication regimens for that patient.

Test score indications of loosening or disorganization of thought processes (preceding item, no. 3) (scale 8 elevated and higher than 7; low K) increase the chances that toxicity is present.

5. *How likely is the patient to be responsive to attention or rest?*

This question concerns both evaluation and treatment planning. Probable high sensitivity to attention and the actions of others is found particularly in any one or combination of three score configurations: elevated 3, elevated 4 and 9; low 10. A high scale 10 is a strong contraindication that attention and social responsiveness of others serve as effective reinforcers for the patient.

6. *How likely are increases in activity to be reinforcing?*

This issue essentially repeats the second part of item 2, that is, it is concerned with measures of energy, restlessness, and activity. It is restated because it bears directly on treatment planning. If other evaluation indications are that there is much operant pain, including reduced activity level, there remains the question of how much help the patient (and his or her immediate environment) will need to maintain treatment gains. In addition to the configurations pointing toward restlessness or surplus energy (high 4 and 9), toward persistence and self-demanding productivity (elevated K and elevated scales 2 and 7), one can add a test profile in which scale 3 is elevated and distinctly above all other scales. Such a person often has a history of job effectiveness and responsibility. He or she often finds activity and productiveness reinforcing.

The foregoing is not intended as a cookbook on how to use the MMPI in relation to evaluating and managing chronic pain. Test profiles need to be viewed in their totality to derive the wisest inferences. The information presented is intended instead to direct attention to the kinds of questions that need to be considered and test analysis methods for dealing with them. They are to be contrasted with approaches that seek to categorize the patient as "hypochondriacal," "conversion reaction," and the like. The data reviewed in Chapter 2 indicate that those kinds of test-based labels fail to distinguish consistently patients with significant physical findings from those without. What is needed is an analysis of the interaction between patient behavior (of which test scores provide one source of description) and environmental contingencies. The latter are, at most, only touched on by test scores.

Selective psychological testing can play other productive roles in patient assessment and management. For example, as part of treatment planning, vocational test appraisals provide helpful information from which to identify appropriate target behaviors. Perhaps the most important and commonly relevant additional contribution of selective testing relates to the question of cortical deficits. Cortical deficits enter in in two ways. One concerns addiction and toxicity; the second concerns other problems for which pain behavior yields time out.

It was noted earlier that significant numbers of older patients reporting pain problems for which physical findings are not clear and definitive are found to have cortical deficits. This also may happen with progressive neurological diseases (for instance, multiple sclerosis). Restrictions in social or vocational activities because of pain yield time out from revealing cortical deficits and the ensuing personal embarrassment.

There is an abundance of evidence (Diller, 1971; Reitan and Davison, 1974) to indicate that an appropriate battery of psychological tests can identify with practical validity the presence of interference in cortical or intellectual activity. That kind of specialized testing deserves to be a frequently used part of the evaluation process in matters of chronic pain. As with any other evaluation procedure, effectiveness of these procedures will depend in large measure on the skill and experience of the person who analyzes the data. If it is a computer memory bank that serves as the repository of the knowledge, the right questions must be asked of that memory bank.

The behavioral analysis guide presented in this chapter serves to identify whether there is a significant amount of operant pain in the picture, what the problems are, and who besides the patient may be involved in perpetuating them. The matter of what to do about these problems involves patient selection. The next task is to transfer evaluation data into patient selection criteria. It is the topic of the next chapter.

7 Patient selection

The objectives of this chapter are to apply patient evaluation data selection criteria for contingency management treatment and to review procedures for presenting the proposed treatment to patients and their families.

Once it has been established that a patient has a significant amount of operant pain, or that, in the case of predominantly respondent pain, activity level or some pain behaviors should be modified, the decision as to whether to proceed with an operant approach is not as straightforward as it might seem. There is, of course, the matter of patient consent to proceed. There may also be questions of funding and third party authorization to be resolved. But there also are critical issues to be considered about whether elements essential to operant-based progress are present. A conclusion that a patient has much operant pain does not mean that an operant-based treatment program will prove helpful.

Patient problems identified as psychiatric, psychological, mental, nonphysical, learned, conditioned, or whatever, are often perceived as somewhat alike by many professionals and lay people. The terms listed in the preceding sentence are not synonyms, nor are problems assigned to one or more of those categories alike. It is often difficult to find elements of similarity, let alone identity. The repeated demonstrations that interdiagnostician agreement often fails to exceed random chance in the placement of patients into psychiatric diagnostic categories is a case in point (Butcher, 1969). Lack of diagnostic reliability occurs in interview, observation, or personality test data, suggesting it is the phenomena that are heterogeneous. The problem is not just lack of precision measuring instruments.

The illusion of homogeneity in human behavior alluded to in this context is fostered additionally by the tendency for professionals carelessly to label their treatment interventions as if they too had somewhat more consistency and definition than they really have. Thus it is that patients are, for example, referred for psychotherapy, as if to imply that that term connotes a precisely definable set of procedures. An illusion of further specification may be offered by identifying the procedure to be used as individual or group psychotherapy. Or, perhaps the specification is in terms of some school or orientation such as neo-Freudian or Rogerian. Similarly, patients are referred for behavior modification, as if to suggest that the term specifies a course of action. As in the preceding example, an illusion of greater specificity may be added by terms such as systematic desensitization or implosion therapy. Each of the treatment strategies or tactics listed here indeed has *some* specifiable characteristics. In some instances (for example, systematic desensitization) procedures can be precisely defined. However, in each example the degree of specification refers to methods and not problems.

The tendency to lump problems and methods (for instance, to refer a patient for psychotherapy) risks working in somewhat the same fashion as would be true if automobile mechanics had one tool, perhaps a crescent wrench. In the analogy, the wrench corresponds approximately to psychotherapy, group therapy, or operant conditioning. If the auto's problem is one for which the crescent wrench is suitable, all is well. If not, little help is to be expected.

The analogy is simple-minded. Clinically, however, one observes repeatedly that chronic pain patients for whom physical findings are lacking are referred for some variant of psychotherapy or now, in more recent years, behavior modification. This is not to suggest that therapists treat all patients and all problems alike. The point is that there must be a specification of the problem and of the criteria by which a given treatment strategy can or cannot be applied with hope of effectiveness. This chapter will focus initially on relating patient evaluation data to procedural selection criteria for an operant or contingency management program. Surgery and psychotherapy are not panaceas. Neither is operant conditioning. Certain criteria relating the problems to the methods must be considered. This will be done within the format of the objectives of the behavioral analysis set forth in Chapter 6.

Patient selection for a contingency management treatment program must consider the following:

A. What pain behaviors or functional impairments are to be decreased or activities to be increased by the patient, spouse, or other?
- Reduce pain behavior
- Increase or decrease activity level (as indicated) and associated well behaviors
- Reduce direct positive reinforcement of pain behavior
- Reduce indirect positive reinforcement of pain behavior resulting from avoidance learning
- Reduce punishment or failure of reinforcement of activity or well behavior

B. What reinforcers hold promise of effectiveness in treatment, particularly in the early phases?
- Rest
- Attention
- Medication
- Signs of progress

C. What posttreatment activity is reasonably to be expected from patient and spouse? Are those behaviors in the repertoires? Are they accessible?
- Vocational
- Leisure
- Retirement (including leisure or avocational involvements)
- Reduce or stabilize pain-related health care utilization behaviors

D. Are spouse and family ready and available to participate in treatment and to support change?

An operant-based or contingency management approach potentially involves each of those questions. They pinpoint behaviors to be changed and the contingency arrangements necessary to bring about and to maintain those changes. Once the behaviors to be changed have been pinpointed (A), there must be the promise of effective reinforcement (B) to bring about change and to maintain it (C and D). The first three elements must be met before the patient is accepted for treatment. The fourth selection element (D) can be ignored only if it is established that the spouse or others are not playing vital roles in regard to any of the pertinent elements of A, B, or C.

Behaviors to be changed

Patients with mainly respondent pain may wish to increase activity for its own sake or in an effort to produce a gating effect, that is, to reduce or inhibit peripherally arising pain impulses. Respondent pain patients may also wish to decrease medication intake or to break a cycle of addiction. The respondent pain patient who actively pursues that kind of help will probably be reinforced effectively by signs of progress. That is likely to be so for two reasons. One is that consequences in the environment are not often significant features in respondent pain problems. Therefore environmental consequences or reinforcers are not likely to be working against progress. The second reason is that active pursuit of help, in the absence of indications that the pursuit itself is a method of seeking social or other reinforcers, suggests that progress and increased activity are likely to be effectively reinforcing.

Rapid and systematic feedback for performance increments, sensitive to fine units of progress, may suffice for respondent pain patients. It is unlikely that significant alterations need to be made between pain behaviors and social consequences they may meet except perhaps to encourage the family to support suitable levels of activity.

The respondent pain patient may not need help to reduce gaps in skills of the well behavior repertoire. Such gaps as may exist will have been shown by the behavioral analysis not to play significant roles in the generation or maintenance of pain behavior. All in all, the problems are conceptually simple although not necessarily easily accomplished. The major task is to lay out a program designed systematically to increase exercise and activity level or, if indicated, to reduce medication intake.

The patient with operant pain presents a more complicated picture. That patient's problem has many complicating ties with the environment. In addition, the operant pain patient often presents difficulties in finding effective reinforcement. Evaluation will have indicated what the problems are, such as direct reinforcement of pain behavior, indirect reinforcement in the form of time-out benefits, or punishment or well behavior. The selection process must then decide which of those problems is currently present and therefore must be treated. This process requires a detailed listing of the pain behaviors and associated functional impairments that will be the subject of change.

Identification of reinforcers

Data from referral sources and from interviews, diaries, and tests should indicate which reinforcers are likely to be effective. Rest, attention, medication (if habituation or addiction is an issue), and signs of progress all have potential. It must be determined that one or more of them is likely to be effective and can be made contingent. It would be the exceptional case to expect success by relying mainly on signs of progress for reinforcement when there is a significant amount of operant pain. Signs of progress, even if having some potentiality as an effective reinforcer for that patient, rarely can be programmed to be sufficiently rapid and effective in the early phases of treatment. Unlike respondent pain, the operant problems are usually too intertwined with other, competing reinforcers.

When activity level is too high, as discussed earlier, a reversal may be considered to make activity contingent on rest and relaxation, instead of the more common reverse pattern. A patient with a too-high activity level might then be selected for help in decreasing that level. Rest or some form of less vigorous activity then becomes the behavior to be increased. Periods of relatively unrestricted activity might be programmed as the reinforcer.

Identification of target behaviors

This aspect of patient selection concerns mainly the optimal acceptable and practical level of outcome deemed appropriate for the patient. Those are treatment goals. Those decisions involve little information in addition to that already developed. The decisions are more a matter of weighing the estimated or probable level of activity the patient can be expected to achieve against how such a person could reasonably be expected to spend his or her time. Financial resources for treatment are another consideration, but those cannot be dealt with here except to note that third-party carriers of treatment costs sometimes need further educating as to the long-term costs likely to result when they express reluctance to fund these broad-spectrum treatment approaches.

If it appears feasible to resume full or part-time employment, a work history and perhaps a more detailed vocational potential appraisal should be obtained. It would be superfluous to describe how to do that here.

Many patients will not be resuming employment, or, if that is the goal, evaluation may have indicated significant deficiencies in leisure-time skills or activities that led to problems and to operant pain. Additional information about past or contemplated recreational patterns may be needed. It can be developed directly by interview of patient and spouse. Items G.2 and G.4 of the behavioral analysis (pp. 135 and 136) bear directly on this matter.

Once significant gaps or skill deficits in well behavior (work or leisure) have been identified, the suitability of an operant program for the patient will depend on the resources available with which to reduce those gaps. Those efforts may be an integral part of treatment or may occur adjunctively through referral to other treatment resources. There are obvious advantages to making those efforts occur concomitantly and coordinated with other phases of treatment. Sometimes that is not practicable. Any plan for utilization of other resources for adjunctive treatment after the operant program should be spelled out at the beginning of treatment so that all parties concerned recognize and accept the deferred component of the overall program as essential.

Additional special problems may arise in this context concerning those patients for whom some variation of legitimated retirement is judged to be the most practical and feasible treatment objective. Many such patients have little skill at becoming effectively involved in leisure pursuits. This can be a problem of gaps in effective well behavior of critical magnitude. It is a problem in how to retire. From a behavioral perspective, the question usually is how to find leisure-time activities providing effective reinforcers. The most common example is the heavy laborer for whom employment is no longer a feasible objective. He probably has limited intellectual and social skills and a history of little opportunity to develop effective leisure of a more sedentary nature. So long as the nature of the problem is understood and its importance to treatment planning is taken into account, there is little merit in trying to spell out behaviorally based ways of identifying these problems. The possible variations are simply too broad. The key point to remember is that specialized assistance (psychiatric, psychological, social service, or community agencies) may need to be called on.

Family readiness to support change

The behavioral analysis by interview of patient and spouse should have made clear what behaviors the spouse and other key family members have been reinforcing or punishing by withholding reinforcement (items C.1, C.2, and G.1 to G.5 of Chapter 6). Families who have been directly or indirectly reinforcing pain behavior or punishing or failing to reinforce well behavior must change their behavior. They must agree to the changes, and the treatment team must be prepared to work with them to accomplish the task, procedures for which are considered in Chapter 12.

The misguided spouse

Spouse reactions to pain behaviors have often been based on misguided notions that reassurance, special attention, assistance, and the like would help the patient improve. Pain behaviors would then have been reinforced in anticipation of such an approach helping to resolve the pain problem. A spouse may also have been discouraging or actively punishing activity and attempts at well behavior for the same reasons. In those cases, spouse behavior was probably being maintained mainly by anticipation of the reinforcer of patient improvement or by patient expressions of appreciation for those behaviors. Not infrequently spouses behave these ways simply because of physician prescription to help limit patient activity. In each of the situations just described, there are few if any other and less obvious reinforcers maintaining spouse overprotective behaviors. It is correspondingly easier to bring about change. Treatment may proceed on the assumption that change is likely to be reinforced, once brought about.

Direct information or instruction given to the spouse to cease reinforcing pain behaviors and to cease inhibiting or deterring activity may suffice. Drawing on the interview data, the precise behavior changes needed should be spelled out, and alternative responses should be discussed. Agreement to proceed in this fashion should be reached with concurrence of the patient in a session in which both patient and spouse are present. How likely spouse behavior will be changed simply by providing information can best be judged by considering how much the spouse is reinforced, directly or indirectly, by the pain behavior or its associated functional impairments (items G.1 to G.5 of Chapter 6).

The reinforced spouse

Where the evidence indicates that the status quo has reinforcing properties for the spouse, change will be correspondingly more difficult. More systematic efforts to promote and to maintain change probably will be needed. Methods for helping with that will be considered in Chapter 12.

Even when the evidence indicates that patient improvement is likely to be reinforcing to the spouse, systematic instruction and rehearsal are often required for the spouse to change effectively. Subtle rather than obvious methods of reinforcing pain behavior or inhibiting activity (items C.1 and C.2 of Chapter 6) are particularly likely to require supervised retraining.

A judgment needs to be made at some point as to how likely the spouse will change and how likely those changes will subsequently be reinforced by the patient or in other ways. This judgment should weigh what the patient and spouse are likely to be doing in the posttreatment era, be it work, leisure, or retirement. A judgment that spouse change is likely or reasonably attainable—and has a reasonable chance of being maintained—crosses another hurdle in patient selection. It is then time for a thorough review with patient and spouse of the probable posttreatment behaviors that each should expect of the other. The steps involved in retraining of the spouse should also be reviewed. Both spouse and patient must be prepared to participate in the ways that have been spelled out. A clear commitment to that effect is a prerequisite to treatment.

Agreement to proceed is sometimes voiced by patient or spouse in an unconvincing fashion. The doubt they convey may reflect their skepticism as to whether the requisite behavior changes can be accomplished. If that is the problem, it is of little importance and may be ignored. Program success or failure do not hinge on confidence, or lack of it. The methods work or they do not. Either or both of them may be ambivalent about changing their own or their mate's behavior. Ambivalence itself need not deter treatment. It is the judgment about the probable quality of participation in treatment and subsequent support of the behavior changes brought about that counts. There may be incomplete understanding of the program or of its rationale. Uncertainties in the atmosphere of the agreement should not be ignored. Additional clarification may solidify their commitment to proceed. If not, it is often helpful to prepare a written statement of treatment objectives and of the general outlines of the program, which both patient and spouse can then examine and sign. That is not some form of legal contract and should not be considered as such. It is a way of helping patient and spouse to identify more clearly where the program plans to go, what will be expected of them, and what they can expect from the program.

However favorable are other signs pointing toward likelihood of success with an operant-based treatment approach, if the spouse does not cooperate and is not available for retraining, the program probably should be abandoned or severely limited. In those instances in which the spouse has been a major (and perhaps *the* major) reinforcer of pain behavior or inhibitor of well behavior, but for one reason or another will not be available for effective participation, treatment probably should not be offered. The exception would be to agree to tackle the limited objective of reducing addiction or habituation to pain medication, though even that circumscribed goal may be impractical because of spouse behavior.

This completes the process of evaluation, patient selection, and determination of treatment goals. The next chapters will focus on methods for implementing treatment for the treatment objectives that apply to a given patient.

SECTION THREE
Treatment

To this point the conceptual and theoretical background for the the use of operant methods in chronic pain and chronic illness have been reviewed. A technology for behavior change has been described. Targets for use of this technology have been discussed in terms of treatment goals and patient selection. Section Three will be devoted to presenting operational details for using these methods.

Before proceeding with methodology, a few general contextual comments are needed to ensure that the procedures are kept in their proper perspective.

The clinical experience from which this book is drawn indicates that the reduction of pain behavior is relatively simple to do and can readily be accomplished in properly selected patients, if the methods are used properly. It is a far more difficult process to help patient and family to replace pain and sick behaviors with effective well behaviors. But, as noted previously in this book, the range of well behavior problems encountered in relation to patients with chronic pain is far too great to permit treating that subject here in operational detail. The necessary compromise is to describe methods by which to reduce pain or sick behavior and to increase exercise and general activity level. In addition, methods for changing immediate environmental interactions that have been serving to reinforce pain behavior, directly or indirectly, and to punish or fail to reinforce well behavior are also dealt with. The behavioral analysis of the problem probably will have pointed to skill deficits in well behavior and to *other* problems the patient has for which pain yields time out. Those issues must also be dealt with. The technology by which to deal with them depends on the particular problem. Since, for the most part, these other problems involve behavior change, the methods described in this book are likely to offer at least equal potential for helping as they do with pain behavior and activity level. The additional procedural details by which to apply them are left for other source materials. Other methods and procedures may be the preferred approach. Both that decision and the methods to which the decision leads are also left for other source material.

The one constraint on methods for dealing with these other problems is that their application must not interfere with the operant program. The matter of potential conflict between treatment approaches virtually always can be reduced to two issues. The first is that other treatment activities should not provide systematic professional activity on a pain-contingent basis. A process should not begin because of a patient's display of pain behaviors, nor should it be omitted by their absence. Equally importantly, the attention or social or professional responsiveness of the therapist should not be pain contingent. It should not violate the procedures set forth in the next chapter regarding professional attention. Briefly stated, therapists concerned with other problems should maintain consistently a posture of social nonresponsiveness to visible and audible displays of pain behavior and, where appropriate to the procedures in which they are engaged, they should be suitably socially responsive to patient activity or well behavior.

Vigilance is required here. Therapists functioning adjunctively to an operant pain program are often improperly oriented and prepared. They may inadvertently work against rather than for the overall program. Chapters dealing with medication management and with exercise contain discussions of how to relate non–pain-related illness events to the operant program. In principle, dealing with those other problems raises the same procedural questions.

The second issue in regard to potential conflict between an operant program and other concomitant therapies is simple to identify. It is that overall scheduling and orchestrating must take into account both the elements of the pain program and these other but related problems as well. The two sets of problems can be tackled concurrently and usually should be. However, someone needs to keep track of the overall scheduling to be sure that the pieces fit together and do not interfere with each other.

The omission of details regarding working with other patient problems in no way implies that they are of somehow lesser importance. They must be dealt with where they play a significant role in the overall picture. It works both ways. If these other problems are ignored, reductions in pain behavior and increases in activity level are not likely to endure. Equally, dealing with the other problems will not suffice unless there is also a systematic effort to reduce pain behavior and increase activity level.

The format of Section Three is first to present a method for orienting patient and family to the treatment process. This is followed by three chapters dealing with each of the major components of the operant program: the use of attention or social responsiveness, management of pain medications, and methods for increasing exercise and activity level. There is next a chapter describing methods for dealing with the special problem of distorted gait produced by pain. These chapters are followed by a chapter on generalization or the maintenance of treatment gains, a topic that receives separate treatment because it cuts across the methods of the chapters that immediately precede it.

8 Patient and spouse orientation

Once the evaluation process has established that a patient is a candidate for an operant-based treatment approach, it is important that the patient and his or her family be presented with a clear explanation of evaluation findings and treatment proposals. It is particularly important to help the patient and family to recognize that the concept of operant pain and a learning-based treatment approach is distinctly different from any implication that the pain is unreal, "hysterical," or "all in your head." Most chronic pain patients share with health care professionals a long tradition of looking at pain in disease model terms. They probably will need special help to recognize that bodily systems can become conditioned without any implication of emotional problems. The orientation process presented below is designed to help them to make that distinction.

Orientation needs also to make clear the treatment objectives, that is, the target behaviors. There should be a description of what the patient and spouse may expect to be able to do at the end of the program. That point refers to patient capabilities or, stated another way, to the degree to which activities will be limited by pain. There should also be a clear statement of what activities (for example, employment or no employment, full or part-time work, retirement) are the goals of treatment. The treatment team cannot decide whether the patient is to return to employment or whatever other posttreatment activity may be at issue. The treatment team can decide which activities can reasonably be expected to be available or attainable. Those should be discussed and agreed on with patient and spouse before treatment proceeds.

Finally, the orientation process should make clear the methods by which treatment objectives will be pursued. This aspect of orientation sets forth what the patient and spouse can expect from treatment and from treatment personnel and what is expected from them, in turn. In this connection, patients, when learning that treatment involves operant conditioning techniques, are sometimes fearful that there will be elements of secret manipulation to the process. It should be made explicit that this will absolutely not occur.

These elements of orientation provide the basis for informed consent by the patient. They also provide an important degree of preparation by the patient and spouse for the specific treatment tasks with which they will be confronted.

Rather than write *about* an orientation approach, one will be spelled out as if it were spoken directly to the patient and spouse in a conjoint interview. The presentation will be shown here with subheadings to facilitate subsequent selectivity as to which elements to include in a given case. This orientation is presented with the assumption that a comprehensive and effective medical evaluation has preceded the behavioral analysis. It is further assumed that a significant element of operant pain has been identified.

Orienting patient and spouse as to possible course of chronic pain and to operant conditioning treatment of it

The evaluation process is now complete, and the evidence is that you have more pain than you need to have. There are ways in which, working together, we can probably reduce and perhaps eliminate how much you suffer, how much your pain interferes with your life, and how much future treatment you will need for it.

First, let's consider what may happen if you do not proceed with treatment along the lines that I will spell out. Chronic pain such as you have usually does not go away by itself. Nor is there some medical or surgical treatment—beyond those you have already received and which did not resolve the problem—that is likely to be of significant further help. Nor does pain medication solve the problem, as you already know. To the contrary, what often happens is that gradually increasing amounts of pain medications are required even to help you to hold your own. The chances are great that sooner or later habituation or addiction will occur or that your system will become toxic or poisoned from the effects of long-time use of pain medications. It is risky stuff. You rarely can get away with using it indefinitely. Moreover, it is often the case that the pain gradually spreads. It hurts more, more often, and interferes more with what you want to do. In short, chronic pain problems do not often remain stable. Usually, either treatment brings improvement or there is a gradual worsening of the problem.

It is important that you understand that no one, and certainly not I, can say there is only one way to treat your pain problem. What I am saying is that the very best evidence we have about your case indicates both that a specialized treatment approach such as I will describe looks promising as applied to your case *and* that we don't see another way to go that offers a better chance of being of help.

Pain as learned behavior

We have said that you have more pain than you need to have. That doesn't mean that your pain is unreal or imaginary. Of course it is real. It is probably true by now —as it is sooner or later for almost everyone with chronic pain—that someone along the way will have said or, at least hinted, that your problem was psychogenic, imaginary, or all in your head. That is a common misconception about pain and it is nonsense. The proper question is not whether or not the pain is real. Pain is what you feel when you hurt. Of course it is real. The proper question is, what are the factors that influence the pain?

Only in recent years have we come to recognize that pain, like a lot of other body processes, is influenced by learning or conditioning. Let's take a look at that for a moment. It is an important point, one you will want clearly to understand.

The easiest way to explain what I mean is with an example. If, as each of you sits there, I begin to talk about a ham sandwich or a piece of chocolate cream pie, or something like that, your mouths will begin to water. The longer it has been since you last ate, or the hungrier you are, the more your mouth will water. If either of you do not happen to care for the foods I named, sooner or later I could name one that you do like and which would cause your mouth to water.

Let's consider what has happened. First of all, the saliva is real. We could put it in a cup and take a picture of it or chemically analyze it. If you put your finger in it, you would feel that it is wet. It is real. Here, we have a basic body process, in this case saliva, that has been influenced by something going on around you: my talking about food.

Notice that salivation occurred whether you wanted it to or not. You could neither turn it on nor turn it off. All you could have done would be to have left the room to avoid hearing what I said. You couldn't have begun to salivate simply by deciding to do so or stop by deciding not to. I had to say something about food. This illustrates a body process that occurs automatically under certain conditions, whether you want it to or not.

Third, notice that the salivation doesn't have anything to do with your personalities. You have different personalities but you both salivated. We could bring in dozens of people and under these conditions each one would salivate. The working of the body process simply does not have anything important to do with personality.

What does control the salivation? The answer is experience or learning. Had I been talking with someone who had never heard of a ham sandwich or piece of chocolate cream pie—say, for example, an Australian bushman–no matter how many times I might have said it, he wouldn't have salivated. Why? Because he had not had certain experiences over and over again in the past, experiences in which the idea of ham sandwich was systematically associated with eating.

The example of salivating illustrates how learning or conditioning can and does influence basic body processes whether we want that to happen or not and regardless of our personalities. All that is necessary is that learning opportunities occur.

Exactly the same point can be made about a number of other body processes. In recent years, the same basic point has been demonstrated about such processes as heart rate, blood pressure, brain wave activity, peripheral blood flow, and others. Learning or conditioning influences them, and learning or conditioning can change them.

One more basic point needs to be understood. We usually think about learning as something we decide to do or not to do. We decide whether to study something or to learn how to do something. Actually, it doesn't work quite that way. We may decide whether to get into a situation in which learning *can* occur. But learning will occur only if conditions are favorable. More than that, learning will occur if conditions are favorable, regardless of whether we want it to occur. For example, we all have learned to be afraid of things we don't want to be afraid of. The fear was learned automatically, regardless of whether we wanted that to occur.

What all of this adds up to is that pain, like many other body processes, can come under control of learning. Pain problems don't start that way, just as yours didn't

start that way. But, once the problem has begun and persisted for a period of time, if learning or conditioning circumstances have been favorable, one's system will have become conditioned. What follows is that the pain comes under partial or total control of learning factors. Keep in mind that that happens automatically. It is not something you decided to do or that you could turn on or off.

The evidence we have indicates that (all, a significant part) of your pain problem is now under control of learning factors. That in turn means that learning—or unlearning—methods can be used to change that. That is what I meant when I said that you have more pain than you need to have. We can, working together, reduce that pain and perhaps eliminate it altogether.

Learning is nothing more than the change of behavior. One of the most effective ways to do that is to change the consequences that immediately follow the behavior to be changed. A behavior or action that is immediately and systematically followed by something pleasant or favorable— positive reinforcement—will tend to be increased or strengthened. If the consequence that follows the behavior is not pleasant or favorable, the behavior will weaken or disappear. That process is called operant conditioning.

Let me take a moment to apply those rules to pain problems. That way you can see how operant conditioning can work to reduce the problem.

Take the example of back pain and doing sit-ups. The person with the pain who is doing the exercise usually works until the pain begins or becomes severe, and then he or she stops to rest. In that arrangement, the action or behavior to be decreased is pain and the behavior to be increased is exercise, in this case, sit-ups. We can diagram it like this (Fig. 17). Notice also that rest—stopping the exercise—is a pleasant or favorable consequence. The person doing the exercise, by working until the pain began or became severe, had arranged things so that the favorable conse-

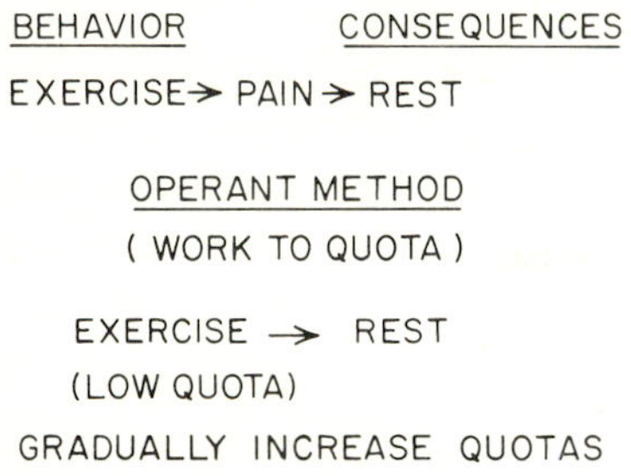

BEHAVIOR   CONSEQUENCES

EXERCISE➔ PAIN ➔ REST

OPERANT METHOD
(WORK TO QUOTA)

EXERCISE → REST
(LOW QUOTA)
GRADUALLY INCREASE QUOTAS

Fig. 17. Usual exercise method (work to tolerance) and operant method (work to quota)

quence, rest, occurred immediately after pain. That was the thing he wanted to decrease, not increase. He was reinforcing the very thing he wanted to get rid of. A simple rearrangement can change that. Instead of exercising until the pain begins, work to a certain point *before* pain begins or becomes severe, and then stop to rest. In that arrangement, rest, the positive reinforcer, now immediately follows the behavior we are trying to strengthen: activity or exercise. Rest, the reinforcer, arrives before the pain but immediately after the exercise. Doing it that way and gradually increasing the amount of exercise done before rest begins helps most patients to increase considerably how much they can do before pain or weakness become a major issue.

That is the basic format of operant conditioning. Essentially the same principles are used in the treatment of chronic pain. The main emphasis is on exercise and activity, on the use of pain medications, and on how those around the patient respond or react to pain and to activity.

The nice part of the program is that it is likely to be helpful in increasing activity or decreasing the amount of interference in your life from the pain problem, regardless of whether your pain is now predominantly learned pain or whether the original or other causes are still the major factor. To the extent that your pain is now controlled mainly by learning factors, we can probably help your system to unlearn it and thereby to get rid of the surplus pain. Even if your pain is not now primarily learned, these procedures can probably help you to

get along with the problem and have a decrease in the amount of interference from it.

Increasing activity or reducing medication addiction/habituation in problems of respondent pain

The evaluation process is now complete. The results indicate that we are not going to be able to do much about the physical problem from which your pain originates. There is a real chance, however, that we can help to reduce how much it hurts and to reduce the amount of limitation or functional impairment you have because of the pain. We may also be able to reduce the amount of medication and medical treatment you will need for it now and in the future and help keep the problem from getting worse. Pain problems such as you have tend not to remain the same. If some form of treatment doesn't solve the problem, usually the pain and the amount of interference in daily activity gradually increase. If much pain medication is being taken, that problem tends also to get worse. A person's system becomes adjusted to the medication so that it takes more and more to produce the same amount of relief. You may become addicted, and your system may become toxic or poisoned by the amount of medication you take. One way or another, even if the physical damage producing the pain can't be changed much, there are probably some things we can do to make it easier to live with the problem and to help keep you from more difficulty in the future.

It is possible for you to train your system not to feel the pain so much. That is, you may be able to train your system to shut down, partly or even substantially, the pain impulses coming from the source of your pain. Your mind is potentially capable of doing that, but it takes a systematic effort to bring it about. A program of selected exercises and activity can be set up and a strict sequence is followed. That is, the amount of activity or exercise done is set by the sequence, and not by the pain. Neither you nor anyone around you is to respond to or pay attention to the pain in any way. The amount of exercise done will start at easy levels, which will gradually increase. Eventually, they will reach amounts that previously triggered considerable pain. Once those levels are reached, you are to continue with the assigned amount of exercise no matter how it makes you feel. In some cases exercises may be held at that level for long periods before increasing further. In other cases it may be judged wiser to increase the amounts done. If you persist faithfully with the program, both a reduction in how much you hurt and an increase in how much you can do have a good chance of occurring.

Pain medications and the pain cocktail—for addicted/habituated patients, respondent or operant

The procedure we will follow to help you reduce the amount of pain medicine you take and need is simple. First let me say that in this part of the program, as in every other part, we will never ask you to do something you cannot do.

For about a week we are going to let you demonstrate how much medication you need. You will decide how often and how much you need. The only restriction is that it must be taken orally. If you are taking medication by injection, we will shift that to oral form, although we will make it strong enough to cover you well. All you must do is to record what you take, how much of it, and when. We will give the medications to the nurses (in the case of an inpatient) or to your husband/wife (in the case of an outpatient) to help keep track of how much is taken. The medication will be there for you whenever you want it. After about a week, we will change to the pain cocktail. That is a procedure in which all of your medications will be incorporated into a single dose, the pain cocktail. The cocktail will contain all of your medications in the approximate amounts you have been taking them. It will also contain a color- and taste-masking substance, perhaps cherry syrup. Once we know how often you need

and take the medications, we will put you on a fixed time schedule, every few hours, around the clock. The time between doses will be *less* than what you used to take. The result is that the pain medication will reach you *before* the pain begins or before it becomes severe. In that way we will break the hookup between hurting and taking medication. Now the medication will come without the pain.

We will gradually reduce the amount of medication in the cocktail, taking it down as far as we can, perhaps to zero. If and when we get to zero, we will tell you. We won't tell you exactly when we have reduced the dosage level because we think it will be easier for your system to decondition if it doesn't know that. You can be certain, however, that we will start you with as much or even slightly more medication than you are now taking. We know that amount will cover you. We will work from there. It usually takes about 7 to 9 weeks to get down to the level we are aiming for.

Use of attention or social reinforcement

Those are the major elements of the program. The plan will be essentially the same for medication and for exercise and rest. We shall also be concerned with how others respond or react to your pain. Make no mistake about it, that makes a difference for everyone. We work with the responses of others—we can call it a form of attention —in two ways. One is that the staff here will tend not to pay attention to pain. We won't ignore it; that could be dangerous. We will be socially nonresponsive: shrugs of the shoulders and that sort of thing.

After about 2 weeks patients in this program sometimes feel that no one around here cares about them. We are more interested in what you think of us after the total program than after 2 weeks. With some people, staff nonresponsiveness is important; with others it plays only a small part. Either way, it can help and so we work with it.

The second way we work with attention is to help your family to respond in ways that will be of the greatest help to you. That is such an important part of the program that we won't agree to work with you unless your husband/wife agrees to participate. We will want to see them perhaps as often as twice a week, for brief sessions. We will work on helping to develop the best ways of responding to pain behavior and to activity. Your husband/wife will have homework to do, just as you will have treatment work to do.

If this program proves helpful to you, it means that at the end of treatment you will be taking little if any pain medication. It also means that there may be little interference from pain in what you do or how you spend your time. We hope and expect you will be able to do much more than you now can do. All of us need to be concerned with how you plan to spend your time. You and our team together must be concerned about that, not because we wish to tell you what to do, but because working with you to plan activities can help you to maintain and even expand treatment gains. We will meet with you and your husband/wife about those matters as the program moves along.

Reduction of gaps in well behavior

Anyone who has been on the sidelines with a pain problem as long as you have is bound to find it difficult to get back into the swing of things. During the course of treatment, we will involve you increasingly in activities similar to things you will be doing after treatment. That will provide you with a chance to prepare yourself at your own pace, instead of all at once. There are probably other things you cannot do so well or problems that make it harder for you to engage in a full range of normal activities. We shall be concerned about those, too. We may work on them directly with you, or it may prove better to let you work with others on those problems. (If evaluation has indicated a clear problem

pattern—something relating to avoidance learning—that can be spelled out.)

General orientation issues

This concludes a sample of patient/spouse orientation. The specificity with which it has been presented is both to illustrate how it might be done and to emphasize the value of candor. There is a myth having some prevalence in human service settings that implies that knowing about behavior-consequence relationships, as they apply to oneself, somehow interferes with their impact. That is not the case. Knowing about the pain cocktail procedure, for example, or of the programming of attention, does not thereby reduce effectiveness of the method. Moreover, patient and spouse participation seems to profit considerably from the candor and completeness of explanation given at the outset. Such an atmosphere serves, among other functions, to help dissipate the suspiciousness and anger that usually accompany long-frustrated efforts at gaining help for a pain problem.

It is often helpful to add to the foregoing orientation a brief description of a typical treatment day and the plan to use passes as a programmed part of treatment.

There should also be a detailed consideration of the question of posttreatment employment, if that is a viable alternative in the picture. The issue of posttreatment employment cannot receive proper attention until there has been clarification with third-party sponsors or with sources of wage replacement or compensation funds as to their plans and expectations. This is often a delicate and complicated issue. It cannot be avoided, and its consideration cannot be delayed beyond the point of considering and offering treatment. If evaluation indicates a reasonable likelihood that the patient will be physically capable of resuming full or part-time employment, a decision is needed as to whether continued compensation is contingent on continued pain behavior and associated impairment. That is, of course, mainly a legal or policy decision to be made by third-party agencies. When employment is concluded to be a viable alternative, all factors considered, it should be made explicit to the patient and spouse that successful treatment will mean that the treatment facility will then certify that the patient is ready for employment and not a candidate for continued compensation. Only when that is made explicit and is convincingly agreed to by patient and spouse should treatment proceed. Alternatively, if the realities of long-time employment, restrictions in employability relating to skill deficits or to medical liability constraints, or the labor market suggest that employment is not a viable alternative—

however successful is treatment—patient, spouse, and funding source need to decide whether to proceed. If the decision is then to proceed, presumably it will be based on the intent to legitimate retirement or, at the least, to strive to reduce anticipated medical costs relating to the pain problem. In either case, it will have been agreed that compensation is not contingent on continued pain behavior and associated functional impairment. These issues have been considered earlier in relation to the genesis of operant pain. The point for now is to clarify the issue in relation to each patient before treatment begins.

9 Managing pain medications

Inpatient/outpatient decision

This chapter concerns patients with medication problems, that is, addiction, habituation, evidence of a currently high level of medication intake, or history of previous heavy medication intake. The procedures outlined may be indicated with chronic pain patients who, while taking moderate amounts of medication, are alcoholic as well. If evaluation points to toxicity from medications or the tendency to develop multiple and surreptitious sources of medication, a period of at least 1 or 2 weeks of inpatient observation is virtually mandatory. The total medication deconditioning program probably will require inpatient observation. Evidence of habituation or addiction also almost certainly requires an inpatient period. The only persuasive contraindication to a period of inpatient care when there is a medication problem is the rare instance in which there is a spouse (or some other person) available virtually full-time for surveillance, and the indications are that the observer is militant, determined, and incorruptible from patient efforts to cheat on a medication regimen.

There is no circumstance in which the pain cocktail deconditioning process can be attempted when medications are injected. The shift to oral intake is a requirement for which there are no exceptions.

The foregoing criteria can be summarized as follows:

1. There must be no injections of distress-relieving medications; analgesics, narcotics, or tranquilizers.
2. There must be an accurate count of every medication taken; what it is, the dosage level, the number of times taken per day, the interval between each dose, and the 24-hour total intake of each. This applies to medications prescribed by all sources and to those taken on a nonprescriptive basis. In short, there must be control over supply, as well as precise records of utilization patterns.

It cannot be stated categorically that those conditions cannot be met on an outpatient basis for the addicted, habituated, or toxic patient. However, the most stringent of performance demands should be placed on both patient and spouse before agreeing to an outpatient trial. Moreover, it should be agreed that evidence of failure to meet these treatment requirements will automatically result either in a shift to inpatient status or end of the program.

The primary objectives of the pain medication regimen are to reduce or eliminate addiction, habituation, and pain medication requirements. There is the additional objective of preparing the patient to follow time-contingent medication regimens in the future to prevent recurrence of medication problems.

The strategy for accomplishing those objectives is to break the pain behavior-medication consequence relationship through extinction. It is a process of deconditioning or unlearning. The behaviors leading to medication intake (visible or audible signs of distress, requests for medication, or reaching for and taking medication) are the pain behavior operants, and the medication and its chemotherapeutic effects are the consequences or reinforcers. The reinforcers are to be withdrawn as systematic consequences to the subset of pain behaviors that previously culminated in medication being taken.

One way to proceed would be simply to withhold all pain medications, to compel the patient to quit cold turkey. That sometimes works, but it does not often produce lasting behavior change. Gradual and systematic change is more desirable. There are the hazards and difficulties of acute withdrawal symptoms to consider, as well.

Procedure

Target behavior: reduce or eliminate asking for and taking pain medications.

Baseline

Patient will have been recording on diary forms during the evaluation phase what pain medications were being taken, in what amounts, and at what intervals. Those data provide a partial basis for determining whether there is addiction or habituation. When there is such a problem, data from diary forms are usually not sufficient to provide a reliable baseline for deconditioning. An additional week (approximately) of professional observation is usually necessary.

In cases where there has had to be a shift from injectables to oral medications, there should be a minimum of a week of baseline recording on the oral regimen to be more sure that a stable baseline level is identified.

Each patient should be instructed to bring his or her medications to admission. They are turned over to nursing personnel for custody. The patient and all relevant nursing personnel should then be informed that the patient is to remain on a strictly *prn* regimen for the baseline period. It is important to emphasize to all that there is no implicit or hidden barrier to taking the medications. Nursing personnel should neither discourage the patient from taking what may be requested nor suggest that it be taken if they observe signs of distress. The patient should be instructed to take what is needed when it is needed.

Nursing personnel should record what is taken, in what amounts, and precisely at what times. Those data should be in a form that readily permits calculating 24-hour in-take totals and the approximate average time intervals between doses.

The patient, having been supplied with additional diary forms, should continue to record the same medication intake information on those forms. The duplication is a backup system, but it also helps to train the patient to record performance carefully and systematically.

Medical prudence in regard to toxicity must always prevail. The free *prn* baseline method assumes that approximately one additional week of essentially unfettered medication intake will not produce significant damage beyond that already produced by prior medication intake. If there is concern about this matter, the procedure can be altered to the extent that 24-hour ceilings and the approaches to them should be communicated to the patient by the nurses as each dose is taken.

There is an area of judgment here that cannot be codified to apply precisely to each case. The importance of determining the naturally occurring baseline of the patient's medication intake, as distinguished from a baseline imposed by the treatment setting, is not to be dismissed lightly. Moreover, as often as not, the newly admitted patient on this kind of baseline regimen will begin by understating his or her requirements. Less medication will be requested than evaluation evidence suggests has been true at home. After a few days of often highly visible suffering, a reminder that the regimen *is*, as stated, one in which the patient should indeed take what is felt to be needed, not what he or she thinks ought to be taken, sometimes results in a sharp increase in intake. When that happens, it confirms that a patient's so-called normal medication pattern is not always readily discernible. A period of observation sufficient to elicit the normal medication pattern is required. The objective of the baseline is to determine what level of medication will provide adequate coverage of distress. If that level is not accurately identified, the early trials with the pain cocktail and deconditioning will not result in pain-free or pain-minimal periods between medication doses, and the opportunity for relearning will have been negated.

If there is pressing concern about lasting damage from toxicity, perhaps the first choice of compromise in the baseline determination method is to shorten the period of baseline observations from 1 week to 2 or 3 days. When that is done, there must be a particularly vigorous effort to encourage everyone involved to promote a normal pattern of unfettered intake for the observation period.

Time-contingent regimen

Baseline data from nursing records and from patient diary forms should be reviewed. The 24-hour totals and the intervals between medication requests are averaged. It is better to be conservative when much variability is observed from day to day or across the week; use the higher dosage levels and the lower time intervals as the baseline values. The guiding rule is to identify what kinds, amounts, and frequencies of medications produce an optimal level of patient comfort or freedom from distress, as shown by the patient's baseline performance. From the learning perspective, it is preferred to err on the high side, medical prudence permitting.

All analgesics, narcotics, or tranquilizers are now combined into a single mix. Due regard should be given to potentiating mixes and to any other dire pharmacological consequences that may result from this procedure. The resulting mix should represent the best reproduction of the baseline intake patterns that is attainable under the circumstances. Where there is essential repetition or redundancy among elements in the mix, that of course can be eliminated by consolidation, but without reducing 24-hour total equivalence.

The pain cocktail

The foregoing mix is delivered in a color- and taste-masking vehicle. Cherry syrup or glyceryl guaiacolate (Robitussin) are the two more commonly used. The total volume of each dose is 10 ml; that is, the active ingredients are supplemented by sufficient amounts of the vehicle to produce a total volume of 10 ml. As active ingredients are gradually reduced, the volume deficit is replaced with vehicle to maintain a constant 10 ml volume. That is Pain Cocktail No. 1.

An alternative procedure is to prepare the mix in capsule form. Each dose is taken in a single capsule. The choice between cocktail and capsule depends mainly on what the pharmacist finds easiest to prepare. Once the choice is made, it should be followed through the entire program.

Delivery schedule

The cocktail is taken at fixed time intervals, around the clock. The cocktail is not pain contingent. It is always taken when scheduled, independently of whether pain is being experienced, a need for medication is expressed, or a need for medication is denied. It is never taken between intervals, should it be requested.

Review of diary and nurse note data will reveal that typical time intervals may vary from one ingredient to another. The lower average interval should then be used from which to set the still lower cocktail interval.

Practical constraints occasionally force deviation from this pattern. Occasional patients will consistently or periodically request medication relief as often as every 1 or 2 hours at times during baseline observations. It is impractical in this kind of program to schedule medications at hourly or even 2-hour intervals for extended periods. Judgment must prevail. The occasional intervals of 2 or fewer hours observed during baseline can perhaps be ignored. A schedule of every 3 hours can be set. The patient is reassured that 24-hour totals will match or slightly exceed what he or she has been taking. Severe pressure for medication occasionally occurs under such a regimen. A modification can be considered. For 2 or 3 days a regimen of delivering the cocktail each 2 hours can be used. This can be followed by a shift to a 3-hour schedule. The 2-day period of demonstrating to the patient a determination to cover his or her medication needs adequately will usually suffice to ease the pressure. If not, an additional day or so on a 2-hour schedule can be carried out.

Adherence to the delivery schedule is important. The interval between doses should be as consistent as can be achieved. The patient's daily activity schedule should be reviewed to ensure that the patient can come for the cocktail at the scheduled times or that it can be delivered.

Fading active ingredients

The objective in fading medications is not simply to eliminate potentially toxic or addictive agents from the patient's regimen at the most rapid rate consistent with avoidance of side effects from acute withdrawal symptoms, seizures, and the like. The objective is to provide opportunity for relearning. The relearning involved is that the pain behaviors making up the signal for medication, or the act of taking it, no longer are systematically reinforced by immediate medication. By providing ample coverage it is the activities previously leading to pain and the request for medication that now are followed by the medication reinforcer before the distress begins. Medication should arrive and be taken in the relative or total absence of the pain behaviors signaling a need for it. Crash programs that replace the active ingredients with methadone and fade the ingredients at the fastest rate that also avoids significant withdrawal symptoms often fail to cope with the relearning tasks. Such crash programs provide little opportunity for the patient to rehearse activity followed by medication relief preceding pain, even when the crash program has set a short between-dose interval. Further, the haste of the program (often 7 to 10 days) means that there will have been, at most, limited opportunity to rehearse taking medication in the relative absence of pain. The fading process seems to work better when carried out in a more gradual way. The period during which high or relatively high medication intake levels are reduced to zero, or close to it, appears from clinical experience to be approximately 7 to 10 weeks. Formal empirical tests of the matter have not yet been carried out.

Fading need not occur at the same rate for each active ingredient. The central pattern is to reduce ingredients approximately once each 7 to 14 days in approximately equal decrements that will approach zero in 7 to 10 weeks. The amounts withdrawn at each decrement can be approximately proportional from one agent to another, unless there are pharmacological contraindications. A sample pain cocktail regimen is provided in Table 1.

The fading pattern may be orchestrated to respond to indications of specific forms of distress during the early fading phases. Muscle relaxants may be faded at a slightly slower rate for the particularly tense patient; tranquilizers may be faded more slowly for an anxious patient, and so on.

The major and most common exception to the foregoing fading pattern concerns antidepressant medications. It is the exceptional chronic pain patient who does not display significant amounts of depression. This was discussed in Chapter 2. Regardless of whether the patient has been taking antidepressant medications, as observed from medical file data and by evaluation and baseline observations, it is often wise to add such a component to the pain cocktail. If there are indications of depression, this step should be taken with vigor.

It is usually not important, from a learning or conditioning viewpoint, whether the antidepressant is incorporated directly into the cocktail or is given separately. Amitriptyline (Elavil) may be used, 25 mgm, *tid* (*not prn*). That agent need not be tapered.

Another antidepressant that may prove helpful is doxepin (Sinequan). This has a usual maintenance dose range of 75 to 150 mg total per day.

Either of those drugs has a significant sedative component and may be given in a single daily *hs* dosage, in which case no other *hs* sedation is given.

The antidepressants usually should be

Table 1. *Sample pain cocktail regimen**

Inpatient days		Pain cocktail format
1-6	*Baseline:*	Patient reports preadmission pattern of ". . . one or two of the 50 mg tablets of Demerol two or three times a day, as needed, at home."
		Physician orders to nurse: "May have Demerol, *prn* pain, not to exceed three 50 mg tablets every 3 hours. Carefully record amount taken."
		Analysis of baseline data: Patient averaged 600 mg of Demerol per 24-hour period, at average of 3 to 4-hour intervals between requests.
7-9 *First cocktail*		
	℞ to pharmacists:	Demerol, 1920 mg
		Bevisol, Plebex, or other liquid B complex, 12 ml; cherry syrup qs 240 ml
	Sig:	Pain cocktail, 10 ml po q3h, day and night, *not prn*
	Nursing order:	Pain cocktail, 10 ml po q3h, day and night, *not prn*
		Since contents of the pain cocktail are not on the label, a copy of the prescription must be kept in a separate pain cocktail book.
10-12		Decrease each daily total by 64 mg, $\frac{1}{10}$ or original amount. A 3-day ℞ is decreased by 64×3 or 192 mg.
	℞ to pharmacists:	Demerol, 1728 mg
		Bevisol, Plebex, or other liquid B complex, 12 ml; cherry syrup qs 240 ml
	Sig:	Pain cocktail, 10 ml po q3h, day and night, *not prn*
	Nursing order:	Pain cocktail, 10 ml po q3h, day and night, *not prn*
13-15	*℞ to pharmacists:*	Demerol, 1536 mg
		Bevisol, Plebex, or other liquid B complex, 12 ml; cherry syrup qs 240 ml
	Sig:	Pain cocktail, 10 ml po q3h, day and night, *not prn*
	Nursing order:	Pain cocktail, 10 ml po q3h, day and night, *not prn*
16-18	*℞ to pharmacists:*	Demerol, 1344 mg
		Bevisol, Plebex, or other liquid B complex, 12 ml; cherry syrup qs 240 ml
	Sig:	Pain cocktail, 10 ml po q3h, day and night, *not prn*
	Nursing order:	Pain cocktail, 10 ml po q3h, day and night, *not prn*
19-21	*℞ to pharmacists:*	Demerol, 1152 mg
		Bevisol, Plebex, or other liquid B complex, 12 ml; cherry syrup qs 240 ml
	Sig:	Pain cocktail, 10 ml po q3h, day and night, *not prn*
	Nursing order:	Pain cocktail, 10 ml po q3h, day and night, *not prn*
22-24	*℞ to pharmacists:*	Demerol 960 mg
		Bevisol, Plebex, or other liquid B complex, 12 ml; cherry syrup qs 240 ml
	Sig:	Pain cocktail, 10 ml po q3h, day and night, *not prn*
	Nursing order:	Pain cocktail, 10 ml po q3h, day and night, *not prn*
37-39	*℞ to pharmacists:*	Demerol 0 mg
		Bevisol, Plebex, or other liquid B complex, 12 ml; cherry syrup qs 240 ml
	Sig:	Pain cocktail, 10 ml po q3h, day and night, *not prn*
	Nursing order:	Pain cocktail, 10 ml po q3h, day and night, *not prn*

(Maintain patient on vehicle for 2 to 10 days; if all is going well, inform patient and ask if continuation of vehicle is desired.)

*The assistance of Barbara J. DeLateur, M.D., in preparing the pain cocktail regimen sample and the related discussion is gratefully acknowledged.

faded at a significantly slower rate and perhaps not at all. At the point in the total program in which the patient has begun to be involved in activities with which he or she is likely to continue after treatment, the antidepressants can begin to be faded or simply discontinued. In behavioral terms, antidepressants begin to fade when the patient has gained access to the reinforcers deemed likely to sustain posttreatment performance.

Long-term fading or maintenance of cocktail regimen

Cocktail ingredients may not reach zero by the time formal treatment ends or may never reach zero, and thus the patient may require an indefinite maintenance regimen. A medication fading pattern extending beyond the limits of treatment more often occurs in regard to antidepressant ingredients or where the respondent element to the pain is significant and essentially unmoved by treatment efforts.

The patient and spouse should have received full explanations of the cocktail rationale and methods. Several weeks of practice with the cocktail will have passed. In the later phases of inpatient treatment, the gradual transition to self-medicating should begin. The early trials at this are most readily accomplished by providing the patient with a weekend pass from the hospital and the precise amount of cocktail sufficient to last through the time of the pass. If the patient has traveled for treatment from a great distance, too far to permit a weekend at home, the spouse should be required to be present to spend a weekend with the patient. There are several reasons for that, as will be discussed in succeeding chapters. One reason is that the spouse provides additional support and supervision of self-medicating with the cocktail, should there be doubt about adherence to the regimen. A report by patient or spouse of difficulties in following the regimen during the weekend means that additional supervised self-medication trials will be needed in the hospital or in additional weekend passes.

Patients who are to be managed after treatment by another physician will require additional preparatory steps. The recommended fading or maintenance regimen should be communicated in detail to the referring physician or whoever will be working with the patient. If he or she is unfamiliar with details of the total program, a copy of the orientation explanation can also be sent. At the time of the patient's departure, a 3- to 6-week supply of cocktail should be provided. This transitional supply ensures that delays in gaining appointments with the home physician will not jeopardize adherence to the regimen.

End of cocktail regimen

The patient should be so informed when active ingredient levels in the cocktail finally reach zero. It is prudent to wait for 1 or 2 days to allow a demonstration of adequate functional performance without assistance from analgesics and the like. The patient can then be informed in a sensitive manner. The patient merits congratulations at having carried him or herself through the conditioning process.

Conditioning is potent. The ritual of taking medication may itself have significant conditioned properties to a patient. Each patient should therefore be offered the option of continuing with the cocktail (vehicle only) for a period of time, should that be desired. This option should be presented in a straightforward manner, as it is not an uncommon choice. A further fading regimen should be worked out if the patient expresses interest in continuing with the cocktail in that form. Since ingredients are now constant, it is time or frequency of doses that can be faded. Intervals between doses can gradually be lengthened: for example, 1 week at each 6 hours, 1 week at each 8 hours, 1 week at each 12 hours.

Medicating strategies for future pain events

Once operant conditioning techniques have been used successfully in bringing medication addiction, habituation, or high utilization under control, the methods become a tool for self-control by the patient. This is also true of other components of the program, as will be discussed in succeeding chapters. The patient now has a method by which to prevent future medication addiction or habituation.

On completion of the total program or the medication aspect of it, it is well to point out to the patient that future pain or illness events (recurrence of the referring problem or separate episodes) can profit from contingency management methods. The patient should be encouraged to strive to use time-contingent regimens. In doing so, he is, at once, serving the pragmatic master of keeping himself out of future medication trouble and exercising self-control methods to help minimize, eliminate, or avoid conditioned pain.

Future pain- or illness-related medication regimens will of course be under medical supervision. If the supervising physician is not conversant with operant conditioning strategies, the patient may need to take some initiative in sharing with that physician the pertinent information.

Common problems or exceptions in pain cocktail regimens

1. *The baseline intervals between doses are as short as 1 or 2 hours.* Neither nursing personnel or the needs of the patient for uninterrupted sleep can long tolerate an around-the-clock 2-hour schedule. After 2 or 3 days of a 2-hour schedule, move to 3 hours, maintaining constant 24-hour intake totals in that shift. If this is tolerated well for a few days, move to a 4-hour interval and hold there.

2. *The patient complains that nighttime cocktails disturb his sleep and he does not have nighttime pain.* Explain to the patient that the deconditioning process requires an initial period of 2 weeks or so of around-the-clock adherence to the regimen. Thereafter, the option to discontinue one of the nighttime doses for a trial period of 3 or 4 nights can be offered; if the patient is on a 4-hour schedule, the 2:00 AM cocktail might be omitted. If the trial results in undisturbed sleep until the dose time after

the omitted dose, this omission may be continued. Subsequently, further nighttime doses may also be omitted on a trial basis in the same fashion and to the same criteria. Alternatively, a trial period of 3 or 4 days may be attempted in which the cocktail is taken each 6 hours, instead of 4, throughout the 24-hour period (or 4 instead of 3, or 8 instead of 6). Should these trials of extending the interval or omitting one or two doses fail, the preceding schedule should be resumed for a few days. Thereafter, if the patient so desires, another trial at extending or omitting may be undertaken.

In each of these variations, the cardinal rule must continue to prevail that the cocktail is taken on a preset schedule and not according to whether need is felt for it at the time it is presented. In short, the cocktail is never pain contingent.

3. *The patient consistently complains of severe pain before the time for the cocktail during the first few days it is instituted.* Assuming that one is satisfied that the baseline data were adequate and the cocktail should be providing adequate coverage, this early complaining behavior represents a shift from time-tolerance pattern noted during baseline observation under comparable levels of medication. The problem probably relates to what often happens when extinction of a strong behavior is undertaken; namely, that the behavior initially increases or rises in intensity.

There are three options. One is to increase active ingredients in the cocktail. That option should not be followed unless there is strong indication that the baseline data were inadequate. There might have been defective recording, the patient might have felt inhibited from requesting adequate coverage baselines, or the physical demands might have increased significantly relative to those of the baseline period. A period of additional analgesic coverage may be required before reconditioning has progressed to where medication needs will have begun to wane.

The second option is to take no action, to wait out the problem. It should be explained to the patient that the increased medication demands are not unexpected. An example can help to make the point clear. When cigarettes are first withdrawn from a heavy smoker, the urge or need for cigarettes at first climbs sharply, although if the withdrawal plan is adhered to, this initial upsurge soon abates. Similarly, a heavy eater, when first beginning a diet, nearly always feels an initial but only temporary upsurge in the longing for food. Either of those examples involves the same learning principle as is the case with the addicted or habituated patient. After this explanation, the patient should be informed that, for several days, the staff will simply ignore his or her requests for early medication. If that does not solve the problem after a few days, the interval will be shortened. If a new schedule is tried, it should be followed for at least a week or so before returning to the original schedule. It can be continued indefinitely.

The third option is to shorten the interval. When the interval is shortened in a new schedule to less than that shown by the patient during the preceding period in which the problem arose and the patient again requests early medication, there is now clear evidence that the problem is the upsurge accompanying the start of extinction. The second option should be reverted to and followed steadfastly: ignore medication requests and wait out the problem.

The kinds of problems described here and the procedures to meet them should be explained to the family. That step helps them to avoid reinforcing the patient's pain behaviors.

4. *After cocktail ingredients have been diminished there is a systematic increase in pain behaviors.* The increase in pain behavior may be respondent or operant. If it is respondent, it may reflect the occurrence of some other pain, illness, or physical defect event. There will usually be other evidence pointing toward that possibility, which should then be explored and followed. Alternatively, the increase in pain behavior may indicate that exercise demands on the patient have reached the point where, given the amount of analgesic coverage presently being delivered, there is respondent pain. This often happens with patients who have presented at evaluation a picture of a respondent pain problem increased or exaggerated significantly by additional operant pain.

The increase in pain behavior may be solely operant in character. The two more common reasons why that might happen during the course of a program that had been moving along satisfactorily are that extraneous cues regarding cocktail levels have been provided or that the approach to success is becoming frightening to the patient and time out is needed.

Check to be sure the cocktail procedure has not been incorrectly altered; it is possible that total volume reduced as ingredients were reduced, there were premature discussions by nursing personnel (or someone) of the current level of ingredients, or delivery was irregular and pain contingent.

Pain behavior increasing as an indication of distress at the approach to post-treatment functional demands can be assessed only by considering the overall picture. Treatment goals may need to be re-examined. The family or treatment staff may not be doing an adequate job of reinforcing activity and of helping extinction of pain behavior by nonresponsiveness.

The possibility that the increase in pain behavior relates to other illness or pain events should first be reviewed. Examination of the patient needs to proceed in such a fashion as to let the special study appear as little pain contingent as possible. This will be described in more detail later in the chapter.

Once it is clear that there is not some new and perhaps unrelated illness event about which one must be concerned, the most direct way of checking whether the question is respondent or operant in character is to manipulate cocktail ingredients. For a period of several doses, perhaps 24 hours, ingredients can be returned to the preceding level, which yielded adequate coverage. If pain behaviors diminish, the problem was probably respondent. If a 24-hour return to the lower ingredient level again produces pain behaviors, further evidence is provided to indicate that the increased pain behaviors are largely respondent in character.

A finding that modifications in ingredient levels do not produce corresponding changes in pain behaviors suggests that the problem is operant.

A conclusion that the problem is respondent usually means that additional reductions in ingredient levels are not likely rapidly to yield either relief or progress. Depending on the patient, the pain problem, and the particular configuration of medications being taken, it may be that the maintenance level currently required has been approached. This level need not be perceived as fixed and immutable. Additional efforts to reduce it should be made, although now at a more gradual pace. Resume the next higher ingredient level, that is, the least amount of medication that yields adequate coverage. Hold at that level for an extended period (perhaps several weeks or months), while exercise and activity continue gradually to increase. If increments in exercise or activity now result in increases in pain behavior, exercises can also be held steady for a lengthy period, perhaps ad infinitum. More optimistically, however, after a period of several days or weeks at stable levels of medication and exercise, further efforts at fading can be resumed. Medications may diminish as exercise holds, medications may hold as exercises increase, or the two may change concomitantly. Whichever pattern is selected, it should be prescribed and should not be based on asking the patient whether to proceed. To ask the patient in this context is to make medication or rest or both pain contingent. Fixed, preset intervals of trials toward further progress (ingredient fading or exercise increases or both) should be scheduled, following which assessment as to whether to continue, retreat, or hold should be made.

A conclusion that the increase in pain behaviors is operant means that there is for the moment insufficient reinforcement for activity and well behavior or excessive reinforcement for pain behavior or both. The procedures described in item 3 should be followed.

5. *The patient requires sleep medication.* Patients may find it difficult to attain sleep for many reasons relating perhaps to the treatment setting and the newly instituted increases in activity, to other problems or worries they may have relating to or separate from the pain problem, or simply because they lack skill at relaxing and moving toward sleep. There is little merit to ignoring the problem in the hope that a few restless nights will suffice and the problem will solve itself. That approach is risky because of the importance of optimizing patient success and relative comfort during early phases of treatment.

Unless there are other medical or pharmacological contraindications, sleep medication may be prescribed and provided in sufficient quantities. This proves in practice to be a simple problem, from a learning perspective. One need not be alarmed at providing additional and potentially addictive medications to the patient because the fading or deconditioning procedures are adequate subsequently to eliminate or control the problem.

Again, assuming that there are not other medical or pharmacological contraindications, aside from the question of addiction or habituation, the procedure is to develop *Cocktail No. 2,* which is Cocktail No. 1 plus the prescribed sleep medications. Cocktail No. 2 is administered at the scheduled cocktail time closest to bedtime. If the sleep problem is sufficiently severe, Cocktail No. 2 can also be programmed for delivery at the next cocktail time, as well. That decision should also be predetermined and should prevail for a preset number of trials (for example, a week) before being abolished.

The sleep medications in Cocktail No. 2 can be faded in the same fashion as with other active ingredients. It again becomes a matter of clinical judgment whether to fade the sleep medications more or less rapidly than other ingredients, or at about the same pace.

Particularly difficult insomnia problems may also profit from adjunctive relaxation training.

6. *Another illness event occurs for which additional medication is needed.* If the newly required medication is clearly not analgesic or tranquilizing in function, there is not likely to be any problem. Proceed without regard to the operant program, taking care to explain to the patient that the additional medication is unrelated to the pain problem.

Should it be necessary for the new medication to be taken for an extended interval, perhaps 2 weeks or longer, it would be prudent to put it on a fixed time schedule. That schedule need not coincide with the cocktail, although it may do so. If it does, the new ingredients need not be incorporated into the cocktail. The point is to avoid another extended opportunity for learning to occur between distress or signs of illness, on the one hand, and the environmental response of illness-contingent attention and medication, on the other.

7. *Additional, nonoral chemotherapy is contemplated.* Three examples are the use of ethyl chloride spray for muscle spasm, lidocaine (Xylocaine) injections to trigger areas of pain or muscle spasm, and nerve blocks, of whatever form.

Any of those procedures may have been used on a trial or diagnostic basis during evaluation. In addition, however, the decision may have been made to give them a therapeutic trial or even definitely to include them in the treatment procedures.

It is beyond the scope of this book to consider when and whether such procedures should be used. If the problem is predominantly respondent pain and those approaches are considered or indicated, they probably should be attempted before embarking on an operant-based approach. In such cases, presumably, the role of the op-

erant program then becomes one of increasing activity level, either for its own sake or in an effort to produce a gating effect to muffle pain.

Given those qualifications, if, for whatever reason, one or more of these procedures or others of similar character accompany the operant program, certain safeguards are indicated to avoid interfering with the learning process. The safeguards are required because systematic and repeated use of those procedures risks providing opportunity for adverse learning or conditioning. The situation is analogous to oral or injected medication. The procedures may provide both specialized attention and potential therapeutic relief on a pain-contingent basis. If that happens, operant pain may emerge, or, if it is already present, it may expand or persist.

The remedy lies in avoiding a pain-contingent arrangement. The criterion by which to judge therapeutic effect should be found in observation of what the patient does, not what he or she says. Instead of asking the patient verbally to report therapeutic effects, the procedure is carried out, and a predetermined, preset period of observation follows, during which patient performance is observed.

Repeated applications of the procedure should be on a fixed time basis, such as twice a day at set times or once a week. Termination of the series should be anticipated at the outset and specified. For example, a series of ten daily ethyl chloride spray trials with concomitant measures of exercise performance is specified to the patient. After these treatments, a clinical judgment is then made as to whether to carry out an additional sequence of trials.

The habituating or addicting potentialities of such procedures should not be ignored. When a routine has been established (for example, injecting a trigger area once each week), consideration should be given to fading the procedure systematically in the same fashion as with the pain cocktail. This can be accomplished by presetting a fading schedule in which the interval between injections will gradually increase on a time-contingent basis, for instance, by raising the interval from 7 to 10 to 15 to 20 days.

If, after a sequence of trials, patient distress continues unabated *and* it appears worthwhile to provide additional trials with the procedure, the resumption itself should not be pain contingent. By waiting a few days before resuming, the time pattern relationship between "how I feel" and "whether I get the procedure" is avoided.

10 Exercise and the increase in activity level

Exercise occupies a special and important place in contingency management treatment of pain, operant or respondent. The concern in this chapter will be with patients having the need to increase exercise and activity, that is, to reduce functional limitations and activity constraints. The alternative case of decreasing excessive activity, a special and atypical problem, will receive brief and separate consideration in a later section of this chapter.

Viewed in learning or conditioning terms, exercise is more than the improvement of physiological tone, body strength, or functional capacity, although each of those is involved. Exercise is, with few exceptions, also a behavior that is incompatible with pain behavior. To increase it is nearly always to diminish correspondingly one or more forms of competing pain behaviors. A period of exercise building also provides essential preparation for entry into long-term activities that will serve to sustain well behavior. If working, gardening, or dancing, to name a random few, are to play important parts in sustaining posttreatment performance, the functionally limited patient will require systematic exercise preparation before those long-term activities are again within reach.

Exercise has another characteristic important to contingency management treatment. The performance of exercise elicits from others responses or reactions much different from those elicted by displays of pain behavior. Stated simply, it is difficult to perceive a person as limited or impaired from pain if he or she is observed to be exercising vigorously and at some length. Moreover, in those situations in which family members have been systematically discouraging exercise, the performance of ex-

ercise provides opportunity for rehearsal by spouse and other family members of the newly reinstituted reinforcement of activity.

For these various reasons, exercise plays a key role in contingency management treatment of chronic pain for patients having reduced and limited activity levels. It is not essential that all exercises prescribed be limited by the referring pain problem, although as many as possible should have that kind of pain relevance. So long as pain, weakness, or fatigue provide some limitation in performance of the exercise, or that the exercise is needed as preparation for an activity or exercise procedure to be practiced later, the exercise can be considered for use in treatment.

In summary, exercise is both a well behavior in its own right and a building block to other well behaviors. As such, it is to be increased by contingent positive reinforcement and by withdrawal of negative or aversive consequences to its performance.

Selection of exercises

There are medical or neurophysiological constraints to exercises, both in performance and in selection. Those constraints take precedence and must prevail. They will not be discussed here as they are not one of my competencies.

There are also medical or neurophysiological considerations for choosing one exercise over another that pertain to functional limitations of each patient and how those may limit functional levels of a treatment program. That kind of information is also beyond the scope of this book. Other sources must be pursued for that information.

This chapter will be limited to considering the use and programming of exercise in relation to learning problems. It is assumed that considerations of medical constraints, prudence, and pertinence of exercise selection to the particular limitations of and objectives for a given patient will serve as precedent-taking guidelines within which the following recommendations will be applied.

So far as learning factors are concerned, an exercise must be pain relevant or limitation relevant, quantifiable, visible, and accessible.

With the possible exception of walking, each exercise should be such that pain, weakness, or fatigue impose at the outset of treatment at least some limitations as to the amount that can be performed without pause. That is what is meant by *pain relevant* or *limitation relevant*. Walking is a potential exception only in the relative sense that patients able to walk as much as 1 or 2 miles without pause may still profit from including walking as a component of the exercise regimen to be prescribed.

The exercise must be reducible to movement cycles that can be counted. The quantification must be in amounts of exercise performed, not in time. To report that a patient has, for example, walked 10 minutes provides no information about how much walking occurred. The amount performed must be recorded in movement cycle terms. The exception to this is, again, in regard to walking or riding a bicycle. Since an individual's strides vary only slightly, it is entirely reasonable to record walking in terms of amount of distance traversed and not in terms of the number of left-right step cycles, so long as the patient is walking (or, in the case of the bicycle, riding) a minimum number of feet without interruption. The special case where walking is being shaped into the repertoire, as will be described in Chapter 11, requires that the number of steps be recorded in the early phases of that process. Later, recording can be as distance walked.

The quantification of exercise can also combine a series of movements into a sin-

gle movement cycle. For example, it is often useful to prescribe in occupational therapy the exercise of weaving at a loom (with weights attached) or using a hand-operated printing press. Sequences of movements can be combined into the units of production for those tasks. In weaving, it can be number of rows completed. In printing, it can be number of pages or pieces printed. The critical distinction must be to avoid relying on time as the measure if at all possible. The unit must be reducible to movement terms.

The criterion of visibility of an exercise is rarely a major issue. Virtually all exercises are visible. The point is that, given a choice, the more visible exercise offers the additional advantage of easier monitoring and of easier social reinforcement by staff and by family.

The issue of accessibility is somewhat more important. Exercises begun in the treatment setting are likely to be continued outside that setting, on weekend passes, at home if the program is an outpatient, or at home in long-term and gradually diminishing extended treatment. The exercises must be accessible to be accomplished. For example, there should not be reliance on extensive level-ground walking as a central part of an exercise program if such an activity is not readily accessible at home because of hilly terrain or restrictions imposed by severe weather conditions. Riding a fixed bicycle may provide an adequate substitute. Walking may be used as part of the early inpatient phase, but the bicycle should be included as well, anticipating that such a device will be acquired for subsequent use at home.

A case example will illustrate a typical range of exercises and activities prescribed as part of treatment. It should be remembered that each patient is different. There is no fixed set of exercises. Those shown are meant only to be representative of those prescribed for some patients with chronic back pain.

The patient was a 41-year-old housewife with chronic low back and leg pain of some 2 years' duration. She had received no surgery. Various treatment programs (exercise, heat massage, ultrasound, and traction) had failed to provide more than temporary relief. The evaluation indicated significant operant pain superimposed on moderate respondent pain. The physical therapy program consisted of:

		Movement cycles
1.	Riding fixed bicycle	0.10 mile
2.	Walking	200-foot laps
3.	Climbing and descending stairs	Flights of 11 steps each
4.	Deep knee bends	Repetitions
5.	Pelvic tilts	Repetitions
6.	Hip extension	Repetitions
7.	Hip abductions	Repetitions
8.	Letbacks	Repetitions

Occupational therapy included:

1.	Turkish knot tying while standing	Rows
2.	Weaving (at loom with weights attached)	Rows
3.	Homemaking (cooking, sewing)	Time

The homemaking element of the occupational therapy program was added in the later stages of treatment. The use of a time measure in the example of homemaking activities is an acceptable compromise with reality demands only when other activities are recorded in performance units, the patient's general activity level has already progressed considerably, and the patient shows steady increases in productivity. If progress is not observed in the homemaking activities, a return to counting units of behavior is needed. For example, the number of salads made or meat courses cooked may suffice.

Procedure for exercise and increasing activity

Exercises are selected and prescribed. They should then be demonstrated to ensure that the patient is thoroughly familiar with their proper performance.

Inpatient baseline. The inpatient is informed that twice-daily exercise sessions will begin in which, for approximately a week, the patient is to work to tolerance at each prescribed exercise. The term *toler-*

ance must be explained clearly. In this instance, the term means that the patient is to begin and continue to perform a given exercise until pain, weakness, or fatigue causes him or her to wish to stop. The patient should make allowances for the other exercises to be performed during each session in assessing fatigue level. Once the exercise is begun, it should be performed continuously until the decision to stop is made. In the case of walking, for example, the patient is to begin walking back and forth on a measured course, without pausing to rest, until deciding that the tolerance limit, as defined above, has been reached. When that limit has been reached, the patient is to stop, immediately record the amount performed in the data kit provided, and rest. After a few moments of rest, the next exercise is to begin and to be carried out in the same manner, stopping only when the tolerance limit has been reached.

During each baseline trial, a staff person (usually the physical therapist) should observe and record patient performance. The surveillance is essential to ensure proper performance of the exercise, continuous performance before stopping, and to ensure accurate recording of amounts performed.

It should be explained to the patient that several baseline trials are necessary because there may be variability in how much can be done, and it is important to determine adequately what the tolerance limits are at the outset of treatment. This reminder helps the patient to feel free to select the stopping point for each exercise during each baseline trial.

It is often useful to remind the patient that baseline trials are for the purpose of determining where to start treatment quotas. Baseline trials are *not* for the purpose of determining how much pain the patient can tolerate or how brave or determined he or she is. The information needed from baseline trials is the approximate amount that can be completed of each exercise before pain, weakness, or fatigue become a major factor *at that point in time*.

Outpatient baseline. The major difference of outpatient from inpatient procedures is that the spouse or some other person becomes the observer and secondary recorder during baseline trials. It is essential that the observer be checked out. The ability to recognize adequate or incorrect performance of each prescribed exercise should be confirmed. Precise times for baseline trials that can surely be followed each day should be agreed on and specified before beginning.

A clinic visit should be scheduled approximately a week after the start of developing baselines. If there is significant doubt as to whether patient or observer will fulfill their assignments faithfully, the clinic visit should be scheduled sooner. The observer must accompany the patient to that meeting. Patient, observer, and clinician review the performance data together. Opportunity for maximum candor in reporting what has transpired should be provided. As part of the clinic visit, the exercise sequence should be repeated in the working-to-tolerance mode. The amounts performed under this professional observation provide additional validation of the adequacy of performance and of recording of baseline trials. Obviously lesser performance while being observed (when the patient had previously been alerted that such observations would be made) strongly suggests questionable patient performance and observer reliability. When that kind of suspicion is aroused, one or more additional weeks of baseline trials should be scheduled, following the same format.

Whether inpatient or outpatient, the observer must be cautioned not to provide encouragement to the patient either to persist or to stop. The judgment and responsibility for determining tolerance limits rests strictly with the patient. Observer comments are social consequences having some influence on patient performance. Those consequences will become a part of treatment later on, but only after essential preparation has been completed.

Initial treatment quotas. The basic objective of the first treatment quota is to provide success in the early treatment (as distinguished from baseline) trials. Quotas that lead to pain, weakness, or fatigue in the beginning trials are too high. Some patients report significant amounts of pain without exercise. When that is the case, starting quotas should be limited to avoid significant increase in pain. Stated in other terms, the objective of initial quotas is to set up a situation in which the patient is sure to win.

The amount performed of each exercise at each baseline trial is noted from therapist records. Patient records serve as a backup system for that information and as rehearsal for recording performance, an activity with which he or she will necessarily become heavily involved as treatment progresses.

Clinical experience indicates considerable variability in baseline value patterns. Many patients, previously reported as having major limitations in activity level, start at modest levels and progress rapidly and in almost linear fashion across baseline trials. Other patients, after an initial burst of activity, display reduced baseline values, which then vary considerably. More often than not, the patient who begins from a low activity level will show a generally upward trend. To do otherwise is not, however, an unfavorable sign.

If the trend of performance during baseline trials has been upward, the average value of those trials is often a prudent starting point. The average will be a value that has been met and exceeded consistently during the latter stages of baseline observations. A patient displaying a highly variable, perhaps almost random set of baseline values presents a different problem. The initial quota for such a patient should be a value exceeded on nearly all trials. It should be a value exceeded on each trial during the last 50% of baseline observations. When in doubt, one should be conservative and set a low quota. The objective is to set a quota that one is confident the patient can and will meet without fail. If there is doubt, lower the beginning quota. There is little merit, however, in setting a quota far below what one is sure the patient can achieve. To do so is to prolong treatment needlessly.

The quota process should have been explained to patient and spouse before treatment began, during orientation. Nonetheless, it is probably wise to reiterate that initial quotas will deliberately be set at levels lower than achieved during many baseline trials. That is not a step backward. It is a specific part of the treatment or relearning process. The intent is to set quotas that the patient can surely reach.

Quotas are never to be exceeded. This also must be made clear to the patient. However easy it may be, the patient is not to work beyond the assigned quota. To do so is to risk working to tolerance. That is to be avoided.

Increment rates. A judgment must be made as to how rapidly the patient is able to increase amounts of exercise performed without being forced to stop because of pain, weakness, or fatigue. There is no set formula for doing this. The guiding principle is to move at a pace that promises a high probability of success for many exercise trials, if not forever. In the inpatient setting, observation by therapists usually suffices to set a realistic increment rate. The rate of increment should also take into account the initial quota or starting point, relative to levels consistently attained during baseline trials. If the first quota is conservatively low, relative to average or typical baseline trials, a slightly more aggressive rate of increment can be considered. If the initial quota is set higher than the baseline average, there is more risk of failure, and a slower increment rate is probably indicated. It should also be remembered that quotas are raised on a programmed basis and never according to how the patient feels. It is easier to begin with a modest rate of increase and subsequently to raise the increment rate after patient performance during the first few days of treatment indicates easy and certain progress

than it is to be forced by persisting increases of pain behavior to lower the increment rate.

Inpatient treatment nearly always provides more social reinforcement for performance and progress than does outpatient treatment. It follows that rates of progress are likely to be greater and ability to meet higher increment rates more sure in the inpatient setting. Outpatient treatment may provide more latitude for extending treatment over a longer time period, thereby making it easier to advance quotas at more conservative rates.

The factors just discussed provide the basis for setting quotas. Increment rates may vary from one repetition per session or per day to one per week, or even more gradual than that. Fixed bicycle or walking increments are in distance terms, such as tenths of a mile on the bicycle or single 50-foot or 100-foot laps or more in walking.

Increment rates for exercises that involve the moving of or pulling against fixed amounts of weight can vary in the amounts of those weights as well as in the number of repetitions. The usual pattern is to take the patient through a cycle of increasing repetitions at a given weight to a predetermined point. Weight is then added, and the number of repetitions is lowered and again systematically increased. A helpful formula to guide how far to lower the number of repetitions is to calculate the product of the number of repetitions times the number of pounds. The new number of repetitions should, when multiplied by the new number of pounds, yield a value slightly below the corresponding product of the preceding repetitions times pounds. For example, for a given exercise a patient may have worked up to ten repetitions at 8 pounds each, yielding a product of 80. The weight is raised to 10 pounds. The new repetition quota could become five, yielding a new product of only 50, well within the load the patient had been achieving. The preceding increment rate is reinstituted, and the patient works up again to ten repetitions before additional weight is added

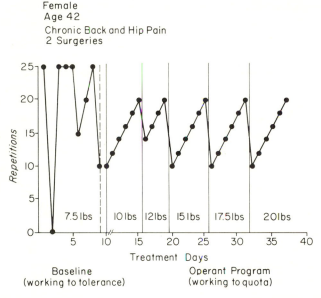

Fig. 18. *Increasing weight and repetitions for quadricep exercise.*

and the cycle is repeated. Fig. 18 illustrates by a case example how quotas of weights and repetitions may be advanced. The first weight was higher than was used in baseline trials, but the quota of repetitions was lower. As weight was increased, the quotas of repetitions were temporarily decreased.

Some patients request more rapid increases in quotas. That is more common in later stages of treatment after much progress has been achieved. An increase in increment rate can be negotiated, if done carefully. The additional increment should not represent a greatly accelerated advance. It should be set for a trial period, such as for 4 days of two sessions a day. During that trial period, the same principles apply as before; rest is contingent on meeting the quota, not on how one feels. If the newly increased increment is successfully met, it can continue. If it is not, it should immediately be abandoned and the preceding increment rate resumed. Moreover, the quota should be lowered to what it would have been under the original increment rate.

Reinforcement for exercise and activity. The quota system provides that rest becomes contingent on and immediately follows the behavior to be strengthened or increased: exercise. That means that exercise sessions need to be planned to provide for intervals of rest immediately completing an exercise quota. In the practical case, after the baseline trials and, at most, a handful of treatment or working-to-quota trials, these rest periods usually can be brief. They rarely need to be timed precisely, as if meeting a quota is to yield *x* minutes of rest. Once the patient has experienced that the therapist will indeed provide opportunity to rest and to prepare for the next exercise, more is rarely necessary. The prospect of a more extended rest after completion of the total set of exercises encourages patients to keep interim rest sessions short so as not to prolong the delay for the more extended rest period.

However, rest must occur initially on a nearly continuous schedule; a brief rest follows when each quota is met, even should the patient indicate a desire to proceed immediately to the next exercise. That kind of eagerness can be dealt with by keeping the interim rest brief. To ensure continuous and immediate reinforcement with rest, it is essential that the therapist be present during early treatment trials. The therapist's presence also ensures immediate delivery of the second reinforcer, attention, also on an initially nearly continuous schedule. Therapists must therefore avoid double scheduling during early phases of treatment. Therapists must be available and militantly ready to deliver the essential reinforcement. Most patients who show consistent treatment progress soon come to the point where they will rest automatically after completing a quota and recording its performance. Once treatment momentum is achieved, as with all thoughtful reinforcement regimens, therapist attention can become intermittent and on a diminishing schedule. A patient can be left increasingly to work somewhat on his or her own, with only periodic checks and attentive responses from the therapist during the course of each session. Even then, however, it is important to ensure that the end of the session is duly noted by the therapist and that consistent attention and encouragement are then delivered.

In the early phases of treatment, exercise sessions themselves need to be spaced through the day to provide sufficient between-session rest periods. In the inpatient setting, occupational and physical therapy sessions need to be separated in time to provide ample rest. Later on, as quotas expand and the work load on the patient increases, less and less rest is likely to be required, relative to the amount of activity or exercise accomplished. Treatment sessions become longer and closer together. The treatment day moves in the direction of a full day's work.

There is no essential difference in the exercise format when treatment is on an outpatient basis. The major difference is that a spouse, other family member, or some other designated treatment observer fills the role of the physical or occupational therapist. The procedures remain the same. Observer presence, undivided attention, and militant surveillance and reinforcement are essential during early trials. It is perhaps more risky to anticipate that the amount of observer involvement and judi-

cious observation can be reduced in outpatient treatment. There are usually fewer collateral cues and reinforcers encouraging full performance at home than in the hospital setting. Accordingly, treatment should be planned in anticipation of the observer needing to be present virtually throughout the treatment program. That constraint may be eased in later phases, if circumstances indicate that the patient is judicious in performing, recording, and spacing of exercise to permit appropriate rest intervals and is deriving sufficient sustaining reinforcement from rest and indications of progress not to require the additional support of observer attention.

Outpatient performance receives additional surveillance and reinforcement from the periodic clinic visits with their exercise sessions under professional observation. The frequency of clinic visits may also be systematically faded according to the situation. A patient whose reliability is subject to doubt or one who has questionable observers as noted previously, may require clinic visits one to three times per week at the outset. Those visits bolster patient and observer performance and provide earlier detection of noncompliance with the regimen. The frequency of clinic vists may be faded as confidence indicates. Interim phone calls from office personnel may provide additional bolstering.

Management of quota failures. The contingent reinforcers for exercise or activity are rest and attention. That means they are delivered when performance occurs *and* that they are not delivered when there is nonperformance.

Most patients sooner or later will fail one or more quotas, although the rate of quota failure tends to be surprisingly low, perhaps as little as 10% or less. Failure to meet a quota may occur for any number of reasons. It may be that the quotas for the exercise have reached and exceeded a practical maximum for that patient or that insufficient rest is being provided between exercises. It may be that on that particular day the patient is simply tired or, for whatever reason, less ready than usual to strive to meet quotas. It may be that the patient is testing whether attention or rest continues to be work contingent or have reverted to the typical pretreatment pain contingent pattern. The possibilities are endless.

The procedure to follow will usually permit one soon to distinguish quota failures representing respondent pain and the patient's having reached a temporary or more permanent practical maximum for the exercise in question, from random failure or failure indicative of ineffective or inappropriate reinforcement. As will be spelled out immediately following, repeated trials in subsequent sessions will provide opportunity to discard random or daily variability as a factor and to check on the adequacy of the scheduling and delivery of reinforcement.

The procedure is straightforward. First, the therapist militantly avoids encouraging or exhorting the patient to try further. Attention is contingent on performance, not nonperformance. With a shrug of the shoulders or some other noncommittal response, the therapist records the amount done and sees to it that the patient does the same. If additional exercises are yet to be accomplished in the session, he or she may say something on the order of, "I'll check back with you in a moment and we'll start the next exercise," and leaves briefly, if only to get a drink of water. She then returns and cues the patient to begin the next exercise, again without comment or encouragement about the importance of meeting the quota for that exercise. Alternatively, she may simply stand by quietly until the patient is ready to proceed with the next exercise. If the next quota is met, it is duly recorded, the rest interval is provided and she makes some attentive or praising comment, although without referring to the previously failed quota. If the second quota is also failed, she repeats the process just described.

If a quota is failed for the final scheduled exercise, the therapist, as before, gives a shrug of the shoulders noncomittally, re-

cords the amount done, and says, "I'll see you (at the time of the next scheduled session)." The patient is then instructed to return to his room (or wherever he or she is next scheduled to be), and nothing more is said about the matter.

Sometimes a patient will indicate before beginning a session or an exercise that he or she cannot meet the quota or, perhaps, that it is doubtful the quota can be met. The therapist response is to avoid special encouragement. He or she might say, "Well, that is up to you, but why don't you go ahead and see what you can do?" If the patient begins to perform, the therapist might make a special effort to remain close by and to maintain casual conversation so long as performance continues, thereby momentarily enriching the amount of professional attention contingent on patient effort. If the patient stops before the quota is reached, that therapist attention is withdrawn in the manner described above. When this kind of additional therapist attention results in increased performance, the evidence is clear that social attention is both potent and essential at this stage of treatment. It should continue to be available until patient progress gains additional momentum.

From the preceding examples, let it be assumed that one or more quotas were not met. Performance may have been partial or not even attempted. At the time of the next session, mindful of the preceding quota failure(s), the therapist is geared to be available. When the patient appears, the session progresses as if there had been no quota failure. There is no exhortation or special encouragement. The quota is as it would have been had there been no failure. The quota is not reduced nor held the same; it continues to advance at the previously determined rate. This is illustrated in Fig. 12 and on p. 71. The procedure remains as before. If quotas are met, they receive the same consequences as before. If they are not met, the procedures just set forth are again followed.

It is important, in the sessions during or immediately after quota failure episodes, that each exercise in the set be presented. In the extreme case, for example, a patient may appear and announce that he or she is unable to perform any repetitions of any of the prescribed exercises. If at all possible the therapist is to endeavor to get the patient at least to set up to try each exercise. There is a fine line here. The therapist should, at this moment, see the objective as one of letting the patient demonstrate nonperformance of each exercise in turn. He or she is neither trying to encourage and promote performance nor to punish nonperformance by compelling the patient arbitrarily to go through a ritual of refusal for each element of the exercise set. Instead, the therapist is providing opportunity for rest and for his or her attention to be applied contingently to each exercise. By requesting the patient to set up at least to approach each exercise, the therapist is also helping to delay rest and time out from exercise so that those reinforcers do not become available so soon after failure to perform. He or she can properly comment to the patient that she understands that there are times when one simply does not feel up to an exercise task. On the other hand, one's feelings are sometimes deceptive, and it may be that the patient may find more can be accomplished than is anticipated. At any rate, it is important to determine that, ". . . and so what I want you to do is to give it a try and let's see what happens. It is up to you as to when you stop, but at least get in position to start each exercise." Partial performance or even simply positioning to begin an exercise is not lavishly praised or socially reinforced. In matter-of-fact style, the therapist stands by while the patient prepares to begin each exercise. Any performance short of meeting the full quota is, as above, responded to in matter-of-fact fashion. The amount accomplished is recorded, and the next exercise is presented. Success at meeting a quota receives special praise: "That's great! Rest a moment and then let's see what you can do with this one."

If there is success at meeting a quota after one or more failures, the quota increment pattern continues without alteration. Performance graphs (Chapter 12) for the exercise will show a gap or temporary drop, but the subsequent resumption of the upward climb (Fig. 12) shows an example of this. The program proceeds as previously scheduled. Fig. 19 illustrates by case example how quotas continue to increase when isolated failures occur. This was also shown in Fig. 12.

Let it now be supposed that the quota for one or more exercises is failed on several successive trials. The number is arbitrary, but three successive failures seems a reasonable reference point. After three successive failures, the quota is deliberately dropped back to a point previously consistently surpassed by the patient. If, for example, baseline data led to an initial quota of eight repetitions of an exercise, to be raised one each 2 days, and the patient had progressed to fifteen repetitions before quota failure began, the newly adjusted quota could well be twelve, with an increment of one each 3 days. It is not always necessary to reduce the increment rate. If clinical judgment raises doubts as to sure patient success, that is a further option by which to provide additional successful exercise trials before the level at which quota failures began is again approached.

When there have been quota failures on more than one exercise, the same procedure is followed with each. The amount by which quotas are lowered and, if done at all, increment rates are reduced, can be orchestrated according to clinical judgment. It need not be the same or even proportional for each exercise with which the difficulties are occurring. The guiding principle is that the patient is being returned to a level at which, by his or her own recent performance, it has been demonstrated that success is assured. From that level the patient resumes working toward higher activity levels.

All of this should be explained to the patient in matter-of-fact terms. Repeated trials of successful exercise sessions, with rest and social response occurring contingent on that success, *do* permit learning or conditioning. A recycling to lower quota levels is simply a convenient way further to facilitate that. The essential elements to the process remain the same: rest and social response are programmed systematically. Working to tolerance is avoided.

When recycling of quotas to lower levels has occurred, eventually the performance barrier previously encountered will again be reached. No special preparation for that point need be made beyond that already carried out. Patients usually move past the barrier uneventfully. If they do not and repeated quota failures occur at or close to the original failure point, a second recycling should be carried out in the same manner as just described. Unless there is some correctable artifact in the situation, the correction of which promises further treatment progress, consistent quota failure at a given performance level strongly suggest that the patient has reached his or her ceiling for that exercise. If it is decided that the exercise should be continued for an indefinite period, for whatever reason, the quota should be lowered slightly to a level of sure success and kept at that level. Alternatively, the exercise may be discontinued.

The more likely correctable artifacts to check for include therapist nonperformance, family failure to reinforce properly, and some other temporary illness event. It may be a physiological limitation that additional rehearsal can be expected to overcome. In the latter case, the quota may be held constant at a level slightly lower than the failure point for a preset period such as a week. The patient having been informed of this at the start of the hold period, the quota can then resume climbing, although the increment rate may be reduced.

The process of adjusting quotas to deal with quota failures is illustrated by the case example material reported in Fig. 19. The patient is the same person described in Chapter 5 in relation to the reduction of moaning behavior. It was necessary to adjust bicycle riding quota plans twice, as shown in Fig. 19. The first quota began at a high level and had too rapid a rate of increase, 0.2 mile/day. After two successful days, the patient began to fail. Performance fell well below baseline levels. Quotas were then reset to begin below the level achieved when she was failing. The new increment rate was also reduced to 0.1 mile/day. This second quota plan was effective for 12 days. It brought her above her base-

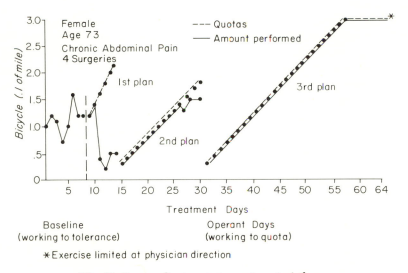

Fig. 19. *Quota adjustments to meet quota failures.*

line average without a quota failure before she again began to fail to reach quotas. This time, as Fig. 19 shows, failures were just below quota levels. When the patient had failed three consecutive trials, quotas were again reset. The therapist was conservative, probably more so than was necessary. She lowered quotas to the beginning point of the second quota plan (0.3 mile) and resumed the 0.1 mile/day increment rate from that point. A starting point of 1.0 might have worked as well, although, when in doubt, it is better to err on the conservative side. At any rate this second recycling of quotas was successful. The patient climbed to a level of 3.0 mile/day, a value more than double her baseline tolerance for the exercise, even while previously high medications were gradually being reduced to near-zero levels. When the 3.0 level was achieved, no additional increments were desired. The exercise was held at that level until completion of the program.

Pervasive and persistent failure to meet a spectrum of quotas may indicate that either a temporary or a more permanent performance plateau has been reached. The plateau may reflect the temporary influence of another illness event. Procedures for responding to that will be discussed. The temporary plateau may reflect an adverse balance between reinforcement for progress and activity versus reinforcement for pain behavior and continued functional impairment. A review of the progress of family retraining and of practicality of treatment goals should then be made. There is always the possibility, as well, that some change in the patient-therapist interaction accounts for the pause in treatment progress. For example, there may have been a reassignment of therapists or a reduction in therapist attention through double scheduling.

Extensive and persisting quota failures, particularly when judged as clinically to be premature, may, however, indicate that the treatment program is unable to arrange sufficiently effective reinforcement in a contingent manner. Reinforcers available for programming within the treatment setting may be insufficient. Sources of reinforcement previously sustaining operant pain behavior may not be sufficiently accessible for adequate change. The prospects to the patient for adequate posttreatment reinforcement may be too dim. Any mix of these may exist and render contingency management treatment inadequate to the task. When that happens, it usually means that there were some miscalculations or estimates in evaluation. Whatever the reason, it is prudent and appropriate to discuss the situation candidly with patient and spouse and to indicate that there is no point in proceeding further unless some change occurs. Treatment should then terminate unless they jointly and voluntarily express interest in an additional trial at treatment. Such a trial can be attempted, but criteria of progress should be specified. Unless certain mileposts are reached at agreed-on times, treatment should be discontinued. These criteria or mileposts must be stated in performance terms, not in subjective judgments by the patient or by professionals as to how the patient feels or how well he or she is progressing. Quotas are met without interruptions or they are not. The criteria or mileposts should represent an extension of the previous treatment plan, although with perhaps a mild lessening of increment rates.

Pervasive quota failures may indicate that the patient has reached an energy expenditure ceiling. That, in turn, may reflect a realistic physiological limit for that person. Occasionally, however, it suggests that antidepressant medications in the cocktail have been reduced too rapidly, resulting in a hopefully temporary limitation in the energy pool, which can be offset by reinstituting a higher level of the appropriate cocktail ingredient.

To summarize the issue of quota failures and what to do in response to them, there needs to be a weighing of several factors: physiological constraints, the adequacy of pacing and reinforcement within the exercise sessions themselves, and the degree to which the increased exercise and activity level achieved is in fact bringing the patient closer to effective posttreatment reinforcement. Some trial and error is often necessary to make these determinations. Trial-and-error explorations should continue to provide for periods of exercise-contingent rest and attention to permit testing the question of whether the problem is better characterized as operant or respondent.

Quota ceilings and movement toward other forms of activity. Ultimately, of course, all exercises will have a ceiling. In all cases, physiological constraints and medical prudence will impose upper limits. Those limits take precedence. So far as possible they should be estimated and defined at the outset of treatment. When they are approached as treatment progresses, ceilings should automatically be imposed. The exercise for which the ceiling has been set may then be discontinued or continued at a constant level.

Within those physiological and medical limits, there are several other factors to consider. A major objective of treatment is to bring each patient to a level of activity that permits entry into the activities or well behaviors expected in the posttreatment period. The exercise program has been a preparation for that and not an end in itself. As target levels of exercise and activity are approached, the program should begin to shift the content of activity. The shift is toward approximations of what the patient is expected to be doing after treatment. This is part of the process of generalization. Details as to its implementation will be reserved for Chapter 13, where other dimensions to the problem can also be brought into the picture. The issue for the moment is to anticipate that exercises will reach ceilings and, in most cases, will also be shifted into different forms to facilitate the maintenance of treatment gains.

Patients expected to have limited posttreatment social or vocational involvement (for example, those in the legitimated retirement group) often profit from an indefinite continuation of exercises. In those cases, prescribed exercise becomes a partial substitute for employment as a sustaining and contingently reinforced activity. In such cases, it becomes a matter of judgment as to whether to keep each exercise at a plateau, to provide for continuing increases in quotas, or even gradually to diminish them. Where exercises should continue to increase, increment rates probably should be extremely slow, such as one additional repetition beginning the first of each month. That sort of arrangement, when monitored by periodic clinic visits and/or by periodic return of diary and performance records for treatment staff review, provides continuing social reinforcement for persistent effort and for the signs of progress inherent in gradually increasing quotas.

Care must be exercised in prescribing posttreatment exercise to take into account the other demands being placed on the patient in the posttreatment environment. The combination of daily activity and prescribed exercise should be held to appropriate totals.

Quota adjustments for other illness events. Illness events will first be considered that are clearly separate from the pain problem, although they may involve pain as well, for example, influenza, a toothache, an ankle sprain, or whatever.

These kinds of problems present for the patient, as well as treatment staff, a task in discrimination learning, such as discriminating the ache of influenza from back pain or the pain of a toothache from joint pain. The discrimination is virtually always easy for both patient and staff. Complications to an operant conditioning program from these other illness events, aside from whatever temporary constraints are imposed on patient activity and participation in elements of the treatment process, usually arise from the medical and social responses they may precipitate. Those responses unfortunately risk being on a pain-contingent or illness-contingent basis. Medications and attention may again become enriched, illness-contingent consequences. Alternatively, the medical response can be matter-of-fact in style, without sacrificing thoroughness. Special procedures, examination or therapeutic, should first be explained carefully as relating specifically to the different or potentially different problem. They should then be carried out so far as possible within a time-contingent mode. (For example, "I am going to do this kind of examination, and if the findings are such and such, we will do this. If the findings are such and so we will do that." The decision derived from the examination is not pain contingent.)

Treatment, particularly analgesics or narcotics, should be on a preset and predisclosed time-contingent basis. (For example, "For this toothache, we will administer such and such medication. You will receive it each 4 hours for *x* days after extraction of the tooth.") Other examination or treatment procedures obviously widely separate from the pain problem can be carried out routinely with little likelihood that they will influence significantly the course of the operant program.

Curtailed activity resulting from other illness events may require the operant program to hold at a given level or even to retreat to an earlier level. If the interruption is brief, activity can probably pick up where it left off. When in doubt, after resolution of the interrupting problem, go back to a lower level. The guiding principle continues to be never to ask a patient to do something he or she cannot do. Stated another way, demands on the patient must *surely* be within reach.

Illness or pain events that may relate to or cannot be readily discriminated from the referring pain problem may be more difficult to handle. The patient referred with back pain, who announces one morning that the back pain is too severe to permit arising to go for treatment, is a case in point. There is always the question of whether the reported pain is the product of some new or altered state in the original pain problem, results from the onset of a new problem at a contiguous site, or is an expression of operant pain. Medical prudence and judgment are again the overriding factors. Further examinations may be carried out in the manner just described. That is, care is exercised to avoid letting especially solicitous attention serve as special encouragement for the patient to proceed with treatment, or to avoid it. Examinations are done matter-of-factly. The findings are then reported matter-of-factly. "The evidence indicates that there is (or may be) an additional problem for which (the following steps) will be carried out." Alternatively, "The evidence indicates that there is not an additional problem about which we must be concerned. There is no need to postpone or alter treatment. We will proceed as scheduled." In this connection, it is often useful, if supported by the available evidence, to remind the patient that it is often difficult to differentiate between pain as a feeling or distress from pain as an indicator that something adverse will happen if activity continues. The problem at hand is one that clearly will not result in further body damage if the prescribed exercise regimen is followed.

Programming pain-related treatment procedures. The issues and methods with pain-related treatment procedures are essentially the same as those described in dealing with noncocktail medications and the like in the preceding chapter. Like ethyl chloride spray or nerve blocks, heat, massage, transcutaneous stimulation, autogenic training, biofeedback-based muscle relaxant training, or other procedures may be used. Most of those procedures are simpler, less costly, and less time consuming than a fully programmed contingency management approach. If they offer promise of resolving the problem, they should probably receive a trial before embarking on an operant conditioning program. If they solve the problem, so much the better. If they do not, they can be abandoned. If they provide significant help but not as much as is hoped for, they may be woven into an operant program and continued, if programmed properly.

The underlying principle remains the same: specialized attention and procedures should not become systematically pain contingent. The procedures listed above, and others like them, used separately or concomitantly, should first receive baseline trials to estimate whether they have any helpful effect. If the evidence is promising, they can then move to a time-contingent schedule. The frequency and duration of the procedure is, from a learning viewpoint, of lesser importance. It can be dictated by the nature of the procedure and its observed or anticipated effects. What is important is that use of the procedure occurs on a preset schedule and not according to whether the patient feels a need for it.

The scheduling format may also be designed to strive for reduced utilization, that is, to work toward fading. The pain cocktail format can serve as a model. Initial sessions with the procedure can occur slightly more frequently than patient distress dictates. Between-session intervals can then gradually be increased on a predetermined schedule. For example, transcutaneous stimulation might have an aggregate daily use quota of x hours, which is to be reduced by 30-minute increments on a weekly basis.

Reducing excessive activity levels (the pacer regimen)

Some patients find relief from pain by movement or activity but in fact overdo, thereby aggravating the problem. Some of these patients with respondent pain problems experience pain and distress beginning only several hours after exercise. The delay of the aversive effects to exercise makes it more difficult to learn precisely how much one can do and still avoid severe pain. But ultimately, virtually every patient does learn that. Among those who experience pain on a delayed basis are some people who are particularly restless and active, perhaps a bit hyperactive. The combination of the lessened inhibitory power of

delayed pain on activity and the strongly reinforcing characteristics of exercise and movement may lead to bursts of activity, which significantly worsen the pain problem. One possible objective of treatment with such patients is to develop more effective restraint or self-control in regard to a harmful exercise or to bursts of excessive activity.

There is a second type of pain problem that has features in common with the preceding example. Tense, restless, hyperactive people may develop muscle tension pain or spasm or both. Emotional tension or the manner in which activity is carried out may directly produce pain or conditions leading to it. Such people often have insufficient ability to achieve meaningful levels of muscle relaxation. If they could relax more effectively, they might ease or rid themselves of the pain problem.

Patients with either of these kinds of pain problems may profit from reduced activity level or its approximate reciprocal, increased effective relaxation. The kinds of problems referred to here were discussed in Chapter 3. The patients were characterized as pacers, that is, people who relieve pain by movement, not rest. They are to be differentiated from recliners, who rest to ease pain. The former group have high uptime values in their diary data and tend not to find rest reinforcing. Activity, even though it may lead eventually to pain, is potently reinforcing. If it were not reinforcing, they would not do it so much. In contrast, recliners have low uptime values in their diary data (less than 80 hours/week), find rest reinforcing, and tend to realize less reinforcement from activity and exercise.

These kinds of problems were also touched on in the context of treatment goals (p. 107). It was pointed out there that relaxation training often has a role to play in treatment of pain. It was also noted at that point that biofeedback methods provide a direct approach to helping patients to achieve more effective and selective muscle relaxation. Generalized relaxation training, with or without use of hypnosis, may also prove helpful. Regardless of whether any one or more of those approaches is helpful for a given patient, sometimes a problem of consistent or episodic excessive activity remains, or the reinforcers by which to keep the patient at the task of mastering deeper relaxation prove insufficient. What remains, in behavioral terms, is the desirability of selectively reducing and controlling activity and of increasing rest and relaxation. A regimen for working toward those treatment objectives will be outlined. It is a regimen that has received only limited clinical use. Little is known about how long the few successful trials with it have persisted. It is offered here with the suggestion that it be used only if the alternatives noted above have failed. It is more costly and time consuming for patient and professional, as well as having a limited clinical experience base.

Procedure for reducing excessive activity

Target behavior. Clinical experience suggests that the target behavior is more often a reduction of overall or general activity level than curtailment of a specific exercise or form of movement. However, either may occur, separately or together. Evaluation makes that determination. These two possibilities will be discussed in parallel here.

Baseline. For baseline information, two or more weeks of diary data identify the overall activity level and the average daily and weekly amounts spent reclining and sitting.

Diary data will serve also as the source of information about how much time is spent in the one or more activities specifically maintaining or aggravating the pain problem. It may be necessary to instruct the patient to record that activity in more detail than other elements of diary recording.

Contingency management program. Stated in the broadest possible terms, the contingency management program for increasing activity and decreasing rest, as outlined in the preceding section of this chapter, arranged things such that rest was earned by activity. Rest, observed to be a high-strength behavior from pretreatment diary data, became, in line with the Premack principle, the reinforcer by which to increase the lower-strength behavior, activity. That process is now to be reversed. Activity, demonstrated by diary data to be a high-strength behavior for the patient, is to be programmed to become contingent on increased amounts of the currently low-strength target behavior, rest and relaxation.

Quotas should be set, based on baseline observations. The quotas are for uninterrupted periods of reclining or sitting (as may be indicated) before unrestricted activity, or access to the particular activity which is contributing to the problem, is permitted. Quota time amounts initially are within the range of quiet sitting or reclining demonstrated in baseline diary data. Quotas may then be raised at a preset rate.

It will be noted that rest or relaxation is almost impossible to measure in movement cycle terms, since, in this instance, it involves doing approximately nothing. It usually suffices in this case to rely on time measures.

Rest and relaxation periods may be enhanced or intensified in their effect by training the patient in relaxation skills and providing that the patient accrue x number of minutes of relaxation at a subjectively estimated level of depth, after which the reinforcer of activity becomes available. For example, a 10-point subjective scale may be developed with the patient. The high point, 10, represents maximum tension, and 1 becomes relaxation so low that it is achieved only by deep sleep. Intermediate points are then defined by the patient. The number 3 may, for example, be designated as a restful and relaxed level at which no muscle tension is felt. Given such a scale, baseline trials of relaxation periods are carried out. At fixed intervals (for example, each 60 seconds) the patient reports the level reached: 8, 6, 3, or whatever. That drill trains the patient to identify levels of relaxation. Subsequently, quotas are set such that, for example, a relaxation period is not to end until there have been a minimum of 10 minutes at level 6 or below. The next quota might be instituted a week later and require 10 minutes of level 5 or below, and so on.

The mechanics of quota setting and increment rates have already been described and should require no further elaboration here.

As intervals of relaxation increase, the undesired activity becomes less and less available. It sometimes happens that a patient may then engage in a furious burst of the undesired activity, using the lessened time available for it but producing as much or more of the disadvantageous effects. That immoderation becomes, however, a self-liquidating problem if the regimen is followed. The immoderation will interfere with reaching the required levels of relaxation during rest. Further extension of relaxation periods will then be required. The patient is forced by his or her own immoderation to pay a higher and higher price in terms of increasing rest and inactivity quotas. If, instead, the patient exercises with prudence during the unrestrained intervals, the success plateau is reached, and it is not necessary to increase further the time spent in rest and inactivity.

11 Distorted gait—a problem of shaping

One form of operant pain behavior that can be particularly troublesome to patients and that often requires a special treatment approach is limping, falling, or knee buckling. These problems may result from a structural or mechanical defect or reflexive (respondent) response to a peripherally arising stimulus. Limping, falling, knee buckling, and other gait distortions are capable, however, of functioning as operants. Once begun, they may persist by virtue of the consequences to which they lead. In short, they may, in a given case, be operant pain behaviors. This chapter will outline procedures that may be followed once medical evaluation and the behavioral analysis indicate that the problem appears indeed to be one of operant pain behavior. Distorted gait under respondent control is unlikely to yield to these methods.

A brief restatement of the critical underlying learning principles should prove helpful at this point. The problem will first be conceptualized in learning terms, the relevant learning principles will be restated, and then procedures for applying them will be presented.

Like other forms of pain behavior, those under consideration here can take many forms, but they have elements in common sufficient to permit consolidation into a single grouping: distorted gait. It will be assumed that the patients now being considered are those for whom normal gait is potentially within the patients' repertoire. The barriers to normal gait are substantially that the distorted gait is amply reinforced, and nondistorted gait is not receiving ample reinforcement. It may also be that the distorted gait has persisted so long that a substantial skill deficit for normal gait has developed. The patient may no longer know how to walk properly. For a variety of tactical reasons, the approach will proceed as if a skill deficit exists, regardless of whether in fact it does so.

Distorted gait, like other pain behaviors, may receive direct reinforcement or may lead to time out and therefore reflect avoidance learning. The time out may be from activities only incidentally related to the original pain problem, such as time out from work, housekeeping, or socializing. The time out may be more specific to the pain problem. For example, a limp may have begun in response to a respondent pain problem. The limp eased or reduced the pain. It was therefore reinforced by the helpful effect it produced. Subsequently, the problem from which the limp originated may have been resolved or reduced to insignificant levels, but the limp persisted. A limp may persist in part because the patient has ceased testing whether the pain will in fact return or increase were he or she to walk some distance without limping. The limp in that case exists in anticipation of pain, not in response to it. In learning terms, cues previously signaling the approach of pain have taken on the properties of the pain itself in that they now elicit the same limp or distorted gait previously elicited by the pain. The limp continues to be reinforced by the failure of the pain to occur. The limp is successful avoidance behavior.

As noted in Chapter 3, this form of avoidance behavior is less likely to persist unless it receives additional reinforcement. A limp or distorted gait that requires extra expenditure of energy for a given amount of walking may take on aversive qualities. It is a form of hard work. For that reason a limp is somewhat less likely to persist beyond the duration of the pain problem it was designed to ease. If, however, the limp, as a form of public display of pain, leads to reinforcing consequences in the environment, it may well persist beyond the duration of the originating pain problem, even if the limp requires arduous effort to walk.

In line with the foregoing, one part of the task is to withdraw reinforcement to limping behavior. Medical evaluation will have indicated, in the cases under consideration here, that the originating pain problem no longer accounts for the limp. The patient can no longer receive periodic reminders of the aversive consequences of normal gait because the organic problem has been resolved. If the problem now is strictly that the cues previously anticipating pain and leading to the limp yield the reinforcement that pain no longer follows, the reconditioning problem will not be difficult. That form of reinforcement is easily overcome. Social reinforcement and other forms of time-out reinforcement also must be withdrawn if they have been playing a role, and that may prove more difficult.

The second part of the task is to ensure that reinforcers such as rest or attention that are programmed within the treatment process to decrease pain behavior and increase activity are utilized with precision. They must be delivered contingent on activity (for example, walking), but only on the forms of activity that are not also pain behaviors. Limping is activity that is also pain behavior. The problem, then, is to arrange for rest and attention to become contingent on normal walking without also becoming contingent on distorted walking.

The strategy that seems to fit this learning problem is to provide for a gradual reinstitution of normal walking into the patient's repertoire. Normal walking is presently occurring at a zero or near-zero rate. Behaviors occurring at zero or near-zero rates can best be restored to one's repertoire by shaping. Shaping, it will be re-

called, is defined as the reinforcement of successive approximations to the target behavior.

The basic strategies and one of several possible procedural outlines were first reported by Trieschmann and associates (1970). Although there are some differences in rationale between their work and what is presented here, the methods themselves are virtually identical. The following procedural sequence draws heavily on their work.

The essential elements of the process are as follows:

1. The distorted gait is not allowed additional rehearsal and reinforcement. Until the patient regains an adequate level of normal gait, all ambulation is by wheelchair.
2. Gait is broken down into its constituent parts, starting with the most basic component: weight bearing on the lower extremities.
3. Starting with the first component, each is rehearsed to mastery, with rest and attention serving as the primary reinforcers. As one step is mastered, the next is added to it and the two rehearsed together, and so on, until full ambulation occurs without significant limp or distortion.
4. Generalization of the newly restored normal gait is then systematically added to the scheme by providing a broadening of amount, time, and place in which walking is permitted to occur.
5. Concomitantly with these steps, as needed, other sources of reinforcement for the distorted gait are withdrawn or reprogrammed, for example, by spouse retraining.

Ambulation training

The following list sets forth one possible analysis of the components to ambulation. This list is adapted from a case plan prepared by Stolov and Patout. To advance to a new step, the patient must perform the preceding step for 2 minutes and be passed by his or her therapist or physician. During each session the patient begins with step 1 and progresses to the current level of attainment, spending 10 seconds at each step in the sequence.

1. Stand in parallel bars for 2 minutes with good posture while holding onto the bars and with weight equally distributed between lower extremities
2. Same as step 1, but holding bars only lightly
3. Same as step 2, but with hands at sides
4. Weight shifting in place from leg to leg, knees straight, feet flat on floor, hands lightly on bars
5. Same as step 4, but with hands at sides
6. Weight shifting in place, knees straight, heels only off floor, hands at sides
7. Weight shifting in place, knees straight, heels and toes off floor, hands on bars
8. Same as step 7, but hands at sides
9. From balanced standing posture, unlock and lock knee of each leg separately with feet always flat and hands lightly on bars
10. Same as step 9, but with hands at sides
11. From balanced standing posture, hands on bars, feet always flat, unlock and lock knees reciprocally (when one knee locks, the other unlocks), weight shifting to locked knee
12. Same as step 11, but with hands at sides
13. Same as step 12, but as knee unlocks, opposite arms swings forward
14. Same as step 13, but heel comes off floor as knee unlocks
15. From balanced standing posture, hands lightly on bars, unlock and lock knee reciprocally with heels and toes coming off floor to produce marching in place
16. Same as step 15, but arms swing at sides
17. Same as step 16, but with slow advance as each leg comes down

Procedure for ambulation training

Each segment of the program is explained to the patient and spouse. The explanation clarifies that it is a gait retraining process, that it is best accomplished by temporarily preventing any rehearsal of the distorted gait, and that the objective is the restoration of full and free ambulation, without significant limp or distortion.

The patient is brought to treatment in a wheelchair, which is then positioned such that when arising to a standing position, he or she will be between parallel bars without having taken steps. The therapist may assist the patient to a standing position. Assuming that the patient can bear weight without falling or slumping, brief intervals (10 seconds or even less if indicated) of quiet standing are rehearsed, interspersed with brief resting periods while seated in the wheelchair. Standing intervals can be set as quotas gradually to be increased in essentially the same fashion as has previously been described in reference to exercise or walking. The starting quota should be slightly less than the patient has demonstrated in a brief baseline observation.

When quiet standing has progressed to uninterrupted success of two minutes' duration, a sequence such as shown in the preceding list can begin.

Just as in other exercises, rest (end of the session) and therapist attention are contingent on performance. Close records are kept. The therapist must be in constant attendance. Her praise and social responsiveness should be used judiciously. It follows performance. It does not precede it in an effort to bolster performance.

In the event that the patient's initial performance capability is even less than simple weight bearing, the process can begin at an even more basic point. For example, on being asked to stand and bear weight between the parallel bars, the patient may immediately collapse and slump to the floor, or be unable to pull him or herself to the standing position. This next lower or more elemental level is first to shape weight bearing. That may be done by use of the tilt table. The patient, strapped to the table and in the horizontal position is gradually elevated toward the upright. Quotas are set, for example, 10 seconds at 70 degrees or, perhaps, 30 seconds at 90 degrees. Quotas are gradually increased; the rate of increment is a matter of judgment, so long as it is predetermined and not pain or distress contingent. Ultimately, the patient should reach the upright (90-degree) position and be able to hold that position without slumping. If there is doubt about ability to stand because of muscle wasting through disuse, preliminary physical therapy exercises can be used to overcome that limitation. Those exercises should not involve walking or standing. When the upright position is mastered on the tilt table, the waist strap can gradually be eased to fade that source of additional support. The patient is now ready for standing weight bearing between the parallel bars.

Ambulation increase and wheelchair fading

Once independent ambulation, essentially free of distortion, has been attained for modest distances (for instance, length of the parallel bars, as in step 17), the amounts of free ambulation can be increased systematically, again using a quota system. When the amount mastered exceeds the amount required to walk from the hospital bed to the treatment area, it is time to begin fading use of the wheelchair. Heretofore, all ambulation outside of the gait-shaping sessions will have been by wheelchair. Now travel to and from treatment occurs without the wheelchair, although that device continues to be used the balance of the day and evening. The following list (Stolov and Simons, 1973) describes a sequence used with another patient, one who had reached a level comparable to that shown at the end of the sequence reported in the previous list.

1. Ambulate full length of parallel bars and return at normal walking speed, three sessions in 1 day
2. Same as step 1 + ambulate 50 feet and return, three times, 1 day
3. Same as step 1 + one 200-foot lap, three times, 1 day, + one 200-foot lap on ward in evening
4. Same as step 3, plus no wheelchair until 8:00 AM
5. Two laps, four times daily, no wheelchair until 10:00 AM
6. Three laps, four times daily, no wheelchair until noon
7. Four laps, four times daily, no wheelchair until 2:00 PM
8. Four laps, four times daily, no wheelchair until 5:00 PM
9. Four laps, four times daily, no wheelchair until 8:00 PM
10. Five laps, four times daily, no wheelchair all day

Return of the distorted gait should lead to resuming use of the wheelchair and a return to the highest level of the gait retraining process that continues to be performed without distortion. The training sequence can then be repeated from that level onward.

Generalization

The gradual expansion of free ambulation periods ensures a certain amount of generalization of the newly retrained gait. Additional and more structured generalization rehearsal should be arranged by moving treatment walking sessions to different locations and by structuring evening and weekend passes to include scheduled walking periods in varied settings. This aspect of treatment will receive additional detail in Chapter 13.

Falling and the incompatible response

There is an additional strategy to be considered in regard to distorted gait, particularly in regard to those patients who are reported or observed occasionally to fall—as if, for example, a knee has buckled. This strategy may also prove useful with patients presenting so-called conversion hysteria paraplegia, that is, patients reportedly unable to walk but for whom there is no demonstrable neurophysiological defect to account for the paraparetic state.

Walking is visible and therefore highly capable of elicting social responsiveness from those around the patient. The quality of the walk can have eloquent impact on observers. A cautious, guarded walk, one that may suggest to observers weakness or vulnerability to collapse, while nominally not distorted by a limp, may nonetheless have effects similar to other visible or audible forms of pain behavior. Observers may be led to punish or otherwise inhibit activity or to provide special attention and protective regard to the patient.

On the other hand, a vigorous and rapid stride is virtually incompatible with weakness, pain, or vulnerability to collapse. For that reason, a vigorous and rapid quality of walking should often be added as a treatment target where falling or knee buckling have been occurring.

Procedure for shaping rapid walking

Walking is brought to a level of approximately 2000 feet of uninterrupted performance, for example, ten laps of 200 feet each. At that point, instead of continuing to expand the amount walked, for a period of time the effort is shifted to working on speed—a variant of vigor.

Baseline. Heretofore in walking trials, it has been distance traversed without interruption for rest that has been measured and recorded. Now, for two walking sessions of ten 200-foot laps, the therapist unobtrusively notes and records the amount of time required to complete the ten laps. If the two time figures are roughly comparable, they may be averaged to give the baseline. If there is marked difference, it is more prudent to start with the greater figure.

Quotas. It is explained to the patient that a period of speed development will assist treatment progress, although distance or stamina will continue to play an important role. To help to achieve gradually greater amounts of speed, optional quotas will be set. For the next trial, for example, it might be stated that the patient has the option of walking twelve laps at his or her own pace or the previous ten laps at 30 seconds less time than the baseline time value. The patient is provided with a stopwatch to carry so that it is possible to keep track of whether the pace is being increased. The patient will also have been informed of the baseline time values and so knows that the time quota is within reach.

If the patient meets the time quota, the next session is given a time quota that is 30 seconds lower, with the option of meeting it or walking fourteen laps at his or her own pace. As the time press becomes greater, the cost of the alternative of proceeding at one's own pace also becomes greater.

The amounts by which time quotas are to be reduced become a matter of judgment, based on knowledge of the patient and the speed of the baseline trials. A practical upper speed limit will soon be reached. That will be marked by repeated time quota failures. At that point, time quotas can retreat to the preceding successfully met level and be held for several sessions before discontinuing speed training and reverting to expanding distance walked.

Intermittent failures at time quotas that do not appear to reflect a practical ceiling on speed are dealt with by holding the time ceiling constant but continuing to increase the optional distance quota. It is to be expected that, sooner or later, the greater distance demands will exceed in personal cost the energy expenditure necessary to meet a not-too-remote time goal. That kind of arrangement seems to help patients to push ahead further toward a faster rate of walking.

Once a rapid stride is achieved and maintained, this should be demonstrated to the family. This can be done by videotaping a walking session and playing it for patient and family together. It can be done

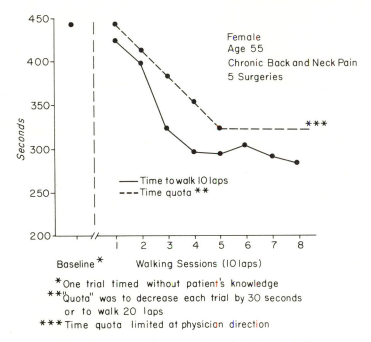

Seconds

450 —
400 —
350 —
300 —
250 —
200 —

Female
Age 55
Chronic Back and Neck Pain
5 Surgeries

***

—— Time to walk IO laps
--- Time quota **

Baseline* Walking Sessions (IO laps)
1 2 3 4 5 6 7 8

*One trial timed without patient's knowledge
**"Quota" was to decrease each trial by 30 seconds
  or to walk 20 laps
***Time quota limited at physician direction

Fig. 20. *Increasing walking speed to inhibit knee buckling.*

by scheduling walking sessions at times when the family can be present to observe. It can be done by arranging for repetition of the speed versus distance option during a weekend pass, in which the patient rehearses treatment at home.

Special effort to provide for extra social reinforcement for speed is desirable. Performance graphs that make prominent the increments in speed are particularly useful.

Fig. 20 portrays results with one patient, using this type of speed training program. The patient was referred to in Chapter 3 and Fig. 12 to illustrate increase in activity when social reinforcement was withdrawn from pain behavior. The patient, as was shown in Fig. 12, increased uninterrupted walking distance from a baseline of 400 feet to more than 4000 feet. Her pace remained moderately slow and she would occasionally waver, as if her knee were about to collapse. Twice, as shown in Fig. 12, walking sessions were interrupted by falling and inability to continue, resulting in quota failures. When an acceptable distance pattern had been achieved (quota of 20 laps of 200 feet each), the knee-buckling problem was attacked by working to de-

velop an incompatible response, that is, rapid walking. Fig. 20 reports the results. A single baseline speed or timed trial provided the starting point. It would have been prudent to time two or more trials, but that was not done. It was explained to the patient that the conditioning process would now seek to eliminate the knee-buckling problem. She was told that that might be accomplished either by extra speed or extra strength and stamina. Accordingly for the next several sessions, she had the option of walking ten laps (2000 feet) initially in 445 seconds (her previously observed baseline) or twenty laps at her own pace. Subsequently, time quotas would be reduced by 30 seconds until a satisfactory speed level was achieved. As shown in Fig. 19, the patient chose each time to work on speed. After five sessions, time was down from 445 seconds to 300. A brisk pace was required to achieve that. It was judged sufficient. Time quotas were held at the 300-second level, that is, one lap each 30 seconds. That pace could not be maintained with wavering or knee buckling. Neither of those were any longer observed.

12 Attention and social responsiveness

Attention or social responsiveness as a reinforcer was given detailed consideration in Chapter 4. This chapter will deal with specific methods and their rationale for working with this reinforcer as a treatment tool.

The objective of working with attention is to let this potentially influential social consequence go to work for rather than against the patient. Insofar as practical, attention should become contingent on behaviors to be increased. It should also be withdrawn as a systematic consequence to behaviors to be decreased.

The discussion in Chapter 4 of attention as a consequence and potential reinforcer asserted that the impact of attention is neither trivial nor childish. It is a reflection of our sensitivity to our environments. In all human service settings, attention is a vital and important force. The matter of attention has another and perhaps yet greater importance in treating chronic pain by the methods described here. People with significant amounts of operant pain have problems that are enmeshed with their environments. Their illnesses often will have presisted and have involved their total situations enough to become a dominating force in what they do. The pain problem will have in many instances become a way of life.

No one relinquishes one well-established and long-rehearsed way of life easily in favor of another, no matter how attractive the new is in comparison to the old. An operant-pain way of life will have been receiving positive reinforcement, perhaps a great deal. Entry into an operant program to change this way means that the patient is asked to give up one set of behaviors

and their attendant reinforcement for another. But if the pain behavior has persisted for a lengthy period, the patient is probably uncertain as to his or her ability to cope with and realize effective reinforcement from resumption of the well behavior now being proffered. As discussed previously, the patient is also likely to face a life of well behavior in which, at the time of entry into treatment, other noxious problems still exist, for which solutions are not yet in sight. There is also the matter of gaps in effective well behavior about which the patient is well aware but for which no solution has yet become tangible. All of these issues can make getting better fall far short of utopia.

In behavioral terms, the issue here can be stated as one in which a person is asked to give up one set of reinforcers to work toward another set that may seem barely or not at all attainable.

The treatment process must provide interim reinforcement to help each patient past the deprivation of reinforcement that almost always accompanies entry into treatment. Interim reinforcement will be needed until the increased activity level begins to pay off. The primary method for providing this interim reinforcement is through professional attention or social responsiveness. Most particularly, the physician-patient relationship should provide a major component of this reinforcement. In behavioral terms, establishing rapport with patients and developing the physician-patient or therapist-patient relationship may be seen in part as a search for interim reinforcement by which to help patients get into and through the treatment process.

Patients entering the kind of treatment

program described in this book can be expected to require and to deserve special attention. They are being asked to give up much for what is for them at that point an uncertain future.

In the earliest stages of treatment, extra effort should be made to check with the patient frequently, to let the patient know by the frequent, although they may be brief, contacts that the health care delivery system is indeed dedicated to helping to achieve the treatment goals. These contacts should not await indications of patient difficulty. They should not be pain or problem contingent. They should come before problems arise. They represent social reinforcement for patient participation in the treatment program. Their special significance at the outset is in recognition of the liklihood that the patient will be in a state of relative deprivation of reinforcement at the very time when new and extra demands are being made.

In addition to the brief contacts just mentioned, one person central to the patient's program should schedule perhaps twice- or thrice-weekly sessions with the patient. These sessions may need to be of only a few minutes' duration. They help to provide coordination in the program and to pick up quickly schedule conflicts or procedural difficulties. More importantly, they ensure that professional attention is directed toward the crucial first small increments of progress. Reviewing with the patient each element of the schedule and the data permits the emphasis of personalized attention on the crucial first treatment efforts.

It is difficult within the health care system to work constructively with attention as a systematic consequence. One reason for the difficulty is that most health care professionals are socially sensitive people who, in addition, are accustomed to being responsive to signs of distress. A display of pain is more sure than a display of well-being to elicit attention from a busy nurse. It is not that the nurse does not want the well behavior but that she is experienced at using encouragement and reassurance as tools for helping to achieve it. In short-term illness, her social attention, as distinguished from more specific procedural interventions, probably makes little difference on treatment outcome or rate of progress. In long-term or chronic illness, the opportunity for nurse responsiveness to have an effect is much greater. There is evidence (Ayllon and Michael, 1960; Berni and Fordyce, 1973; Fordyce and associates, 1973) that nurse responsiveness can work to the disadvantage of the patient, since it is often contingent on illness behaviors and systematically reinforces them. A second reason for the difficulty of programming attention relates to tradition. Health care professionals often fail to recognize the potential impact of their attention and so use it indiscriminately. A program that proposes that social responsiveness be withheld on occasion in the interests of greater patient progress is sometimes received with skepticism and even outright hostility. A major source of reinforcement for professional performance is peer approval. Efforts by one or a handful of professionals to change a component of the professional role may lead to a deprivation of reinforcement. Their professional peers may question the change and withhold approval. As a result, the innovators are at a special disadvantage.

These considerations make it important to prepare a treatment staff in the methods and their rationale before undertaking an operant program. Information about the methods should be provided. It remains no less true here, however, as elsewhere, that giving information by itself is not a reliable method for changing behavior. Rehearsal and, most important of all, intensive interim reinforcement to the staff who embark on these methods are essential. The methods should eventually yield their own reinforcement, making the task easier. Ultimately, the methods require less rather than more time. They make it possible to help patients otherwise not helped. They also tend to help the commonly abrasive, suspicious, hostile, and reluctant chronic pain patient to become a more pleasant person to be around. But it takes time for those effects to emerge. Effective reinforcement of the early efforts to achieve them is imperative.

Clinical experience suggests yet another problem in this context. When a patient expresses distress of a bodily complaint, physicians and nurses, for example, are not only responsive but also have well-developed repertoires of responses appropriate to the situation. These same health care professionals sometimes prove to be less adept at attentiveness and effective social responsiveness when a patient is not communicating illness or distress. Treatment personnel need to give some thought to their repertoires of reactions to activity and well behavior. One of the nice features about performance graphs displayed prominently at the bedside is that they provide a subject for discussion and professional attention that is activity contingent and not illness contingent.

Procedures for contingent attention

Unlike the case with medications and exercise, contingent attention is necessarily programmed with considerably less precision. It is imperative that both patient and spouse receive thorough explanations of the role of attention in treatment so that this process does not take on the characteristics of a socially reprehensible behind-the-scenes manipulation. There is no baseline and no counting by professional staff except in rare and extreme circumstances (for example, the patient described in Chapter 5 who aspired to reduce the rate of her moaning). The basic plan is that each staff person interacting with the patient should be geared to recognize and discriminate the audible or visible pain displays from the patient, which are behaviors to be reduced. When those pain behaviors are displayed, the staff person adopts a neutral, nonresponsive style. He or she does not seek to ease the distress by comment or by physical action. If it is a nurse or an occupational therapist, for example, in tran-

sit elsewhere at the time of encountering the pain behaviors, he or she continues. If the therapist is engaged in some activity with the patient, he or she should be as noncommittal in word and deed as possible. If the therapist is involved in a conversation with the patient or engaged in some interruptible task, and the complaints of pain are persistent, the therapist can say, "You don't seem to be feeling well. I'll come back a little later when you are feeling better," and can then withdraw. If this latter course is followed, it is important to return soon to test whether pain behaviors have subsided. The prompt return ensures that there is rapid social reinforcement for the patient for terminating pain displays.

Often the professional is engaged in a task that must continue. The task should go forward unless the pain behavior specifically interrupt or prohibit that. This possibility was dealt with in Chapter 10 on exercise management. During the interval before resuming a task interrupted by pain behaviors, there should be neither casual conversation nor therapist efforts to distract the patient from the pain. To do that is to make attention pain contingent. Instead, the therapist simply waits quietly until resumption is indicated, then proceeds with the task and picks up with whatever socializing may have been going on before the interruption. In that manner, he or she has made the attention activity contingent.

Attention as a consequence can be minimized during physically close interactions by breaking eye contact and by quietly subsiding in conversational efforts.

One of the major difficulties in the use of contingent attention regimens is that traditional patient-therapist interactions are often designed to elicit comments or demonstrations of pain and distress. There may, at times, be a self-fulfilling prophecy to this. On ward rounds, the physician often asks, "How do you feel?" or "How is the pain today?" Statements like that signal to the patient that professional attention is potentially contingent on pain and distress. There is the implicit possibility that if there were no pain, there would be no (or reduced) physician presence. Moreover, if pain is present, there is professional attention. The prestige of the physician and of other health care professionals makes for potent social reinforcement. Slight and not difficult changes in the approach can put this attention to work as a tool for behavior change. Fig. 13 provided an illustration of the influence of professional attention on patient readiness to express pain behaviors.

The approach to the patient should begin by directing attention toward behaviors to be increased, not decreased. In this context, it is exercise and activity that are to be increased and pain behaviors (verbal and otherwise) that are to be decreased. Therefore the opening comment on ward rounds might be, "How did it go yesterday?," rather than, "How are you feeling?" The opening question can be specific to any of the exercise elements of the program, for example, "How many letbacks were you able to do yesterday?" Alternatively, if it is honestly indicated, one might say, "You look great!" or "You know, you are really looking better." In the earliest stages of treatment such comments usually evoke a patient objection that the pain is still bad. Do not argue. Shrug the shoulders and say, "OK, but you are looking better."

There is nothing in the preceding comments to imply that pain or indications of illness or physical distress are to be ignored. The health care professional should not diminish at all his or her vigilance toward indications that some form of assistance or intervention is needed. It is the particular set of pain behaviors associated with the patient's operant pain problem that are the special concern. Moreover, it is not essential physical assistance that is being withheld but social (some would say psychological) responsiveness. The set of pain behaviors about which to be concerned here may be narrow or broad, depending on the patient. Those pain behaviors may be specific to a body site at which the pain problem arose, or they may have generalized to widely disparate forms of expressions of

bodily distress. Their character and extent should have been identified in the evaluation process and communicated to all treatment staff. New or unexpected indications of illness or some form of body crisis should receive the same kind of professional concern as would be indicated in any treatment setting.

Withholding social responsiveness to pain behavior should not result in a net reduction in the amount of contact with the patient. The regimen calls for attaching social responsiveness as much as possible to activity and well behavior. It is when the patient is *not* engaging in pain behavior that treatment staff should be making special efforts to interact and to provide social stimulation.

During professional interventions such as exercise in the physical therapy room or delivery of medications on a nursing unit, therapists should be making special efforts to converse, to be friendly, to be interested, to be responsive. If the patient then begins to talk about pain or to display distress, a posture or style of social nonresponsiveness should begin. But if the patient discusses something other than pain and does not display distress, the therapist reinforces that behavior with attention.

Contingent attention is of greatest importance in the early phases of treatment. Treatment staff who follow the regimen well are likely to find that their efforts have far more rapid and pervasive effect than they might expect. Moreover, as progress is observed, social interactions with the patient can become increasingly natural. The rate of pain displays, often after an initial upsurge, soon begins to diminish.

Even though patients have read descriptions of the program and have received orientation to it, they often will behave as if the contingent attention element is unexpected. One may find, for example, on morning rounds on a ward, that a patient will respond to the physician's question, "How is it going?" with, "Well, I'd like to tell you about my pain but I know you don't want me to talk about that." A variation of this is, "I'm hurting just as much (or more), but I know I'm not supposed to say so." One way to handle that kind of interchange is to listen impassively, perhaps shrug the shoulders or smile a bit, and then say, "OK, but how far were you able to walk in physical therapy yesterday?"

It is a temptation in episodes of the sort just described to use the evidence from performance graphs and other sources to try to convince the patient that he or she is getting better. When the patient complains of as much or more pain, the tempting countercomment is, "How can you say you are no better when you are able to do more with less medication?" That is not a wise choice. It tends to force the patient to defend the previously stated position that indeed pain is being experienced. The countercomment can readily be interperted by the patient as a challenge to the authenticity of the pain. A wiser choice for response would be to pause a moment after the patient's expressions of pain and then to say, "You are doing a nice job. The program is coming along very well. We are very pleased at your efforts. We hope you are pleased, too."

Attention from visitors and other patients

A later section of this chapter will deal with family retraining. That section will deal with family visits to the patient. There may be other visitors. When the picture with a given patient indicates that attention has been a major factor in maintaining operant pain behavior, the number of untrained visitors should be held to a minimum during the first 1 to 3 weeks of treatment. They might provide intense reinforcement of pain behavior, and that is to be minimized. If this prohibition results in too much isolation for the patient, a compromise may be sought. The compromise can work in either of two ways. One is to instruct the visitors not to talk about pain. If the patient brings up the subject, say nothing, pause, and then change the subject. The second way is to instruct the patient

in how to limit discussions of pain during the visit. One way to do that is to assign the patient the task of counting the number of times he or she discusses pain during each visit. If it appears desirable, visitors can also be asked to count. The act of counting in this context has the major function of reminding those who must count of what behaviors are the concern and are to be reduced. If counting is employed, a nurse or someone else must retrieve the count. The information will help to determine whether the visits have worked to the disadvantage of the patient, as well as indicating more about how effectively the patient is changing the rate of pain behavior displays. If the rate of pain behaviors during such visits continues to be high, a greater effort to remedy the situation is needed. For example, visits might be limited in time or frequency. One simple rule that might help would be to contract with the patient that visits must end when a certain number of pain behaviors have been displayed as counted by patient or by visitor. This does not mean that the visits must last that long but only that they must not exceed that limit.

As with all other elements of the program, these steps in relation to visitors should first be discussed thoroughly with the patient. It is usually best to offer the patient the choice of counting or of having visitors count. Similarly, if counting is not used and simple prohibition of talk about pain is the remedy, the patient should again be offered the option of withholding talk about pain or of staff discussing the matter with visitors.

The impact of specialized attention from other patients is often a more difficult problem. It is neither possible nor desirable to impose limitations on interactions between patients, except in a limited way. A nursing unit that houses a large number of operant pain patients at one time could consider imposing a restriction on discussions about pain as a ward rule. It would probably be rather difficult to enforce unless the patients felt strongly favorable toward such a rule, but it might be helpful.

The presence of a small number of other pain patients at the same time seems not to raise many problems. If two patients entering the program both give evidence that the attention factor has been a major force, it would seem unwise to place them in the same or nearby rooms, at least until there has been treatment progress. A patient well along in the program may be a positive or a negative force. If that advanced patient is doing well, he or she can, by example, be positive force to a newly admitted patient. This question of whether to put two pain patients together should rest on judgments about how readily and in what direction influence is likely to flow from one to the other. If the newly admitted patient appears more likely to be the dominating force in the pairing, the advanced patient may lose ground. If the flow of influence is in the other direction or perhaps not likely to be strong in either direction, pairing the patients may pose no problems.

Overall, patient influence is usually much less than staff influence. Physician and other health care professional attention is likely to have more impact than that of a lay person in the context of hospitals and chronic illness. It follows that interactions among patients seem not to have great effect one way or the other on the operant program. The major exception to this is the easily influenced and somewhat passive follower patient who is highly sensitized to and responsive to virtually everyone. That kind of patient may require special management with regard to room assignments and other patient interaction opportunities.

Outpatient management of attention

The concern here is with treatment programs attempted solely on an outpatient basis. Inpatient programs that later have an outpatient phase were dealt with in the preceding section.

Treatment that is on an outpatient basis from the beginning is seriously threatened in those instances in which spouse atten-

tion appears to have been playing an important part in reinforcing pain behavior or in failing to reinforce well behavior. Treatment attempted strictly on an outpatient basis requires that the family retraining component of the program set forth in the last section of this chapter receive intensive attention in the first few weeks of treatment. Family responses to pain and well behavior require careful attention early in the program even when the evidence suggest that those responses have had only minor roles. The reason for that is that the project at hand is to change pain behaviors, not to intermittently reinforce them. Gradual change in family response, when the patient is at home, provides intermittent reinforcement of the wrong patient behaviors during the change phase.

There are two pathways one may follow in working with contingent attention on an outpatient basis. One involves retraining family members. That will be dealt with later. The other is to work directly with the patient to help the patient to be his or her own behavioral engineer. It is an exercise in self-control akin to self-medicating.

When working directly with the patient, there are two strategies. One is to reduce the rate of pain behavior displays. The second is to alter the social consequences those displays (or the displays of activity and well behavior) receive. Either or both may be used.

Self-control of pain behavior displays

The procedures are, in principle, the same as with any other behavior change project. The target behaviors are pinpointed. It should be remembered that the objective here is to reduce pain behavior displays in the presence of people who reinforce them to the disadvantage of patient progress. This makes the task easier. Once it is known who provides the adverse reinforcement, pinpointing and counting can be restricted to those periods when the pain behavior reinforcers are present. Private and nonreinforced pain behavior displays are usually of no importance and may be bypassed entirely. In an interview with the patient, the roster of ways in which pain is communicated to others is developed. Next, a baseline observation period of up to a week is set in which the patient counts and records each time one of the pain behaviors occurs. Third, reinforcers are selected, optimally by discussion with and choice of the patient. Fourth, reinforcement schedules are set up. This usually can most easily be done by setting quotas and arranging that the reinforcers become contingent on meeting the quotas. The following hypothetical example will illustrate. Pain behaviors identified for elimination or reduction are (1) talking about pain, (2) rubbing the sore back, (3) asking for medication or a heat pad, (4) grimacing or moaning, and (5) asking for help with a task, the performance of which is inhibited by pain.

Baseline

The patient acquires a wrist counter (sporting goods stores sell them to golfers) and is trained in its use.

The five pain behaviors are considered of equivalent importance. During the baseline week, their collective daily rate is counted. If the program focuses solely on interactions with the spouse, counting is only during presence of the spouse.

Reinforcers

It is a temptation to rely solely on signs of progress, as in graphs displaying change. That is risky. They should be used, but, at the outset, additional contingencies should be explored. One of the simplest is that the predinner cocktail (not pain cocktail) or postdinner TV become contingent on meeting a performance quota for the preceding 24-hour period. If more precision is needed, a point or token system can be set up; for example, each unit of one reduction in pain behavior count over the preceding day yeilds x number of minutes of TV time. A more detailed review of point systems is provided on pp. 94 and 95.

Reinforcement schedules (quotas)

Once the baseline is known, a starting quota should be set that is clearly within reach. The first quota can be at or even above the daily average rate. It is much preferred to achieve a modest gain than to fail at a more ambitious one. Quotas can then be lowered in either a preset rate or by negotiation during weekly clinic rechecks.

Patient modification of spouse behavior

The procedures are the same in outline as in the self-control approach just described.

Pinpointing target behaviors

In a conjoint interview with patient and spouse, spouse reinforcers for pain behaviors or discouragements of activity are identified and listed.

Baseline

For a week the patient counts and records by wrist counter the collective daily rate at which the spouse is noted to express the target behaviors listed.

Reinforcers

The same procedure as in the preceding example can be followed. The spouse selects the reinforcer. The reinforcer is to become contingent on meeting a performance quota to be monitored by the patient. That is, the spouse has a quota of reinforcements of patient pain behavior or of discouragements of activity to reduce.

Reinforcement schedule

Quotas are set initially at approximately baseline levels. They may be reduced at a rate agreed on by the spouse at the outset or by negotiation at weekly clinic contracts.

• • •

It may be apparent that a third variation can be used, one in which the spouse monitors or counts patient pain behavior displays. That is a possibility for use from the outset of a totally outpatient program. Although it may appear logically as straightforward as the other two procedures outlined, it is often not so easily accomplished. The greater difficulty arises because the spouse is often receiving some form of reinforcement for the status quo. The treatment program will not yet have changed that. As a consequence, spouse efforts to bring about behavior change may not receive adequate reinforcement. Spouse effort may therefore prove to be ineffective. The issue will receive more attention in the last section of this chapter.

Reinforcement and feedback from performance graphs and records

The distinction was drawn on pp. 12 to 14 between what is said and what is done. This distinction has special importance in regard to the contingent management of attention. What one says is one set of behaviors, what one does is another. Each set encounters consequences in its own right. Sometimes the consequences are the same. Often they are different. Because what we say and what we do usually encounter different consequences, they can be expected to diverge. The practical effect of this is that a person may make statements reflecting one set of affairs and may take overt actions reflecting a different set of affairs. A chronic pain patient, for example, may make statements about the status of his or her pain problem that convey that the pain is unchanged or even worse than previously reported. Within the same day, and perhaps only seconds away from such statements, the patient may engage in overt actions that convey that the pain problem has apparently changed for the better. Logically, of course, the opposite pattern may also occur. The patient may talk as if the problem is better and act as of it is not.

The importance of this distinction between what is said and what is done has already been considered in regard to pa-

tient evaluation. It is also important in the operant treatment program.

The likelihood that patient statements about pain will receive at least some continuing special attention is inherent in the social complexities of the hospital setting. Untrained or unalert professionals will periodically let their attention be pain behavior contingent. Visitors, other patients, and hospital employees can be expected to display solicitousness and special attention when pain is communicated. One common result is that what chronic pain patients in an otherwise effective operant program say about the pain tends to change at a slower rate than what they do. The regimens described in Chapters 9 and 10 dealing with medication and exercise or activity level management usually produce rapidly discernible results with properly selected patients. Medication intake goes down, and exercise performed and tolerated goes up. Meanwhile changes in what the patient says about the pain lags behind.

If asked about the level of pain, a patient may insist that it is unchanged or even that it is more severe as compared with the beginning of treatment. Concomitantly, the patient may be observed routinely to exceed by increasing amounts a range of exercise quotas larger than could be tolerated during baseline observations. Further, the increased performance is accompanied by significantly less pain medication than was ostensibly required to make possible the lesser performance observed at the beginning of the program. The semantic debate as to whether it is pain that is improved or something else ("how one lives with the pain" or "how one acts in the presence of pain") has already been discussed (p. 103) and will not be considered further here. It can be stated again that exercises and activity levels noted previously by direct observation to be limited but now occurring at significantly higher rates represent behavior change. The significance of that change is yet greater when it occurs despite reduced medication intake.

The special significance of this point here is that the chronically ill patient may be improving without knowing it. This certainly appears to be the case with many chronic pain patients. That is understandable. One reason is the previously mentioned differential reinforcement of verbal versus performance actions. Performance behaviors are usually more effectively reinforced, and so they change more rapidly. Another reason is that changes are often gradual, subtle, and not readily discernible. As in an example used earlier, snapshots taken 6 months previously reveal to a person changes in the succeeding 6 months not noticed by peering into the bathroom mirror each morning.

One of the implications of this is that precision recording and display of performance graphs and other methods permits rapid and precise feedback to the patient and to others as to what is happening. It is difficult to judge on a Monday morning whether one's pain is significantly better than was true the preceding Monday. It is somewhat easier to observe changes in a performance graph that reports that walking has increased by 1000 feet, and each of seven exercises has increased by five repetitions during the preceding week. This distinction applies to patients and to others. That is, both patients and others can detect performance changes, whatever a patient may be saying and subjectively experiencing about pain.

Procedures for recording and graphing

The data kit. At the time of entering the program, the patient should be presented with a data kit. A hardbound folder in which is a packet of multicolored pens, 2 weeks of diary forms, several performance record sheets (Fig. 21), and an ample supply of graphs suffices. The patient's name can be shown on the cover of the folder. Fig. 21 illustrates how quota and performance data can be recorded for later transfer to graphs.

Instruct each patient in how to use each component of the kit. There should also be a reminder about the importance of bringing the kit to every treatment session. This instruction should be supplemented by directions to all treatment staff to check at the beginning of each session to be sure the kit is present. If it is not, the patient should be sent back to get it.

Diaries. Diary forms will have already been completed during the preadmission evaluation phase and so will be familiar. Diary recording continues in the same fashion, although a new diary form is begun on the day of admission.

Performance records. Each exercise and other treatment activity prescribed for the patient heads a column of the performance records. Rows correspond to treatment sessions. For the first day or two as each exercise is completed, the therapist can help the patient to record the amount accomplished before proceeding to the next exercise or procedure. During baseline trials the amounts accomplished represent a measure of current tolerance. Later, performance is recorded as amount done and the quota to which it relates. For example, if the exercise of deep knee bends has reached a quota of 12 and the quota is met, the proper cell of the form shows 12/12. If the quota was failed and only 10 were achieved, 10/12 would be recorded. Exercises involving pulling weights record the weight; for example, 9/9, 5 pounds. Exercises in which the left and right upper or lower extremity perform separately should also be recorded and graphed separately. Recording left and right separately has several advantages. The principal gain is that it permits one to identify and record differential performance between the left and right side. It also makes it easier to portray different quotas and quota-increment rates when that applies. Fig. 22 describes such an instance. As shown in the baseline values, there was considerable disparity between her left and right hips on the abduction exercise. In the earlier phases of treatment, one side worked to move heavier weights than the other, although the number of repetitions and the increment rate were the same. Eventually the weaker side improved to where the thera-

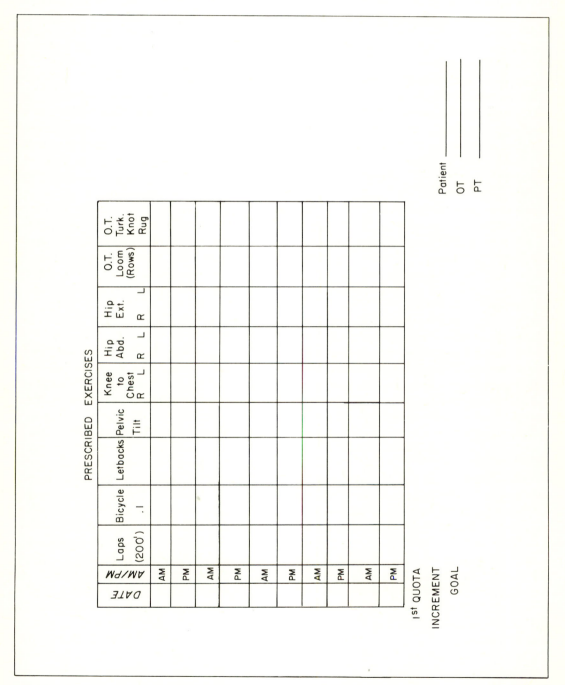

Fig. 21. *Recording exercise quotas and performance.*

Continued.

PRESCRIBED EXERCISES

DATE	AM/PM	Laps (200')	Bicycle .1	Letbacks	Pelvic Tilt	Knee to Chest R L	Hip Abd. R L	Hip Ext. R L	O.T. Loom (Rows)	O.T. Turk. Knot Rug
	AM	8/8	1.5/1.5	6/6	12/12	10/10 10/10	6/6 9/9 5# 8#	8/8 10/10 7.5 10	16	12
	PM	8/8	1.5/1.5	6/6	13/13	10/10 10/10	7/7 10/10	9/9 5/5 12.5	16	12
	AM	9/9	1.6/1.6	7/7	14/14	11/11 11/11	8/8 5/5 10#	10/10 6/6	17	13
	PM	9/9	1.6/1.6	7/7	15/15	11/11 11/11	9/9 6/6	5/5 7/7 10	17	13
	AM	10/10	1.7/1.7	8/8	16/16	12/12 12/12	10/10 7/7	6/6 8/8	18	14
	PM	10/10	1.7/1.7	8/8	17/17	12/12 12/12	5/5 8/8 8#	7/7 9/9	18	14
	AM	11/11	1.8/1.8	9/9	18/18	13/13 13/13	6/6 9/9	8/8 10/10	19	15
	PM	11/11	1.8/1.8	9/9	19/19	13/13 13/13	7/7 10/10	9/9 5/5 15	19	15
	AM	12/12	1.9/1.9	10/10	20/20	14/14 14/14	8/8 5/5 12.5#	10/10 6/6	20	16
	PM	12/12	1.9/1.9	10/10	20/20	14/14 14/14	9/9 6/6	5/5 7/7 12.5	20	16
1st QUOTA	8		1.5	6	12	10 10	6 9	8 10	16	12
INCREMENT	1/Day		.1/Day	1/Day	2/Day	1/Day				
GOAL	30		3.0	20	20	20 20	20/20# 20/20	20/20#	16	

Patient _____
OT _____
PT _____

Fig. 21, cont'd. For legend see p. 199.

pist brought the two quotas into alignment. Performance of the two hips are shown in the figure as superimposed on each other to display the quota differences more clearly. In practice, the right and left graphs were maintained separately.

As was discussed in Chapter 10 on management of exercise, prescribed exercises must be quantifiable in performance terms. This issue sometimes requires careful review of therapist procedures. It is a point that is not always well understood. Working at a loom or with wall weights is not to be measured in time units but in numbers of units of completed performance: rows of weaving at a given width or repetitions at a given weight.

Many physical therapy exercises involve lifting or holding against weights of varying magnitude. Graph recording of performance for such exercises should reflect both the number of repetitions and the amount of weight against which force is exerted. Fig. 22 illustrates the scalloped effect produced by such graphs. It will be noted from Fig. 22 that the therapist's initial quota began with the weights used in baseline trials. The disparity between left and right sides continued for some time before quotas were equalized.

There may be two potential exceptions to the performance-versus-time rule, but they may arise only in later stages of treatment after considerable progress will have occurred. The first exception relates to job station assignments. It is often difficult and logistically impractical to develop precise movement cycle units for job stations. Output and progress at the job station would be better monitored and rate of improvement would probably accelerate if the time were taken to analyze jobs in those terms. But that is often impractical. A compromise that can be hazardous is to record job station activity in time units. If review of a job station assignment indicates a reasonably steady rate of the job activity, performance may be recorded in time units. Should monitoring of job station performance suggest a general lagging of patient effort, the additional step of developing measurable production units should be resorted to. When that is done, the usual quota procedure can be applied. In noting this exception, it should be remembered that job stations enter into the picture only after there has been considerable patient progress in a range of activities all having quantifiable movement cycles. This point is important because it means that rest and

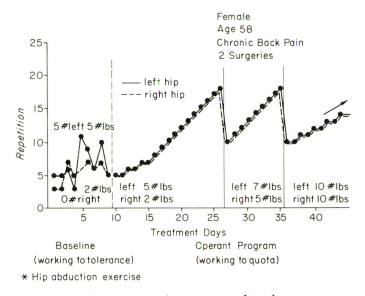

Fig. 22. *Quota variation for asymmetrical involvement.*

attention will have been made contingent on performance, not time, and will have brought the patient to a point of intermittent and diminishing rates of reinforcement. At that point, the time method, a fixed interval schedule, is appropriate. The behavior has been established and rehearsed. Interval schedules tend to yield durable behavior, although they are less effective in generating a behavior. A similar exception was noted on p. 170 in relation to cooking or homemaking activities in occupational therapy. The exception is justifiable only after considerable treatment progress has occurred.

Graphs. The performance figures shown throughout the book were prepared from patient performance graphs. At the close of the baseline period, graphs can be posted at the bedside, and the transfer of data from performance records to graphs should begin. Graphing is not begun before that time because to do so would risk adding social reinforcement as a systematic consequence to performance during the baseline trials. Those baseline trials are strictly for the purpose of determining patient performance when he or she is left free to respond to inner cues or subjective experience.

Most professionals have at least some experience at constructing and reading performance graphs. Many patients do not have that experience. It is therefore important to follow up the initial instruction as to how to transfer performance data to graph form. After the first postbaseline treatment day, someone should go through the process with the patient to be sure the graphs are constructed properly. This first session of graph construction should include retroactive graphing of baseline trials, followed by display on each graph of the first quota or treatment sessions. Subsequently, daily ward rounds provide built-in monitoring of upkeep of graphs.

Graphs should be posted in a fashion that permits extension of performance of each precedure onto second and subsequent graph forms as they are needed. The display of a row of walking performance graphs from baseline tolerance trials, perhaps describing ability to go no more than a few hundred feet before resting to topped-off quotas of up to 1 or 2 miles, can provide an intensely rich reinforcement to patient, family, and staff.

General activity level as recorded in diary forms should also be displayed in graph form for both daily and weekly units. The graph showing weekly cumulative uptime (sitting plus standing or walking) is often one of the most readable indices of patient progress, particularly when it displays preadmission performance, the week of baseline observations, and subsequent achievements.

Fig. 23 shows daily uptime totals for one severely impaired patient who had had seven surgeries and many significant neuromuscular deficits associated with those procedures, as well as severe distress from pain. Fig. 24 reports the weekly totals from the same patient's diaries of sitting, standing or walking, reclining, and the sum of sitting and standing or walking: uptime. There are several things to be noted about these figures. The daily uptime totals reflect the gradual trend upward of her activity level, but it is difficult to discern the extent to which she changed. The second graph, Fig. 24, which reports weekly totals of each of the kinds of activities, yields both a more evident and a more precise picture of where the changes are occurring. Keeping the daily uptime graph helps the patient to focus attention on activity level. Keeping the weekly totals graph makes the major trends more evident and shows the changes from preadmission data to the present. Finally, this patient was severely involved. It was a long and arduous task for her to reach a significantly higher level of performance. Most patients will show changes in activity level sooner than those shown in Fig. 24. The patient discussed on p. 58, whose weekly uptime totals were shown in Fig. 7, represents one of the more rapid rates of increase in activity level.

One person within the treatment facility

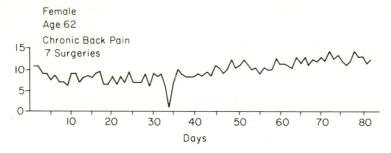

Fig. 23. *Daily uptime (sitting and standing or walking) graph.*

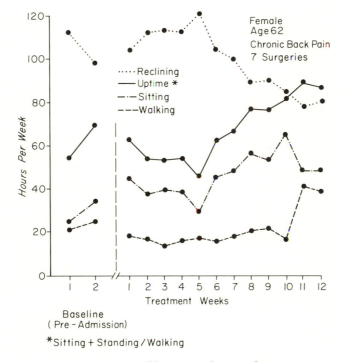

Fig. 24. *Weekly activity diary totals.*

should be designated as the source for replenishment of diary and graph forms. The patient can then assume the responsibility for going to that person to receive additional performance, diary, and graph forms, as needed.

Reinforcement function of graphs. Reinforcing functions of graphs can be listed briefly.

1. Graphs provide rapid and precise report of performance, permitting patients to make more sensitive judgments of change.

2. Graphs help patients more precisely to communicate to spouses and others what is being accomplished in treatment.

3. Graphs provide reinforcement to spouse and other family members for their efforts in behalf of the program. These records of change often pick up progress more rapidly than casual observation.

4. Graphs demonstrate to treatment personnel whether their efforts are having an effect. Upward curves on

graphs are tangible demonstrations of the effectiveness of therapist effort as well as that of the patient.

5. Graphs have indirect as well as direct reinforcing functions. When displayed prominently, graphs provide cues to people interacting with the patient to be prudent about the use of attention and social responsiveness. Graphs remind visitors, professional and nonprofessional, to be selectively responsive and also provide them with information about activity or well behavior to which they can respond.

Measurement of progress (and of pain)

On pp. 20 and 21 there was a limited discussion of the measurement of pain. It was noted there that this book would not offer definitive measures of pain. The present chapter is concerned with procedural and not theoretical matters, but since the recording of progress and change is being discussed, a few additional comments about the matter of pain measurement are in order.

The procedures described here measure what people do who are identified as having functional limitations associated with chronic pain. If it is assumed that pain is an inner event, a subjective experience whose presence or absence depends on the verbal report of the person, the procedures described here do not measure pain. They do measure aspects of what the person does who has the pain problem. More particularly, these measurement procedures record changes in what the person does of those behaviors identified at the outset as limited by the pain problem. When the activities recorded (for example, diary data or exercise performance) indicate change, it is moot as to whether pain has changed, as well. Sometimes patients continue to state that the pain is unchanged. They are not surely correct. They may or may not be. The only data are patient statements about an alleged or inferred inner event. Similarly, patients may state that the pain is now im-

proved or has disappeared altogether. That, too, may or may not be a correct statement.

The contingency management approach to chronic pain works with what people do, their actions or behavior. It is true that some attention is directed toward modifying what patients say about their pain. Those efforts necessarily lack precision and therefore lack as much effectiveness as other elements of the program. They are not intended to change anything more than what is said. It is not contended that helping a person to change what he or she says about pain changes inner, subjective experience.

What this comes down to is that the methods described in this book are directed at what people *do*. The measures used record changes in what they do. The behaviors of concern relate to reported pain problems, but it is not known whether behavior changes produced represent changes in unobserved and unmeasured inner events such as subjectively experienced pain.

Spouse and family training

The procedures described in this section are for use with the spouse or whatever other person may be indicated. The person is selected who has played and is likely to continue to play a significant role in the direct or indirect reinforcement of pain behavior or the discouragement or punishment of activity and well behavior. The recipient of training is nearly always the spouse. Sometimes other family members such as a parent or in-law living within the home or adolescent or older progeny also participate. Occasionally, when the patient is unmarried, a girlfriend or boyfriend participate.

The social responsiveness of others as an important element in the picture usually relates to but one key person. Modification of that one person's behavior in relation to the pain problem usually suffices. Typically the contributions of others are peripheral and, if warranting action at all, may be accomplished with a single contact or by preparing the spouse (or other key person) to be the agent for change of these others.

The procedures to be described are presented with the spouse as the key person.

Some member of the treatment team with interviewing and interpersonal skills as well as knowledge of the operant program's methods should be selected to carry out spouse training. In multidisciplinary hospital settings this might be a psychologist, psychiatrist, social worker, nurse, or some other health care professional. Selection is a matter of judgments about knowledge, skill, and interest, not professional identity.

Training procedures will need to be scheduled with a number of factors in mind. Assuming that the spouse or other recipient of the training is within reasonably easy commuting distance of the treatment setting, sessions probably should start with twice-weekly contacts of 20 to 40 minutes each. As progress occurs, the frequency can usually be reduced to once-a-week sessions.

Due allowance must be made for other commitments of the spouse. On the one hand, the procedure is clearly an integral part of treatment. The sessions should have been made an explicit requirement. Failure to agree to this participation ordinarily should result in refusal to accept the patient for treatment. On the other hand, scheduling should interfere as little as possible with the spouse's employment and family responsibilities. Sessions may have to occur in the early or late parts of the day, as well as perhaps evenings or weekends. Those details need to be agreed on before treatment begins.

The operant program is specialized. Patients often come from great distances, far beyond commuting distance. In those cases, it is imperative before beginning treatment to clarify both the scheduling and the funding of spouse contacts. Special negotiations with third-party treatment sponsors may be required to get them to recognize that spouse visits are an integral component of treatment, without which the whole enterprise may be fatally compromised.

The spouse who must come from afar will require a different schedule pattern.

The minimum indicated by clinical experience is that the spouse come with the patient at time of admission, remain for 1 to 3 days, return at least once during the inpatient phase for 2 to 3 days, and return again for approximately a week during the last part of the outpatient phase. Daily spouse contacts should be scheduled during that outpatient week.

Ideally, the spouse who lives at a distance should be seen each 2 or 3 weeks. He or she may come for a late afternoon session, visit the patient that evening, and have another training session the next morning before departure for home.

Concomitant with modification of spouse responses to pain behavior and to activity, the treatment program may use these sessions to help plan posttreatment activities. Joint sessions with patient and spouse should be scheduled for that purpose. In addition, problems indirectly related to the pain problem may also become a focus of spouse contacts. For example, a patient's pain may yield time out from activities that, were they engaged in, would lead to marital strife. Spouse training sessions might then also have the character of marital counseling. The choice depends on whether these other problems are to be dealt with by the immediate treatment team. If they are to be treated by adjunctive therapists, that enterprise should proceed apace and with intercommunication with the treatment team.

It is of utmost importance to provide for coordination between the person working with the spouse and the rest of the treatment team. For example, evening visits, recreational activities, and weekend passes often involve the spouse. Those activities provide opportunity to rehearse steps in the training process. The activities must be made available at the proper times.

Pinpointing target behaviors

In consultation with the spouse, a list of pain behaviors that the patient displays with some frequency is identified and written out. These are the ways in which the spouse is made aware that the patient has a pain problem or functional impairment associated with pain. A typical list includes:

- Talks about pain.
- Moves in guarded fashion.
- Grimaces or rubs or touches a painful area.
- Reclines (or sits in a particular position) at a point in time when, were there no pain problem, it would not occur.
- Asks for medication or some other palliative procedure (heat pad, massage).
- Asks to be excused from or relieved of some activity because otherwise pain will occur or be aggravated.

The list may not include all of these, but most of them are common. The final list should probably have about five to ten items. More than that is excessively detailed. Items can be grouped into homogeneous clusters. Fewer than five or six items probably indicates lack of effective observations by the spouse, and further observations during subsequent visits should be required.

Counting pain behaviors

By negotiation with the spouse, a fixed amount of each spouse visit with the patient is committed during which pain behaviors will be covertly counted. A balance needs to be found. The time should be long enough to provide a reasonable behavior sample but not so long as to stretch beyond practical limits the spouse's ability simultaneously to visit and to count. Experience indicates that a 20-minute counting period is usually adequate. A longer counting period is often superfluous and excessively burdensome. Shorter counting periods may lead to inadequate spouse vigilance or recognition of the importance of the task.

Doubt about the spouse's readiness or ability to handle a 20-minute counting period may require a shorter interval initially. This can perhaps be increased at a later time when more mastery has been developed.

Counting periods should be constant in length, so for as possible, to permit meaningful comparisons across visits.

During each of the first several visits, the spouse is assigned the task of counting the number of times any one or combination of the pinpointed pain behaviors occur. It is not necessary, except in rare instances, to record the rate of each pain behavior separately, only the number of times any one or more of them occur. At the end of the counting period, the spouse should be prepared to state with some precision how many pain behavior display events occurred. Moreover, the spouse should keep a record so that the number for each visit is retrievable. It should be made clear to the spouse that at the next session he or she will be expected to report specific numbers; for example, Tuesday evening, six; Wednesday evening, eight; Saturday afternoon, five.

The counting task can be made easier by pointing out to the spouse that a new pack of book matches provides a convenient counter. Each time a pain behavior is displayed, the spouse can bend a match from the book while it is held in a pocket or unobtrusively in the hand. It is a simple matter to count at the end of the visit how many matches have been bent.

The spouse should also record the count of verbal pain behaviors during the length of telephone conversations with the patient, and the records should note that it pertains to a telephone conversation. For lengthy telephone conversations, the same 20-minute limit can be used. For shorter calls, the compromise with necessity is to rely on the length of the call as a reasonable basis for an estimate.

More often than not, spouses will underestimate the counting task. At the time of the second session, the spouse will report that counting was forgotten or that "there were a lot of (or few) pain behaviors." Additional counting sessions must be carried out until there is a consistent reporting of numerical values by the spouse. The numbers themselves need not be consistent, but the counting of them must be.

Keeping a covert count of one's spouse's behavior while also visiting with that spouse understandably can raise difficulties in interpersonal communication. In practice, this proves less of a problem than one might expect. In the first place, both patient and spouse will have been informed before treatment that there would be a training program for the spouse concerned with his or her reactions to pain and to activity. In addition, however, the issue of making a covert count of one's mate's behavior should be discussed explicitly with the spouse. There is no critical reason why the counting must be kept a secret. It should be emphasized that if the spouse wishes to tell his or her mate that the counting is going on, it is perfectly all right to do so. The telling will in no way obstruct the program. Once that is made clear, it can also be added that "it is usually easier in terms of your communication with your spouse that you say nothing about your counting. However, if for any reason you feel you should tell him/her, by all means do so. Otherwise, we recommend that you simply not discuss it until later in the program." The handful of times in which the spouse has reported to the patient that he or she was counting did not lead to any untoward difficulties.

The function of the count is not to develop some form of quota. The baseline rate of pain behaviors displayed to the spouse can be used as a reference point against which the rate at later points in treatment can be compared. But that rarely proves necessary. The data are there, however, and should the spouse need special encouragement, later counts can be taken. The major reason for counting is that to do so forces increased vigilance. The reported count is a method for determining when the spouse has developed skill at discriminating pain behaviors from other ongoing patient behavior.

Fig. 25 shows counts by a husband of his wife's pain behaviors. Their home was several hundred miles away. The husband accompanied her to her admission. After a

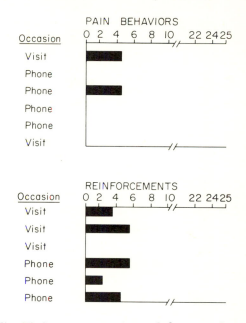

Fig. 25. *Spouse count of pain behavior and reinforcement of activity.*

brief instructional session, he counted pain behaviors the first 20 minutes of a visit with her on the ward the second day of her treatment. He returned to his home and his work but again visited 2 weeks later and again counted. Between those visits he counted pain behaviors during telephone conversations with her. Those counts are shown in the upper part of the figure. This patient's operant pain related in part to deprivation of reinforcers from her preoccupied husband. In later phases of treatment, when the husband appeared to have mastered discriminating pain behaviors and his own responses to them, the psychologist working with him in the retraining process assigned him the task of counting his reinforcers of his wife's activity. For the first 20 minutes of each visit or telephone conversation, the husband counted the number of times he provided some word of praise, encouragement, or approval to his wife when she engaged in movement and activity. A sample of those counts is shown in the lower part of Fig. 25.

Fig. 26 portrays the trend of a patient's pain behaviors observed and counted by his wife during the first 20 minutes of her

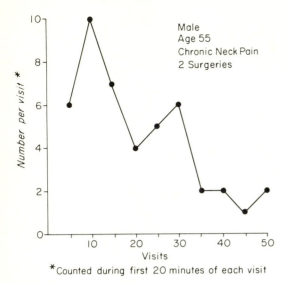

*Counted during first 20 minutes of each visit

Fig. 26. *Pain behavior counts by spouse.*

numerous visits with him. In this particular case, the wife continued to count pain behaviors throughout the program because her efforts in his behalf seemed to realize considerable reinforcement from observing the continuing reduction in what had once been virtually incessant complaints of pain.

Pinpointing spouse responses

Once mastery of counting patient pain behavior has been demonstrated, it may be discontinued or held in abeyance to be resumed only if further need for it should arise. The next step is to train the spouse to identify his or her own responses to patient pain behavior and to patient activity.

The objective of this second step is to make it easier for the spouse to begin to change. What is to change first needs to be identified.

One procedure for the second step is to instruct the spouse to note precisely what he or she does in the first seconds after a display of pain behavior by the patient. The spouse can be instructed that during succeeding visits with the patient, for each of the first three pain behavior displays, the spouse is to make a mental note of exactly what he or she does. This instruction is often helped by the explanation, "It

is as if we were going to videotape what you do while the patient is displaying pain. What would the tape show you doing, and what would we hear?"

A session with the spouse should be scheduled soon after the first attempts at self-observation to help firm up the efforts and to gain better recovery of the spouse's recall. It usually takes several visits before mastery over this task emerges. As noted in the earlier discussion on patient evaluation, the spouse cannot do "nothing" in response to a pain display. "Nothing" takes many forms. A rather consistent pattern of spouse behaviors that follow pain displays usually emerges.

The self-observation task is difficult to do with precision. If the process is not moving ahead well, it is often useful to schedule a joint appointment of patient and spouse in which each tries to identify both his or her own and the mate's responses. The patient develops a list of pain behaviors and another list of spouse reactions to them. The spouse develops a list of patient pain behaviors and of spouse reactions to them. These two pairs of lists can then be compared and discussed within the session. Such a session nearly always breaks the logjam and helps the spouse better to pinpoint.

The same sequence is followed in regard to the step of training spouse responses to patient exercise or activity. This step can sometimes be lumped with the second step, the work on the responses to pain behavior, and dealt with simultaneously. If that seems too difficult, they can be treated consecutively.

Withdrawing attention to pain behavior

Consistency of spouse reports as to what he or she did after pain behavior and activity displays during visits with the patient is an indication of mastery over the self-observation pinpointing task. When that mastery has occurred, the next step is to examine the roster of spouse responses to pain behaviors, one by one, and to develop alternatives appropriate to treatment objectives. When the spouse has been discouraging patient exercise or activity, alternatives for those behaviors also need to be developed.

In the case of spouse reactions to pain behaviors, the major objective is to develop skill at being socially nonresponsive. Ways of doing this have already been discussed in relation to staff training. A simple and usually adequate remedy to the problem is to instruct the spouse, when pain behavior is seen or heard, to first break eye contact. Shifting one's gaze from eye contact to the patient's shoulder, for example, is a specific action, easily done, and easily remembered. The spouse can then be instructed to pause for a couple of seconds and then to ask the patient a question about some aspect of activity. The graphs displayed at the bedside offer a most convenient selection of topics or questions on which the spouse can draw.

Changing well-habituated ways of behaving after the occurrence of pain behavior is more easily described than accomplished. The task can be made easier by providing specific rehearsal sessions within the spouse training sessions. This kind of role playing helps the spouse have confidence and more precision.

Two or three visits during which these responses are rehearsed with the patient are usually required before moving on to the final step in the process.

Spouse reinforcement of activity and well behavior

The roster of ways in which a spouse has been discouraging activity is reviewed. The first change in that may simply be the admonishment not to do it, but that is rarely enough. The spouse's task is made easier and the marital relationship is furthered if the spouse has a generally supportive response to offer at the appropriate moments.

A roster of ways to express support or approval is easily developed in a few moments of discussion, should that be needed. The task is to increase the use of these responses at the proper times. To accomplish that, the next spouse assignment can be to count the number of times that he or she reinforces the patient for activity or well behavior.

By the time this phase of training is reached, the patient will almost surely be ready for evening and weekend passes. As with the earlier counting of pain behavior by the spouse, counting periods can be set up. For an evening pass, it might be the first hour. For a 2-day weekend pass, it might be 30-minute counting periods during each morning, afternoon, and evening. During those counting periods, the spouse is instructed to count the number of times he or she reinforces the patient for activity. The only constraint is that reinforcement is not to occur contiguous to pain behavior. There should be ample opportunity for reinforcement, since the patient is bound to be doing something.

One might properly question whether a spouse will simply lavish arbitrary praise on the patient for doing essentially nothing, and thereby build up the count; for example, "It's sure good to see you sitting there reading the newspaper," said three times in 5 minutes. That kind of frivolous effort should, in the practical case, offer no hazards. Even a modicum of rapport with the spouse in the training sessions should be enough to avoid that kind of sloppy effort.

Spouse visits to and observations of physical therapy or other treatment sessions provide additional and convenient opportunity for rehearsal of the reinforcement of activity.

It is sometimes helpful to arrange for programmed mutual reinforcement of patient and spouse during the course of a pass or an evening recreation program. A spouse may have the mission of counting the number of times he or she reinforces the patient for activity. The patient may have the task of counting the number of times he or she receives reinforcement for activity. This mutual reinforcement can be done covertly or with mutual awareness that it is underway. Perhaps some will be surprised to observe that effectiveness rarely appears to be diminished by both parties being aware that the counting is going on.

There is no formal target number of reinforcements for activity to be attained. It becomes strictly a matter of judgment as to when the spouse has mastered adequately the task of avoiding pain-contingent social reinforcement and of providing sufficient intermittent reinforcement of suitable activity or well behavior.

13 Generalization and the maintenance of performance

The concept of generalization was defined and illustrated in Chapter 4. The importance of generalization to contingency management treatment of pain was discussed there and in Chapter 5 in relation to treatment goals. This chapter will be concerned with providing illustrative detail of methods for helping treatment gains to generalize, that is, to broaden in scope and to persist across time and into other environments. The central issue is the maintenance of treatment gains.

The sequence for this chapter will be first to identify strategies for generalization and then to describe and illustrate their application.

The reason for concern about generalization is contained in a principle of learning stated in Chapter 3: ". . . conditioning effects are somewhat specific to the stimulus conditions in which they arose. A behavior acquired in one setting is likely initially to occur only in that setting or closely similar ones." Generalization may occur to overcome that specificity by providing for systematic and effectively reinforced practice in other settings. Generalization is also helped by enhancing access to reinforcers naturally occurring in home and work settings that may maintain performance.

There are three broad strategies by which to promote generalization. These were described and illustrated in Chapter 4 and so will be restated only briefly. They are first to prepare the patient for self-control, to become his or her own behavioral engineer. In that approach the patient tries to arrange or program his or her sustaining reinforcement. A second approach is for the treatment facility to work with the patient's natural environment to arrange sustaining reinforcement for patient performance. A third way to bring about generalization is to increase access to naturally occurring reinforcement for the newly established behaviors deriving from treatment. Each of the three may have a role in a patient's program. The third approach provides, in most cases, the greatest potential long-term benefit and ease of implementation. It will receive the greatest attention here.

Generalization should not be left to chance. It should be designed as an integral part of treatment to ensure that it receives the care and attention it deserves. A concerted effort should be made to promote the maintenance of treatment gains.

Methods for achieving generalization include prescribing variations in place and time of activity and well behavior rehearsal by passes, home visits, and shifting of exercise and activity sites. Broadened combinations of activities that involve exercise building in treatment and that relate to posttreatment activity plans (such as simulated and real work situations or structured and unstructured recreational activities) may also be assigned. Providing planning and, where needed, placement assistance for vocational and leisure activities anticipated to follow formal treatment is yet another way to help bring about generalization.

Patients who enter treatment addicted or habituated to pain medications often provide a prototype of the problem of generalization. Addicted patients will have developed a network of cues and associations in their home and work environments that initiate the chain of behaviors culminating in taking medication. The potency of these stimuli or cues, or, stated another way, our sensitivity and responsiveness to them, is often greatly underestimated. Addiction and habituation are thought of as residing within the person, as being something he or she *has*, similar to a motivation. They do, of course, reside in the person in the sense that the cortex is the repository of learning effects. In the particular case of physiological addiction, the process also resides within the person in the sense that internal, neurophysiological cues deriving from tissue deprivation can and often do occur independently of environmental stimuli or cues. But environmental cues may still elicit or enhance body demands for more of the agent to which one is addicted. Habituation has a much closer bond with environmental cues. Breaking a habit is not to be understood as stopping doing something. Breaking a habit consists of *changing* what is done in the presence of cues previously initiating the sequence of behaviors making up the habit. A different behavior is made to occur in response to those cues. If the cues themselves could be eliminated, the habit-breaking process would be much easier, but that is often not possible. We are not often able to radically change our environments. Therefore it becomes essential in habit breaking to learn and to rehearse adequately different and more acceptable behaviors in the presence of the cues that have been eliciting the unwanted habit behavior. A behavior change or habit-breaking process that pays insufficient attention to the role of environmental cues and to the importance of learning *and rehearsing* new responses to those cues will lose much of its effectiveness.

Let it be supposed that the pain cocktail regimen has brought a patient to zero or near-zero and diminishing medication intake levels. For the period of weeks under the cocktail regimen, the patient will have been learning and rehearsing different responses to cues previously leading to taking medication. The learning will have been taking place virtually exclusively in the hospital setting. There will have been little or no exposure to and practice at different responses in the presence of the cues at home and work that previously preceded taking medication. Absence of rehearsal of nonreinforcement (extinction) of the old medication-taking behaviors and absence of reinforcement of the new non–medication-taking behaviors in home and work settings increases the probabilities that the medication habit will be resumed. Systematic rehearsal of new behavior patterns in the environments in which they are to continue to occur is essential. The medication problem just described is virtually identical to that of a heavy smoker who lives in one environment but goes to another to learn to quit smoking. The treatment environment in which he learns to quit is likely to be somewhat different from his natural environment. When he returns home, the desire for a cigarette is likely at first to be acute. The old cues previously long associated with and leading to taking a cigarette are still present. New behaviors have not been rehearsed in their presence. Even a long period of no smoking in the treatment environment is not enough. The upsurge of desire for a cigarette can be expected to be great when the patient returns to the old environment. Environmental cues have potency. We are responsive to them. That dimension to the learning process needs to be taken into account. The person who would break a habit or change behavior needs to practice the new behavior in the presence of the old cues.

Generalization of modified medication-taking behavior

One treatment objective is to maintain the level (from moderate to zero) of pain medication anticipated to be needed in the posttreatment years. Helping the patient to avoid imprudent regimens associated with future illness or pain episodes is a related treatment objective.

Generalization for an inpatient

A patient will begin to go home for intermittent evening and weekend passes in the later stages of inpatient treatment. Alternatively, if the patient's home is too distant, the spouse may come to spend weekends in the vicinity of the treatment setting. In that sense, an element of home will have been brought to the patient. During passes, there is rehearsal of taking the current level of medication outside of the treatment setting. If medication has been faded to zero and the cocktail has been discontinued, the zero level will be experienced in the presence of more normal activity and social interactions than was true in the hospital. When the cocktail is still being taken, although presumably at reduced levels of active ingredients, the new levels of medication will also be rehearsed in a broadening range of company and activity. Patients will have a later phase of outpatient treatment, permitting still more exposure to the old cues previously associated with taking medication. But now there is supervised rehearsal at doing something else, that is, at not taking medication and engaging instead in the activities that have been the objectives of treatment.

Patients who have come from afar for treatment will almost certainly require a period of outpatient treatment after the inpatient phase. This should be close enough to the hospital to permit adequate supervision and feedback. The outpatient phase, all or part of which occurs with the spouse also present, provides for a critically important additional element of generalization rehearsal. This is true in regard to medication behavior as well as other elements of treatment.

The final step to help generalization occur in regard to the taking of medication is to prepare for future pain and illness episodes. Each patient and spouse should receive detailed explanation regarding the time-contingent medicating strategy to be used in the event that future analgesic needs arise. In addition, the referring physician should receive appropriate information and recommendations concerning future management of medications.

Generalization for an outpatient

Freeing a patient of addiction or habituation is considerably more difficult to accomplish on an outpatient basis. True addiction or a strong medication habit ensures that the medication-taking behavior is strongly tied to and triggered by cues in the environment. Patients are often overwhelmed by the strength of the medication-taking response when cues for it arise, either as internal neurophysiological tissue demands or as external habit triggers. On those rare occasions when the task has been tackled on an outpatient basis and with enough success to have brought the patient down to little or no medication intake, the generalization problem may then become easier. Because the patient has continued to reside in his or her natural environment, the medication fading process will have been receiving continuing rehearsal in that environment. Relationships between cues and medication-taking responses will have been diminished and perhaps broken. What remains to be accomplished mainly is to work toward long-term follow-up to be sure that the gains are maintained. Instead of seeking special outpatient rehearsal, arrange for extended follow-up contacts with patient and spouse to ensure maintenance of the reduced intake of medication.

It might happen that treatment was strictly outpatient but outside the patient's normal environment. In that event, the final phase of the program should include a period spent with the spouse but under continuing treatment observation and feedback before the patient returns home.

Generalization of exercise and activity

Generalization of exercise and activity is a two-level problem. The first and narrower level is to establish and maintain a specific exercise program (for example, walking, deep knee bends, pelvic tilts, let-backs) after treatment. The problem is one of helping a particular set of exercises to be continued across time and into other environments. The second level is to broaden the scope of exercise and activity. Exercises prescribed in the early phases of treatment are building blocks or prerequisites to broader activities. The generalization problem is often to encourage the continuation of activity and movement, although not the specific exercises prescribed earlier. A comprehensive contingency management approach to chronic pain will certainly involve this second and broader level of generalization. The first level of generalization will also be involved if selected exercises have been prescribed to continue indefinitely. These will be dealt with separately, although they are closely related.

Continued exercises

Continuation of an exercise program is a straightforward problem. It is likely to be a part of the total treatment approach in any of several situations. One is where a particular exercise or series of exercises is to be continued for an extended period, perhaps indefinitely, in behalf of a particular physical restoration objective. For example, the surgically weakened function of a knee joint may continue to require a particular exercise. A second reason for prescribing posttreatment exercise might be that a long delay is anticipated before a patient will gain access to the broader activities contemplated as promising to keep him or her going. A third possibility is where it is apparent that the posttreatment environment will not provide sufficient stimulation and activity to maintain treatment gains or that the patient's physical status precludes adequate participation in those activities. A case of legitimated retirement illustrates.

The problem here is simply to decide what forms of reinforcement will most effectively (and cost-effectively) maintain an exercise regimen. A patient may realize pleasure or satisfaction at mastering exercise quotas. In that event, all that is likely to be required is to provide the patient with the materials and methods for recording and graphing performance. That step ensures that there will be immediate and precise feedback to the patient as to amount accomplished, for it is delivered by himself.

Additional steps might be taken to involve the spouse in graphing patient performance. That step adds the spouse's (and other family members') reinforcement to patient performance. Graphs can be posted in the home to elicit appropriate social reinforcement from people around the patient.

Continuing although diminishing professional social reinforcement can be built into such a program by providing that performance graphs or some form of performance feedback periodically be sent to the physician. Simple checklists on which the patient reports weekly totals of prescribed exercises completed, mailed bi-weekly to the treatment setting, may suffice. A brief note can be sent back to the patient to provide appropriate encouragement and acknowledgement of effort put forth. Periodic clinic visits will provide yet additional and probably even more potent continuing reinforcement.

The more common method of obtaining continuing performance feedback is for the patient to continue to record on the regular diary forms after treatment, although on a diminishing schedule. Diary recording may be scheduled initially for alternate weeks. The interval between weeks of recording can gradually be lengthened. Some patients find diary recording too demanding a task when they return home and resume more normal activities. In that event a simple checklist may suffice. Fig. 27 portrays one of the early feedback checklists returned by the patient with vulvar pain described on p. 62 and in Fig. 8. The range of activities she reported at the time of follow-up received general confirmation from other

Please check each day which of the activities listed you engaged in.

Week of October 8-14, 197_

	MON	TUES	WED	THUR	FRI	SAT	SUN
1. VISITING							
Came to visit:							
Relative(s)_ _ _ _ _ _ _ _ _ _		✓	✓	✓		✓	✓
Others _ _ _ _ _ _ _ _ _ _ _ _	✓			✓	✓		✓
None _ _ _ _ _ _ _ _ _ _ _ _ _							
Went out to visit:							
Relative (s) _ _ _ _ _ _ _ _ _		✓	✓	✓		✓	
Others _ _ _ _ _ _ _ _ _ _ _ _	✓				✓	✓	
None _ _ _ _ _ _ _ _ _ _ _ _ _							
2. OUTSIDE HOME TRIPS							
Sight-seeing excursion _ _ _ _ _			✓				
Movie, ballgame, concert, etc._ _							✓
Attended meeting _ _ _ _ _ _ _ _				✓			
Shopping _ _ _ _ _ _ _ _ _ _ _	✓	✓	✓	✓	✓	✓	
Other_ _ _ _ _ _ _ _ _ _ _ _ _							
None _ _ _ _ _ _ _ _ _ _ _ _ _							
3. INSIDE HOME ACTIVITIES							
Calls made to relatives/ friends/neighbors_ _ _ _ _ _ _ _	✓	✓	✓	✓	✓	✓	✓
Calls you received from relatives/friends/ neighbors_ _ _ _ _ _ _ _ _ _ _	✓	✓	✓	✓	✓	✓	✓
Reading_ _ _ _ _ _ _ _ _ _ _ _	✓	✓	✓	✓	✓	✓	
Television _ _ _ _ _ _ _ _ _ _	✓	✓	✓	✓	✓		
Radio/records/tape _ _ _ _ _ _ _	✓	✓	✓	✓	✓		
Hobbies - handicrafts_ _ _ _ _ _	✓	✓	✓	✓	✓	✓	
Others _ _ _ _ _ _ _ _ _ _ _ _							
None _ _ _ _ _ _ _ _ _ _ _ _ _							
4. WALKING QUOTA_ _ _ _ _ _ _ _ _ _ _	✓	✓	✓	✓	✓	✓	✓

Fig. 27. Activity diary.

family members. They indicate a marked increase in performance over that reported before admission.

Longer-term arrangements for continued reinforcement of exercise should be preceded by gradual introduction of the exercises into the home setting. Weekend passes in which the exercise regimen is carried out at home in the presence of the spouse make up part of that effort. In the special case of walking, even before the use of passes to promote generalization, efforts should be made to arrange for walking to occur in an ever wider range of settings. The distances to various reference points within the hospital and in the vicinity of the building should be estimated and noted. When the number of laps walked without interruption in a measured course within the treatment setting becomes sufficient, the patient can then begin walking to landmarks or reference points at distances approximating the walking quotas presently achieved. This arrangement offers many advantages. It breaks the monotony of the walking to make the task more pleasant. It provides rehearsal of walking in the presence of others—strangers —thereby permitting further practice of walking without pain behavior displays in public. It lets the naturally occurring stimulus variety inherent in walking over new courses or paths help to take over as sources of sustaining reinforcement. For all of these reasons, cues or stimuli more like the home environment can now be experienced but in the presence of walking instead of pain behavior.

The methods just described illustrate combinations of the patient as his or her own behavioral engineer or reinforcement programmer working with the patient's environment to provide continuing reinforcement of the target behaviors: exercise. In the illustrations, the exercises were ends in themselves and not antecedents to broader ranges of behavior. Had they been the latter, naturally occurring sources of reinforcement might have begun to take over to maintain performance.

Generalization through broadened activities

The prescribed exercises of the early stages of treatment must be linked to the broader behavioral clusters making up post-treatment activity. The overall plan is to exchange exercise, narrowly defined and prescribed at the outset of treatment, for meaningful vocational and avocational or leisure activity. The exchange process should be gradual and programmed systematically to ensure that there is adequate reinforcement to maintain performance during the transitional phase. As a patient becomes established in the target activities and they begin to yield sustaining reinforcement, the interim reinforcement provided by the treatment team can be faded out.

Some broadening of activity is a natural and inherent by-product of the increased activity level generated by treatment. In the hospital setting, for example, as activity level climbs, a patient will almost inevitably begin to interact with more other patients and more hospital staff than was true at the outset. Strolls to the lobby and visiting areas, visits to other patient rooms, coffee in the cafeteria, all are likely to yield some pleasure or stimulus variety and therefore reinforcement for the walking and body movement they involve. But the matter should not be left to chance. Active programming may be needed to ensure that these and other broader activities occur. Which elements of those discussed in the following sections are to be used will depend on the resources of the facility. All of them can be helpful and, where possible, should be used. Each of these avenues toward generalization requires certain minimum performance levels or stages of progress before they can be used prudently and effectively. Particularly, no activity should require a greater amount of energy or physical mobility than presently has been attained by the patient. A patient who can walk but 600 feet without interruption should not have a grounds pass extending more than 300 feet from the ward. A second qualification is that none of the activities discussed should expose the patient to more than casual and incidental reinforcement for pain behavior. The exception is where treatment has progressed to where the special attention of others to pain behavior no longer appears to deter patient activity. For example, two pain patients, each prone to commiserate with the other about the difficulties of walking, should not be allowed to stroll together until each has demonstrated the withholding of commiserating behaviors.

Recreation

Organized recreational programs within the hospital setting are most useful. The recreational therapist needs to be informed of the general nature of the treatment program and of the importance of avoiding social reinforcement or solicitousness at displays of pain behaviors. The approximate amount of uninterrupted standing, walking, and other exercise that the patient is presently able to perform should also be described. The therapist can then be encouraged to engage the patient in recreational activities within the prescribed physical limits.

Many patients long restricted by their pain problems are initially reluctant to enter into recreational programs. It becomes a matter of judgment as to how vigorously to pursue the matter. Sometimes the activity should be prescribed. Make clear that it is an essential part of treatment and not a casual or frivolous effort to entertain the patient. When it is prescribed, and the patient follows the prescription with at least some semblance of cooperation, a particular effort should be made the following day to provide additional acknowledgement and praise for that effort.

Recreational programs can also provide a useful medium in which to promote more effective patient-spouse interaction. The spouse may, for example, rehearse ignoring or tuning out pain behavior and providing social reinforcement for well behavior. Spouse participation in the recrea-

tional program can be invited and even prescribed.

Job stations

The term *job stations,* as used here, refers to unpaid work within the hospital or related facilities. Hospitals, particularly large ones, have within their organization a broad range of jobs routinely being performed. Those work situations or stations provide an important potential opportunity to promote generalization and maintenance of treatment gains.

Questions have been raised about the fairness of using patients as unpaid employees. However, it is important to distinguish between patients in essentially custodial or long-term institutionalization and short-term or transient hospitalization. Some mental hospitals illustrate long-term care. Utilization of patients for extended periods to perform institutional tasks may be exploitative in these kinds of settings. Exploitation is a particular hazard if the work assignment does not have a substantial and clearly stated therapeutic objective.

The situation is different in relation to an operant pain program. Patients are in the institution for brief periods (5 to 7 weeks) and are assigned to job stations for even less time (1 to 5 hours a day for 2 to 4 weeks). More importantly, job station assignments have specific therapeutic objectives. Were there no such therapeutic objectives to job station assignments, no assignments should and would be made. Job stations are essential elements to the process of generalization. Job stations are not for the purpose of replacing paid with unpaid personnel, nor do they exist to help the hospital. Job station assignments help patients.

Before dealing with treatment tactics in relation to job stations, a few administrative matters need to be considered. Administrative approval for developing a job station program requires first that the insurance carrier for the facility be contacted to clear the activity in regard to medical and accident liability matters. The assignment of a patient to clerk in the hospital gift shop, to clean tables in the cafeteria, or to fold sheets in the laundry is a prescribed aspect of treatment. In the medical and accident liability sense, any of those assignments is the equivalent of sending a patient to the x-ray unit for some laboratory procedure or to the occupational therapy room to work at a loom. In each case, accidents could happen. In each case, hospital employees and patients should receive equivalent protection from liability. In each case, the hospital employee is expected to do only his or her normal job; no more, no less. Coverage for patient and for employee should continue in job stations as they do in x-ray units or any place else.

Once administrative approval is obtained and liability coverage is established, the roster of potential job stations needs to be reviewed in regard to the physical demands they provide. Finally, job station supervisors need to be prepared to respond selectively to pain behavior and to activity or well behavior. Only then should patients be assigned.

Job station assignments should be reviewed in relation to posttreatment objectives as well as physical demands and activity generalization. The issue of posttreatment employment is often a sensitive one. There may be legal, financial, and emotional implications that need to be considered. These issues were discussed in Chapters 3 and 5. The immediate issue is that job station assignments may be indicated even where posttreatment employment is not anticipated. Job stations provide useful rehearsal at activity and movement in varied settings apart from any vocational implications. The patient who anticipates that he or she will not be employed and who further anticipates that wage replacement funds are contingent on not working may understandably feel threatened by the prescription of a job station assignment. The precise objectives of that assignment must be made clear. Third-party carriers may also require clari-

fication on this point. A first objective of job station assignment is to provide a graded and controlled level of physical activity of a known character in settings sufficiently varied from the formal treatment setting as to promote generalization. Any vocational implications to the assignment may be totally irrelevant for a given patient. It is also true that job stations *may* provide the additional feature of exposure to and rehearsal at some particular form of work or working condition. A decision to expose a patient to a particular kind of work *may* be part of the preparation for posttreatment employment. If so, that, too, should be made explicit at the outset.

One implication of the various potential functions of job stations is that a given job station assignment need not be consistent with either the patient's posttreatment vocational plans or his or her particular vocational interests. The more a job station assignment does fit in with interests or future plans, the more reinforcing it is likely to be. But exposure to the physical demands of a job station can be a sufficient reason for the assignment in a given case. That, too, needs to be made clear to everyone involved.

Care must be exercised in use of job stations that the total physical load imposed on the patient by the assignment is consistent with what is currently achieved in treatment. Prescribed exercises may be reduced and replaced by corresponding amounts of job station activity. Prescribed exercise may be leveled off and job station load gradually expanded in the movement toward increasing activity levels. Specific limitations of each patient need also to be considered. For example, the patient who presently walks 1000 feet twice per day should not be assigned a job station 1500 feet away.

It is often helpful to deliberately shift a patient from one job station to another to promote additional variety and exposure.

Patients may eventually reach a point during an inpatient or outpatient program in which virtually the whole day is spent on job station assignments. A few days, perhaps a week or so, at such a level is often vital to establish appropriate activity levels. Such a schedule should not be discontinued until the patient seems capable of maintaining an equivalent activity level after treatment. At that point, job station assignments can begin to be faded, replaced by time at home, at work, or in pursuit of employment, depending on the goals of treatment. By that time, formal exercise may have been reduced to token levels or eliminated altogether. Posttreatment exercises to be done on a daily basis should be a part of the overall schedule.

Passes

Passes should become a specific and planned part of inpatient treatment. Other hospital treatment programs provide for passes that are diversionary or at the convenience and wish of the patient. This distinction needs to be made at the outset.

Passes provide learning opportunities. They provide access to generalization. They provide opportunity for rehearsal by patient and family of the behaviors that make up the objectives of treatment. It follows that adequate preparations are essential before passes can be put to work on behalf of treatment objectives.

The generally applicable preparations for the assignment of passes can be stated briefly. There may be additional specific preparations in individual cases, an illustrative few of which will also be noted.

1. Patients coming with problems of addiction, habituation, medication toxicity, or a recent history of utilization of multiple and surreptitious sources of pain medications should not receive passes until there is adequate control over supply and level of intake. That in turn, means that there will have had to be a minimum of a week of inpatient baseline medication observation and an additional week in which to stabilize the pain cocktail schedule. If the first cocktail schedule is more frequent than once each 4 hours, further time will

be needed to bring the patient to a 4-hour schedule. Moreover, family training sessions should have advanced (Chapter 12) to the point that monitoring of intake and supply of pain medications will be effective during the life of a contemplated pass. In short, passes outside the hospital setting should not occur until there is assurance that the cocktail regimen will be strictly adhered to.

2. The physical demands of the pass must be continuous with those presently true in treatment. A pass should result in neither significantly higher nor lower physical demands. For the purposes of this program, a pass is not time out from treatment; it is an extension of treatment. This in turn means that patient recording and spouse observation of activity level and demands during the pass need to be assured. It also means that the pass cannot require performance levels not yet attained in treatment. The most common example of this issue pertains to the patient with distorted gait or who, for other reasons, has thus far achieved only limited amounts of adequate free ambulation. A patient who can walk but 500 feet should not go on a pass that requires 800 feet to the car or from the car to the house. If a patient is in a gait-shaping program providing for interim use of a wheelchair and it is decided to prescribe an evening or weekend pass (rarely a wise decision when the patient is still wheelchair-bound), there must be assurances that the same restrictions on walking prevail during the pass as apply in treatment. Patient and spouse need to agree to these constraints.

3. Patients who have spouses or other family members who previously effectively reinforced pain behaviors or inhibited activity and well behavior should not go on passes with those people until progress has been made in spouse or family retraining. The first pass should be deferred until the spouse has progressed in the retraining program (Chapter 12) to where patient pain behaviors are effectively counted, recorded, and tuned out. Thereafter, passes become

rehearsal opportunities for the stages of spouse training currently reached.

Exceptional circumstances may arise that warrant authorizing a pass when the preceding three criteria are not met. Those circumstances should, however, pertain to matters outside the domain of treatment, for example, urgent family business. Pressing requests for a pass from patient or spouse because someone is lonely or "the patient needs to get away from the hospital for awhile" should not be acceded to. If the pass means that much, it can be considered a reinforcer to be made contingent on some element of performance. A patient who has been progressing slowly in, for example, the increase of uninterrupted walking, may find extra incentive for those efforts by knowing one requirement for a pass may be to walk 1000 feet without pausing. Determined effort by a patient toward the first pass may even justify a slight increase in daily walking quota increments.

The planning of a pass should incorporate immediate treatment issues. The pass is a learning and rehearsal opportunity. What is to be rehearsed or learned should be thought through and provided for. The possibilities are endless. Some of the more common examples concern arranging that a particular activity occur, commensurate with currently attained exercise levels. A patient having difficulty riding more than 20 miles in a car may be ready for a 25-mile ride. That ride can become a prescribed part of the pass. A patient having difficulty sitting more than an hour may be ready for a 2-hour movie. A patient having difficulty standing at a sink or kitchen table to prepare a meal may be ready for a 30-minute stint at preparing each of the weekend dinners.

Each pass should be followed up by a session with the spouse from which to gain feedback as to whether performance assignments and constraints set for the pass were met.

Before departing on a pass, each patient should be checked to ensure that there is an adequate supply of pain cocktail for the length of the pass and that diary forms and other performance recording supplies are taken along.

The role of the spouse in the pass as part of the spouse retraining program and of the patient in regard to that program was considered in Chapter 12.

The end of treatment: final phase of programmed generalization

The transition from intensive inpatient care to final termination of treatment should be as gradual and continuous as practically possible. The inpatient phase should be followed by a minimum of a week of outpatient care in which the patient remains committed to the treatment program virtually full time. He or she should spend most of each day at job stations or in exercise and other prescribed activities. A patient who lives at a distance can reside in a hotel or rooming house facility within easy commuting distance from the hospital during the outpatient phase. As noted previously, the spouse should be present for much and, if possible, all of that outpatient week. During that interval evenings are programmed, just as if they were evening passes from the hospital. Spouse retraining and feedback sessions continue, usually on an intensified basis, perhaps with daily sessions.

Patients living within commuting distance of the hospital may reside at home during the outpatient phase. The first week of that phase should have a nearly full-time treatment schedule; the patient comes daily and spends most of the day at the various treatment activities. That in turn means that the home schedule will have to be regulated such that the patient does not resume significant additional demands at home. For example, if the patient is the wife, during the first outpatient week the family should continue with whatever homemaking arrangements were made during the patient's absence for inpatient treatment. Typically, the outpatient load can begin to diminish rapidly. As treatment time and load is reduced, it should be replaced by corresponding amounts of nontreatment activity. The fading pattern by which treatment time is reduced may take many forms. Often the easiest is for the patient to come 3 days the second week of outpatient treatment and 2 days the third. The third week may begin with a final outpatient recheck and, if no further intervention is indicated, treatment ends, except for periodic follow-up clinic rechecks.

Parallel with the fading of formal treatment, there should be a continuing concern with implementing access to posttreatment activities. Vocational training or placement efforts may be underway. An increasing range of social or recreational plans may be receiving repeated rehearsals.

The demarcation between outpatient treatment and long-range follow-up is often arbitrary. Some patients may require indefinite periodic clinic visits to bolster the patient or spouse or to assess the maintenance of gains. Other patients may require protracted, although infrequent, clinic follow-up to help maintain momentum until long-range objectives become accessible, for example, until job retraining is completed or job placement succeeds.

Patients will sometimes experience flareups of the pain problem many months after treatment. These episodes may necessitate reinstituting elements of formal treatment. The clinical experience thus far accumulated indicates that these later episodes usually require but a few days of treatment. The patient returns for a brief inpatient period. Exercise quotas can be reinstituted. Increments usually can proceed at a much more rapid rate. Spouse training is reviewed and perhaps brushed up.

More often than not, these flare-up episodes relate to some failure of performance by others in the patient's home or work setting. Job objectives failed to materialize. Leisure and recreational objectives did not prove to be as accessible as had been anticipated. The patient's spouse had not maintained effective reinforcement of activity. The patient's home physician, failing adequately to appreciate the importance of avoiding pain-contingent rest, medications, and special professional attention, had responded to pain behaviors (or some other illness episode) in ways that fostered a resumption of operant pain problems.

A review of the situation usually reveals the source of the renewal of operant pain. A few days of treatment are usually sufficient to reestablish treatment gains and to work through the problems and the remedies with the other people involved.

Bibliography

Albee, G.: Give us a place to stand and we will move the earth (president's message), Clin. Psychol. **20**:1-4, 1966.

Ayllon, T., and Michael, J.: The psychiatric nurse as a behavioral engineer, J. Exp. Anal. Behav. **2**:323-334, 1960.

Baer, D., and Wolf, M.: The entry into natural communities of reinforcement in achieving generality of behavioral change, Symposium presented at meeting of American Psychological Association, Washington, D. C., Sept., 1967.

Bandura, A.: Behavioral modifications through modeling procedures. In Krasner, L., and Ullmann, L. P., editors: Research in behavior modification, New York, 1965, Holt, Rinehart & Winston. pp. 310-340.

Bandura, A., and Walters, R.: Social learning and personality development, New York, 1963, Holt, Rinehart & Winston, Inc.

Beecher, H. K.: Measurement of subjective responses: quantitative effects of drugs, New York, 1959, Oxford University Press.

Berni, R., and Fordyce, W.: Behavior modification and the nursing process, St. Louis, 1973, The C. V. Mosby Co.

Birk, L., editor: Seminars in psychology: biofeedback: behavioral medicine, vol. 5, no. 4, New York, Nov., 1973, Grune & Stratton, Inc.

Bonica, J. J.: The management of pain, Philadelphia, 1953, Lea & Febiger.

Bonica, J. J.: Fundamental considerations of chronic pain therapy, Post-Grad. Med., **53**:81-85, May, 1973.

Bonica, J. J., editor: The management of pain, ed. 2, Philadelphia, 1975, Lea & Febiger. (In press.)

Bond, M.: The relation of pain to the Eysenck Personality Inventory, Cornell Medical Index, and Whitely Index of Hypochondriasis, Br. J. Psychiatry **119**:671, 1971.

Butcher, J. N., editor: MMPI: research developments and clinical applications, New York, 1969, McGraw-Hill Book Co.

Christopherson, V.: Socio-cultural correlates of pain response, final report of project no. 1390, Vocational Rehabilitation Administration, Washington, D. C., 1966, U. S. Dept. of Health, Education, and Welfare.

Clark, W. C., and Hunt, H. F.: Pain. In Downey, J. A., and Darling, R. C., editors: Physiological basis of rehabilitation medicine. Philadelphia, W. B. Saunders Co. 1971, pp. 373-401.

Clark, W. C., and Mehl, L.: Thermal pain: a sensory decision theory analysis of the effect of age and sex on d', various response criteria, and 50 per cent pain threshold, J. Abnorm. Psychol. **78**:202-212, 1971.

Dahlstrom, W., Welsh, G., and Dahlstrom, L.: An MMPI handbook, rev. ed., Minneapolis, 1972, University of Minnesota Press.

Diller, L.: Cognitive and motor aspects of handicapping conditions in the neurologically impaired. In Neff, W., editor: Rehabilitation psychology, Washington, D. C., 1971, American Psychological Association, pp. 1-32.

Engel, G.: Psychogenic pain and the pain-prone patient, Am. J. Med. **26**:899, 1959.

Ferster, C.: Classification of behavioral pathology. In Krasner, L., and Ullmann, L., editors: Research in behavior modification, New York, 1966, Holt, Rinehart & Winston, Inc.

Ferster, C., and Skinner, B. F.: Schedules of reinforcement, New York, 1957, Appleton-Century-Crofts.

Fordyce, W.: An operant conditioning method for managing chronic pain, Postgrad. Med. **53**:123-128, 1973.

Fordyce, W.: Treating chronic pain by contingency management. In Bonica, J., editor: Advances in neurology, vol. 4, International Symposium on Pain, New York, 1974, Raven Press, pp. 585-87.

Fordyce, W., Brena, S., DeLateur, B., Holcombe, S., and Loeser, J.: Diagnostic judgments of chronic pain and MMPI and activity level measures. (In press.)

Fordyce, W., Fowler, R., Lehmann, J., and Delateur, B.: Some implications of learning in problems of chronic pain, J. Chron. Dis. **21**:179-190, 1968.

Fordyce, W., Fowler, R., Lehmann, J., Delateur, B., Sand, P. and Trieschmann R.: Operant conditioning in the treatment of chronic clinical pain, Arch. Phys. Med. Rehab. **54**:399-408, 1973.

Fowler, R. S., Jr.: Biofeedback in the treatment of pain. In Bonica, J. J., editor: The management of pain, ed. 2, Philadelphia, 1975, Lea & Febiger. (In press.)

Gannon, L., and Sternbach, R.: Alpha enhancement as a treatment for pain: a case study, J. Behav. Ther. Exp. Psychiatry 2:209-213, 1971.

Gendlin, E., and Rychlak, J.: Psychotherapeutic processes, Ann. Rev. Psychol. 21:155-190, 1970.

Green, D. M., and Swets, J.: Signal detection theory and psychophysics, New York, 1966, John Wiley & Sons, Inc.

Green, E., Green, A., and Walters, E.: Self-regulation of internal states. In Rose, J., editor: Progress of cybernetics, Chapters VII-XVI, Proceedings of the International Congress of Cybernetics, London, 1961, London, 1970, Gordon & Breach Science Publishers, Ltd.

Hass, H., Fink, H., and Harfelder, G.: Das Placeboproblem, Fortschr. Arzneimittel forschung 1:279-454, 1959. Translation of selected parts in Psychopharmacol. Service Center Bull. 2:1-65, 1963.

Herman, R. M., Krusen Research Center, Moss Rehabilitation Hospital, Philadelphia, Pa.: Interview, 1973.

Hilgard, E. R.: Pain as a puzzle for psychology and physiology, Am. Psychol. 24:103-113, 1969.

Hill, H. E., Kornetsky, C. H., Flanary, H. G., and Wilder, A.: Effects of anxiety and morphine on the discrimination of intensities of pain, J. Clin. Invest. 31:473-480, 1952.

Janis, I.: Psychological stress, New York, 1958, John Wiley & Sons, Inc.

Kamiya, J.: Operant control of the EEG alpha rhythm and some of its reported effects on consciousness. In Tart, C., editor: Altered states of consciousness, New York, 1969, John Wiley & Sons, Inc.

Kanfer, F. H., and Goldfoot, D. A.: Self-control and tolerance of noxious stimulation, Psychol. Rep. 18:79-85, 1966.

Kast, E. C., and Collins, V. J.: A theory of human pathologic pain and its measurement: the analgesic activity of methotrimeprazine, J. New Drugs 6:142-148, May-June, 1966.

Kolb, L.: The painful phantom: psychology, physiology and treatment, Springfield, Ill., 1954, Charles C Thomas, Publisher.

Krasner, L., and Ullmann, L.: Research in behavior modification, New York, 1966, Holt, Rinehart & Winston, Inc.

Lasagna, L.: Clinical measurement of pain, Ann. N. Y. Acad. Sci. 86:28-37, March, 1960.

Lazarus, A.: Learning theory and the treatment of depression, Behav. Res. Ther. 6:83-90, 1968.

LeShan, L.: The world of the patient in severe pain of long duration, J. Chron. Dis. 17:119, 1954.

Lewinsohn, P., and Atwood, G.: Depression: a clinical-research approach, Presented at Washington-Oregon Psychological Associations joint meeting, Crystal Mountain, Washington, May, 1968.

Lindsley, O.: Interview, 1969.

Livingston, W. K.: Pain mechanisms, New York, 1943, The Macmillan Co.

Loeser, J. D.: Neurosurgical relief of chronic pain, Postgrad. Med. 53:115-119, May, 1973.

McGlashan, T., Evans, F., and Orne, M.: The nature of hypnotic, analgesia, and placebo responses to experimental pain, Psychosomatic Med. 31:227-246, 1969.

Meldman, J.: Diseases of attention and perception, Elmsford, N.Y., 1970, Pergamon Press, Inc.

Melzack, R.: The perception of pain, Sci. Am. 204:41-49, Feb., 1961.

Melzack, R.: Pain. In Sills, D. L., editor: International encyclopedia of the social sciences, vol. 2, New York, 1968, The Macmillan Co., pp. 357-364.

Melzack, R., and Chapman, C.: Psychological aspects of pain, Postgrad. Med. 53:69-75, May, 1973.

Melzack, R., and Wall, P. D.: On the nature of cutaneous sensory mechanisms, Brain 85:331-356, 1962.

Melzack, R., and Wall, P. D.: Pain mechanisms: a new theory, Science 150:971-979, 1965.

Mendell, L. M., and Wall, P. D.: Presynaptic hyperpolarization: a role for fine afferent fibers, J. Physiol. 172:274-294, 1964.

Merskey, H., and Spear, F. G.: Pain: psychological and psychiatric aspects, Baltimore, 1967, The Williams & Wilkins Co.

Miller, N.: Learning of visceral and glandular responses, Science 163:434-445, 1969.

Mischel, W.: Personality and assessment, New York, 1968, John Wiley & Sons, Inc., pp. 146-147.

Mortimer, J. T.: Pain suppression in man by dorsal column electroanalgesia, Ph.D. dissertation, School of Engineering, Cleveland, 1968, Case Western Reserve University.

Nesbitt, R. and Schacter, S.: Cognitive manipulation of pain, J. Exp. Soc. Psychol. 2:227-236, 1966.

Neuringer, C., and Michael, J., editors: Behavior modification in clinical psychology, New York, 1970, Appleton-Century-Crofts.

Noordenbos, W.: Pain, New York, 1959, American Elsevier Publishing Co., Inc.

Pilling, L. F., Brannick, T. L., and Swenson, W. M.: Psychologic characteristics of psychiatric patients having pain as a presenting symptom, Can. Med. Assoc. J. 97:387-394, 1967.

Pilowsky, I.: Dimension of hypochondriasis, Br. J. Psychiatry 113:89, 1967.

Premack, D.: Toward empirical behavior laws: I. Positive reinforcement, Psychol. Rev. **66**:219-233, 1959.

Reitan, R., and Davison, L. A., editors: Clinical neuropsychology: current status and applications, New York, 1974, Halsted Press, Division of John Wiley & Sons, Inc.

Sachs, L. B.: Comparison of hypnotic analgesia and hypnotic relaxation during stimulation by a continuous pain source, J. Abnorm. Psychol. **76**:206-210, 1970.

Shealy, C. N., Mortimer, J., and Hagfors, N.: Dorsal column electroanalgesia, J. Neurosurg. **32**:560-564, 1970.

Skinner, B. F.: Science and human behavior, New York, 1953, The Macmillan Co.

Sternbach, R.: Congenital insensitivity to pain, Psychol. Bull. **60**:252-264, 1963.

Sternbach, R.: Pain: a psychophysiological analysis, New York, 1968, Academic Press, Inc., p. 5.

Sternbach, R., and Fordyce, W.: Psychogenic pain. In Bonica, J. J., editor: The management of pain, ed. 2, Philadelphia, 1975, Lea & Febiger. (In press.)

Sternbach, R., Murphy, R., Akeson, W., and Wolfe, S.: Chronic low back pain: characteristics of the "low-back loser," Postgrad. Med. **53**:135-138, May, 1973.

Sternbach, R., Wolf, S., Murphy, R., and Wolfe, S.: istics of the "low-back loser," Postgrad. Med. S.: Aspects of low back pain, Psychosomatics **14**:226-229, 1973.

Stolov, W., and Patout, C.: Unpublished case study, Department of Rehabilitation Medicine, Seattle, 1972, University of Washington.

Stolov, W., and Simons, D.: Unpublished case study, Department of Rehabilitation Medicine, Seattle, 1973, University of Washington.

Swenson, W. H., Pearson, J., and Osborne, D.: An MMPI source book: basic item, scale, and pattern data on 50,000 medical patients, Minneapolis, 1973, University of Minnesota Press.

Szasz, T.: Pain and pleasure: a study of bodily feelings, New York, 1957, Basic Books, Inc.

Tinling, D., and Klein, R.: Psychogenic pain and aggression: the syndrome of the solitary hunter, Psychosom. Med. **28**:738, 1966.

Trieschmann, R., Stolov, W., and Montgomery, E.: An approach to the treatment of abnormal ambulation resulting from conversion reaction, Arch. Phys. Med. Rehab. **51**:198-206, April, 1970.

Ullmann, L., and Krasner, L., editors: Case studies in behavior modification, New York, 1965, Holt, Rinehart & Winston, Inc.

Ulrich, R., Stachnik, T., and Mabry, J.: Control of human behavior, Glenview, Ill., 1966, Scott, Foresman and Co.

Wall, P. D.: The origin of a spinal-cord slow potential, J. Physiol. (Lond.) **164**:508-526, 1962.

Welsh, G. S., and Dahlstrom, W. G., editors: Basic readings on the MMPI in psychology and medicine, Minneapolis, 1956, University of Minnesota Press.

Woodforde, J., and Merskey, H.: Personality traits of patients with chronic pain, J. Psychosom. Res. **16**:167, 1972.

Appendix A

DIARY ANALYSIS FORM

Name _____
Hosp. Number _____

Week in ___ out ___ No. ___	Sitting	Walking	Uptime	Reclining	Don't Know		Week in ___ out ___ No. ___	Sitting	Walking	Uptime	Reclining	Don't Know
TOTAL							TOTAL					
Avg/Day							$\bar{x}$/Day					

Week in ___ out ___ No. ___	Sitting	Walking	Uptime	Reclining	Don't Know		Week in ___ out ___ No. ___	Sitting	Walking	Uptime	Reclining	Don't Know
TOTAL							TOTAL					

Appendix B

DAILY DIARY PAGE

Day of Week _____

Date _____

Midnight	SITTING Major Activity	SITTING Time	WALKING Major Activity	WALKING Time	RECLINING Activity	RECLINING Time
12 - 1						
1 - 2						
2 - 3						
3 - 4						
4 - 5						
A.M. 5 - 6						
6 - 7						
7 - 8						
8 - 9						
9 - 10						
10 - 11						
11 - 12						
NOON 12 - 1						
1 - 2						
2 - 3						
3 - 4						
4 - 5						
P.M. 5 - 6						
6 - 7						
7 - 8						
8 - 9						
9 - 10						
10 - 11						
11 - 12						
TOTAL						= 24

Index

A

Acquisition of operant pain, 41-73
Activity(ies); *see also* Exercise(s)
  changes in, as result of pain, 133-136
  diary of, 215
  discouraging of, in behavioral analysis of pain
    behavior, 128-129
  generalization of, 213-216
  increasing, in respondent pain, 153-154
  levels of; *see* Activity level(s)
  modification of, by pain patients, 134-135
  -pain time interval, 130-131
  pain-free plans for, 135
  reinforcement for, 173-174
    and pain behavior, spouse count of, 207
  of spouse
    modification of, 135-136
    reinforcement of, and well behavior, 209-210
Activity level(s)
  definition of, 109
  increase in, 109-111
    exercise and, 168-183
      procedure for, 170-181
    reduction of excessive, 181-183
      procedure for, 182-183
  treatment goals related to, 110
Addiction
  managing pain medications and, 157-167
  reducing, in respondent pain, 153-154
Ambulation
  generalization of, 187
  increased, and wheelchair fading, 187
  training in, 185-187
    procedures for, 186-187
Amitriptyline (Elavil), 160
Analgesia; *see also* Medication(s)
  hypnotic, 21, 22
  placebo effects and, 22
Anger as response to pain in childhood, 30
Antidepressants, 160-161
Anxiety
  and depression in pain, 29-31
  and pain
    discrimination between, 31-32
    level of, 15
    perception of, 23
Attention
  contingent, procedures for, 192-195

Attention—cont'd
  outpatient, management of, 195
  as reinforcer, 87-89
  and social responsiveness, 154-155, 190-210
  from visitors and other patients, 194-195
Attentional approach to pain, 20
Aversive consequences and avoidance behavior,
    60-61
Aversive learning and treatment goals, 118
Avoidance behavior
  pain behavior as, 64-69
  persistence of, 61
Avoidance learning, 60-69

B

Baseline(s)
  in assessing behavior change, 81
  for exercise and increasing activity
    inpatient, 170
    outpatient, 171
  in patient modification of spouse behavior, 196
  for reducing excessive activity, 182
  for self-control of pain behavior displays, 196
  in shaping rapid walking, 188
Behavior(s)
  attention-seeking, in illness and pain, 20
  avoidance, 60-69
    pain behavior as, 64-69
  change in, 77-98; *see also* Behavior change
  chronic illness and, 3-4
  counting of, 80-82
  decreasing or weakening, 79-80
  definition of, 1, 76
  and environmental events, relation between, 41
  expressions of pain as, 1
  generalization of new, 43
  increasing or strengthening of, 79
  learned, pain as, 151-153
  medication-taking, modified, generalization of,
    212-213
  nurturant parental, pain-contingent, 47-48
  as operants, 44
  pain
    as avoidance behavior, 64-69, 109, 127-128;
      see also Operant(s)
    avoidance learning and, 60-69
    compensation as reinforcer of, 52
    cost factors in, 113-115

Behavior(s)—cont'd
  pain—cont'd
    counting of, and attention and social responsiveness, 206-208
    current reinforcement of, 50-60
    decreasing roster of, 78
    in describing pain, 28
    direct reinforcement of, 45, 128
    distorted gait as, 184-185
    environmental effect of, 107-108
    exercise and activity as reinforcer of, 57-60
    family responses to, as current reinforcement, 50-52
    increasing activity levels and, 109-111
    legitimation of, 113-114
    medical diagnosis and, 120-121
    medication as reinforcer of, 53-57
    as operants, 38
    and pain, distinction between, 103
    -pain stimulus linkage, 28
    and personality traits, differentiation of, 121
    physician's behavior as reinforcer of, 53-57
    reduction of, 105-109
      and functional impairment, 109-111
    reinforcement of; *see* Reinforcement
    self-control of displays of, 195-196
    spouse count of, and reinforcement of activity, 207
    systematic, and environmental consequence sequences in search for operant pain, 124
    target, for behavior change, 105; *see also* Behaviors, target
    treatment goals and, 103-119
    verbal and nonverbal, 12-14
      conditioning and discrepancy between, 12-13
    withdrawing attention to, 208-209
  pain as, 76
  pain-related health care utilization, reduction of, 111-117
  pinpointing of, 76-77
  respondent, distinguished from operant, 36-37
  of spouse, patient modification of, 196-197
  target
    for behavior change, 105
    identification of, in contingency management treatment programs, 143-144
    in patient modification of spouse behavior, 196
    in reducing excessive activity, 182
    of spouse and family, in attention and social responsiveness, 205-206
  well
    definition of, 117
    effective, promotion and maintenance of, 117-119
    failure of, to receive positive reinforcement, 45
    gaps in, 143-144
    increasing range of, 78

Behavior(s)—cont'd
  well—cont'd
    nonreinforcement of, 69-72
    positive reinforcement of, 42
    punishing of, 128-129
    reduction of gaps in, 155
    reinforcers and maintenance of, 118
    spouse reinforcement of activity and, 209-210
Behavior change; *see also* Behavior analysis; Contingency management treatment program(s)
  activity level as indicator of, 109-110
  analysis of problems in, 77-78
  in chronic illness, 3-4, 6
  baseline in assessing, 81
  and behavioral analysis, techniques of, 74-100
  counting behavior and, 80-82
    movement cycle in, 80-81, 82
  decreasing or weakening behavior and, 79-80
  ethical issues in, 74-75
  family readiness to support, 144-145
  and functional impairment, reduction of, 109-111
  generalization and, 95-98
  increasing or strengthening behavior and, 79
  increasing well behaviors and, 78
  in pain-related health care utilization behaviors, 111-117
  programming environment to maintain performance and, 97
  programs of, monitoring and evaluation of, 98-99
  and promotion and maintenance of effective well behaviors, 117-119
  reduction of well behaviors, 105-109
  reinforcers and; *see* Reinforcement; Reinforcer(s)
  self-control and, 96-97
  schedules of reinforcement and, 89-94
  shaping behaviors and, 78-79
  target behaviors and; *see* Target behaviors
  treatment goals in, 103-119
  vocational counseling and, 117-118
Behavior modification; *see* Behavior change; Contingency management treatment program
Behavior influence factors
  behavioral model, 38-40
  motivational model, 36-38
Behavioral analysis
  of activity-pain time interval, 130-131
  and behavior change, techniques of, 74-100
  changes in activity as result of pain and, 133-136
  of chronic pain, 45-46
  direct reinforcement of pain behavior and, 128
  discouraging activity and, 128-129
  disease model and, 120-122
  diurnal time patterns and, 127
  environmental responses and, 128-129
  episodic pain and, 125
  family role in, 123-124
  interview guide for, 125-137

Behavioral analysis—cont'd
  interviewer set in, 122-137
  issues determined by, 124
  modeling in, 49-50
  nocturnal awakening and, 126
  nocturnal medications and, 126-127
  nocturnal time patterns and, 125
  pain activators and, 129-131
    roster of, 130
  of pain behavior, 120-140; *see also* Pain be-
      havior
  pain diminishers and, 131
  patient diaries and, 123, 137
  psychological tests and, 137-140
  punishing of well behavior and, 128-129
  reasons for performing, 120-122
  respondent pain and, 120-121
  schematic criteria for patient selection in, 121
  supplemental data for, 137-140
  tension and relaxation in, 132-133
  of time patterns of pain, 125-127
Behavioral concepts
  biofeedback and, 5
  and chronic pain, conceptual background, 9-
      100
  health care system and, 103-119
  and mental illness and retardation, 4-5
  and pain, relationship between, 1
Biofeedback, 5
  in reducing respondent pain, 106-108

C

Childhood pain experiences, 29-30
  direct and positive reinforcement of pain be-
      haviors in, 46-50
Chronic illness; *see also* Chronic pain
  and chronic pain, 3
  conditioning and, 6
Chronic pain; *see also* Pain
  activators of, 129-131
    roster of, 130
  activity-pain time interval in, 130-131
  anxiety and, 15, 29, 30-31
  behavior and; *see* Pain behavior(s)
  behavioral analysis of, 45-46
  behavioral concepts and, 1-2
  changes in activity as result of, 133-136
  and chronic illness, 3
  as clinical problem, 11-25
  conceptual background, 9-100
  conditioning and, 6, 26; *see also* Conditioning
  cost factors in, 113-115
  cultural identity as factor in response to, 15
  depression and, 29, 30-31
  diminishers of, 131
  disease model perspective and, 33-36
  episodic, 125
  evaluation of, 101-146
  family involvement and, 8; *see also* Family(ies)
      of chronic pain patients; Spouse(s) of
      chronic pain patients

Chronic pain—cont'd
  as form of chronic illness, 6
  health care system and, 53-60, 103-119
  increased emotional distress accompanying, 35-
      36
  medical diagnoses of, as probability statements,
      120-121
  nocturnal awakening in, 126
  nocturnal medications and, 126-127
  orienting patient and spouse to treatment of,
      150-153
  patients with; *see* Pain patients
  reporting of, 11-14
  tension and relaxation in, 132-133
  time patterns in, 125-127
    nocturnal, 125
  treatment of, 147-221
  verbal reports of, 14
Chronicity
  behavior change and, 3-4
  conditioning and, 26
  learning opportunities attendant on, 6
  legitimating process and, 113-114
Cold pressor test, 19
Communications problems in behavior analysis,
    122-123
Compensation as current reinforcer, 52-53
Conditioning
  as aspect of chronicity, 26
  childhood pain experiences and, 29-31
  in chronic pain, 6
  and discrepancy between verbal and nonverbal
      pain behaviors, 12-14
  discrimination and, 115
  effects of, as temporary, 42
  exercise viewed in terms of, 168
  history of, in pain perception, 18-19
  operant
    explanation of, to patient and spouse, 151-153
    principles of, 38
    time-limited characteristics of learning and,
        42
  prior emotional, in diagnosis of pain, 29-32
  stimulus-specific effects and, 42
  systematic, in reducing respondent pain, 105-
      108
Contingency management treatment programs; *see
    also* Behavior change
  behaviors to be changed in, 142-143
  for distorted gait, 184-189
  exercise in, 168-183
  family readiness to support change and, 144-145
  for reducing excessive activity levels, 182-183
  and reinforcers, identification of, 143
  selection of patients for, 141-145
  target behaviors in, 143-144
Contingent attention, 192-195
Continuity and change, personal, 7
Cost factors in chronic pain, 113-115

Counter-stimulation in reduction of respondent pain, 105-106
Counting behavior, 80-82
  movement cycle and, 80, 81, 82
Cultural patterns and response to pain, 23-24
Current reinforcement of pain behavior, 50-60

D

Data kit for performance graphs and records, 198
Decreasing or weakening behavior, 79-80
Delayed reinforcement (token or point systems), 94-95
Depression, 72-73
  and anxiety in pain, 29-31
  and pain perception, 23
Diaries, patient
  of activity, 215
  in behavior analysis, 137
  daily, sample page of, 226
  form for analysis of, 225
  medication data from, 158
  for performance graphs and records, 198
Diminishing ratio schedule of reinforcement, 91-93
Direct and positive reinforcement of pain behavior, 46-60, 128; *see also* Reinforcement; Reinforcer(s)
Discrepancies between verbal and nonverbal pain behaviors, 12-14
Discrimination learning, 115-116
Disease model perspective on pain, 35-36
  in behavioral analysis, 120-122
Distorted gait
  ambulation training in, 185-187
  falling and the incompatible response in treatment of, 187-189
  as operant, 184
  as problem of shaping, 184-189
Distress and feeling states, 31
Doxepin (Sinequan), 160

E

Elavil; *see* Amitriptyline
Environmental responses and chronic pain, 128-129
Episodic pain, 125
Ethical issues in behavioral modification, 74-75
Ethyl chloride spray, 166
Evaluation, 101-147; *see also* Behavioral analysis
  and behavioral analysis of pain, 120-140
  data from, related to patient selection criteria, 141-145
  disease model and, 120-122
  monitoring behavior change programs, 98-99
  pain patient expectations of, 122
  and patient selection, 141-145
  treatment goals and, 103-119
Exercise(s); *see also* Activity(ies)
  accessibility of, 169
  and activity, as reinforcers of pain behavior, 57-60

Exercise(s)—cont'd
  continued, 214-216
  generalization of, 213-216
  and increased activity levels, 168-183
    procedure for, 170-181
  increment rates and, 172-173
  initial treatment quotas, 171-172
  inpatient baselines for, 170
  management of quota failures in, 174-179
  medical or neurophysiological constraints to, 168
  outpatient baselines for, 171
  pain-relevant, 169
  programming pain-related treatment procedures, 180-181
  quadricep, 173
  quantification of, 169
  and quota adjustments
    to meet quota failures, 177
    for other illness events, 179-180
  quota ceilings, in movement to other forms of activity, 179
  quotas and performance, recording of, 199
  reduced to movement cycles, 169
  reduction of excessive activity levels, 181-183
    procedure for, 182-183
  reinforcement for, 173-174
  selection of, 168-181
  tolerance for, 170
  typical range of, 169-170
Expectations and perception of pain, 20

F

Fading, 93-94
  of active ingredients in management of medications, 160-162
  wheelchair, and increasing ambulation, 187
Falling and the incompatible response, 187-189
Family(ies) of chronic pain patients; *see also* Spouse(s) of chronic pain patients
  and attention and social responsiveness, training in, 204-210
  current reinforcement and, 50-60
  direct reinforcement of pain behavior by, 128
  discouraging activity (punishing of well behavior) by, 128-129
  readiness of, to support change, 144-145
  reinforcement and, from performance graphs and records, 197-204
  role of, in behavioral analysis, 123-124
Fixed interval schedules of reinforcement, 90
Functional impairment, reduction of, 109-111

G

Gaining access to naturally occurring reinforcers, 97-98
Gait, distorted
  ambulation training and, 185-187
  as operant, 184
  as problem of shaping, 184-189

Gate control theory of pain, 16-18
  in reduction of respondent pain, 105-106
  time dimension of, 16-17
Generalization, 95-98
  of exercise and activity, 213-216
  for inpatients, 213
  job stations in, 217-219
  and maintenance of performance, 211-221
  methods for achieving, 211
  of modified medication-taking behavior, 212-213
  for outpatients, 213
  passes and, 219-220
  programmed, final phase of, 220-221
  of recreation, 217
  through broadened activities, 216-220
Glyceryl guaiacolate (Robitussin) in pain cock-
    tail, 159
Graph(s), 202-204
  and performance records, reinforcement and
    feedback from, 197-204
  reinforcement function of, 203-204

H

Habituation
  managing pain medications and, 157-167
  pain medications and
    management of, 157-167
    pain cocktail for respondent or operant pain,
      154
    reducing, in problems of respondent pain, 153-
      154
Health care system
  attention and social responsiveness in treatment
    and, 190-210
  behavioral concepts and pain related to, 103-119
  and health-contingent payoffs, 116
  pain-related use of, reduction of, 111-117
  and reinforcement of pain behaviors, 53-60
Hypnotic analgesia, 21, 22
Hypochondriasis, 30

I

Iatrogenic reinforcement, 53-60
  medication as, 53-57
Illness
  attentional approach to, 20
  chronic, and conditioning, 6
  chronicity and, 3-4
  mental, and retardation, behavioral concepts ap-
    plied to, 4-5
Increasing activity level (reduction of functional
    impairment), 109-111
Increasing or strengthening behavior, 19
Increment rates for exercise, 172-173
Indirect but positive reinforcement of pain be-
    haviors, 60-69
Inpatient(s)
  baselines for, in exercise and increasing activity,
    170
  generalization for, 213
Interviewer set in behavioral analysis, 122-137

J

Job stations and generalization, 217-219

L

Learning; *see also* Behavior change; Conditioning
  automatic character of, 31-32
  avoidance, 60-69
  discrimination, 115-116
  modeling as source of, 49
  time-limited character of, 42
Learning model approach, 39-40
Lidocaine (Xylocaine), 166

M

Measurement of pain, 21-23
  signal detection theory of, 21
Measurement of progress (and of pain), 204
Medication(s)
  antidepressants, 160-161
  as iatrogenic reinforcer, 53-57
  management of, in treatment, 157-167
    baseline in, 158-159
    data from patient diaries and, 158
    delivery schedule and, 159-160
    fading active ingredients and, 160-162
      long-term, 162
    inpatient/outpatient decision in, 157-158
    pain cocktail and, 159
      common problems and exceptions in use
        of, 163-167
      end of regimen for, 162
      maintenance of regimen for, 162
      simple regimen for, 161
    procedures for, 158-162
    and strategies for future pain events, 162-163
    time-contingent regimen and, 159
  nocturnal, 126-127
  pain, and pain cocktail for addicted/habituated
    patients, 154
  pain behaviors and, 112-113
  as pain diminishers, 131-132
  reduction of addiction/habituation in respon-
    dent pain, 153-154
  -taking behavior, modified, generalization of,
    212-213
Mental illness and retardation, behavioral concepts
    applied to, 4-5
Minnesota Multiphasic Personality Inventory
  as adjunct to behavioral analysis, 137-140
  findings in, and chronic pain patients, 35
MMPI; *see* Minnesota Multiphasic Personality In-
    ventory
Modeling
  in behavioral analysis of pain, 49-50
  as source of learning, 49
Monitoring and evaluation of behavior change
    programs, 98-99
Movement cycle, 80-81, 82
  reduction of exercise to, 169

N

Natural versus exogenous reinforcers, 86
Neurophysiological approach to pain, 9, 14-18
Nocturnal awakening in behavioral analysis, 126
Nocturnal medications, 126-127
Nocturnal time patterns, 125
Nonreinforcement of well behaviors, 69-72; *see also* Reinforcement
Nonverbal and verbal pain behaviors, 12-14

O

Operant(s); *see also* Pain behavior(s)
  definition of, 37
  distorted gait as, 184
  environmental setting and, 38
  illness, and environmental reinforcement of, 44-45
  pain behaviors as, 38
  reinforcers and, 42
  and respondents, distinctions between, 41-42
Operant conditioning; *see also* Behavior change; Contingency management treatment programs; Operant-based treatment approach
  explanation of, to patient and spouse, 151-153
  principles of, 38
  time-limited character of learning and, 42
Operant pain
  acquisition of, 41-73
  analysis of; *see* Behavioral analysis
  discrimination of, 124-127
  key element in search for, 124
  medications and pain cocktail, 154
    as reinforcer of, 54
  modeling as influence in, 49-50
  reduction of, 107-109
Operant-based treatment approach; *see also* Behavior change; Contingency management treatment program
  exercise, rest, and attention in, 154-155
  increasing activity or reducing medication addiction/habituation in respondent pain in, 153-154
  orientation of patient and spouse to, 150-156
  and pain medications, 153-160
  reducing gaps in well behavior and, 155
Orientation of patient and spouse, 150-156
  general issues in, 155-156
  increasing activity or reducing medication addiction/habituation in respondent pain and, 153-154
  to pain as learned behavior, 151-153
  to possible course of chronic pain and treatment, 150-153
  reducing gaps in well behavior and, 155
  to use of exercise, rest, and attention, 154-155
Outpatient(s)
  baselines for, in exercise and increasing activity, 171
  generalization for, 213
  management of, and attention for, 195

P

Pacer regimen, 181-183
Pain
  activators of, 129-131
    roster of, 130
  activity changes as result of, 133-136
  activity-pain time interval, 130-131
  anxiety and, 29-31
    discrimination between, 31
    levels of, and pain intensity, 15
  behaviors of; *see* Pain behavior(s)
  as behavior, 76
  and behavioral concepts, relation between, 1
  behavioral analysis of, 120-140; *see also* Behavioral analysis
  in childhood
    anger in response to, 30
    associations with, 29-30
  chronic
    behavioral analysis of, 45-46
    behavioral concepts and, 1-2
    and chronic illness, 3
    as clinical problem, 11-25
    conceptual background of, 9-100
    conditioning and, 6, 26
    cost factors in, 113-115
    cultural identity as factor in response to, 15
    episodic, 125
    evaluation of, 101-147
    family involvement in, 8; *see also* Family(ies) of chronic pain patients; Spouse(s) of chronic pain patients
    as form of chronic illness, 6
    health care system and, 103-119
    increased emotional distress accompanying, 35-36
    medical diagnoses of, as probability statements, 120-121
    orienting patient and spouse to possible course and treatment of, 150-153
    patients with; *see* Pain patients
    reporting of, 11-14
    responses to
      anxiety and, 15
      cultural factors in, 15
    tension and relaxation in, 132-133
    time patterns in, 125-127
      nocturnal, 125
    treatment of, 147-221
  as clinical problem, 11-25
  communication of environmental effects of, 107-108
  depression and, 29-31
  diagnosis of, emotional factors in, 29-32; *see also* Behavioral analysis
  diminishers of, 131
  disease model perspective on, 33-36
  elicited by environmental events, 31
  episodic, 125

Pain—cont'd
  evaluation of, 101-146
    learning model approach to, 39-40
    experimental and clinical, differentiation be-
      tween, 26-27
    as stimulus-response paradigm, 26
  expression of, as behavior, 1
  -free activity plans, 135
  gate control theory of, 16-18
  as learned behavior, 151-153
  measurement of, 21-23
  medication and; *see* Medication(s)
  modeling in behavioral analysis of, 49-50
  neurophysiological approach to, 9, 14-18
  nocturnal awakening and, 126
  nocturnal medications and, 126-127
  operant
    acquisition of, 41-73
    key element in search for, 124
    medications and pain cocktail for addicted/
      habituated patients and, 154
    reduction of, 107-109
    and pain behavior, differentiation between, 103
  patients with; *see* Pain patients
  patient perception of, 11-14
  pattern theory of, 14, 15-16
  perception of, and distractions, 19
  and progress, measurement of, 204
  psychogenic, 26-40
    assumptions underlying diagnosis of, 32-40
    behavior influence factors
      behavioral model, 38-40
      motivational model, 36-38
    definitions of, 27
    disease model perspective of, 33-36
    learning model and, 39-40
    psychodynamics of pain and, 29-32
    results of psychotherapy in, 41
  -related health care utilization behavior, reduc-
    tion of, 111-117
  -related treatment procedures, programming of,
    180-181
  -relevant exercise, 169
  respondent
    behavioral analysis and, 120-121
    behaviors to be changed in, 142-143
    increasing activity in, 153-154
    medication addiction/habituation in, 153-154
    reduction of, 105-108
  responses to; *see* Responses to pain
  social context of, and response to, 20-21
  social and interpersonal effects of, 1-2
  specificity theory of, 14-15
  tolerance of, 46
  treatment of, 147-221; *see also* Treatment
    goals in, 103-119
  verbal reports of, 14
Pain behavior(s), 64-69, 109, 127-128; *see also*
    Operant(s)
  avoidance learning and, 60-69

Pain behavior(s)—cont'd
  compensation as reinforcer of, 52
  cost factors in, 113-115
  counting of, and attention and social respon-
    siveness, 206-208
  current reinforcement of, 50-60
  decreasing roster of, 78
  in describing pain, 28
  direct reinforcement of, 45, 128
  distorted gait as, 184-185
  environment and, 107-108
  exercise and activity as reinforcer of, 57-60
  family responses to, as current reinforcer, 50-52
  increasing activity level and, 109-111
  legitimation of, 113-114
  medical diagnosis and, 120-121
  medication as reinforcer of, 53-57
  as operants, 38
  and pain, distinction between, 103
  -pain stimulus linkage, 28
  and personality traits, differentiation of, 121
  physician behavior as reinforcer of, 53-57
  reduction of, 105-109
  reduction of functional impairment and, 109-111
  reinforcement of; *see* Reinforcement; Reinforcers
  self-control of displays of, 195-196
  spouse count of, and reinforcement of activity,
    207
  systematic, and environmental consequence se-
    quences, 124
  target, for behavior change; *see* Target be-
    havior(s)
  treatment goals and, 103-119
  verbal and nonverbal, 12-14
  conditioning and discrepancy between, 12-13
  withdrawing attention to, 208-209
Pain cocktail, 154, 159
  common problems or exceptions in use of, 163-
    167
  delivery schedule for, 159-160
  end of regimen for, 162
  maintenance of regimen for, 162
  sample regimen for, 161
Pain patient(s)
  activity modifications and, 134-135
  addicted or habituated, medications for, 154
  avoidance behaviors of, 60-69
  behavioral view of, 2-3
  behaviors of; *see* Pain behavior(s); Well be-
    havior(s)
  behaviors to be changed in, 143
  childhood pain experiences of, 30-31, 48
  repression and, 72-73
  diaries of, in behavioral analysis, 123, 137
  discrimination between anxiety and pain by,
    31-32
  effects of chronicity and, 3-4
  -environmental interplay, 124-128
  environmental responses and, 128-129
  expectations of evaluation of, 122

Pain patient(s)—cont'd
  families of; *see* Family(ies) of chronic pain
      patients
  functional status of, assessment of, 109-111
  histories of
      and direct and positive reinforcement of pain
          behaviors, 46-50
      nonreinforcement of well behaviors in, 69-71
      pain behavior as avoidance behavior in, 64-65
  interview guide for, in behavioral analysis, 125-
      137
  as losers, 122
  Minnesota Multiphasic Personality Inventory
      scores of, 35
  modification of spouse behavior by, 196-197
  orientation of, to operant-based treatment ap-
      proach, 150-156
  -physician relationship as reinforcer, 190
  preoccupation of, with pain, 19-20
  reliance of disease model perspective as risk to,
      111-112
  selection of
      for contingency management treatment pro-
          gram, 141-145
      schematic criteria for, 121
  spouses of; *see* Spouse(s) of chronic pain pa-
      tients
  vocational counseling for, 117-118
Passes for inpatients, generalization and, 219-220
Pattern theory of pain, 14, 15-16
Performance graphs and records
  data kit for, 198
  patient diaries in, 198
  procedures and, 198-202
  reinforcement and feedback from, 197-204
Personality traits differentiated from pain be-
      haviors, 121
Physician(s)
  behavior of, as reinforcer of pain behavior, 53-
      60, 112-113
  -patient relationship as reinforcement, 190
  self-interest of, and pain behaviors, 116
Placebos as analgesics, 22
Premack Principle, 85-86
Programming of environment to maintain perfor-
      mance, 97
Programming pain-related treatment procedures,
      180-181
Promotion and maintenance of effective well be-
      haviors, 117-119
Psychodynamics of pain, 29-32
Psychogenic pain, 26-40
  behavior influence factors
      behavior model, 38-40
      motivational model, 36-38
  definitions of, 27
  diagnosis of, assumptions underlying, 32-40
  disease model perspective and, 33-36
  learning model and, 39-40
  psychodynamics of pain and, 29-32
  results of psychotherapy and, 41

Psychological tests in behavioral analysis, 137-140
Punishing of well behaviors, 128-129

Q

Quantification of exercise in contingency manage-
      ment treatment programs, 169
Quota(s)
  adjustment of
      to meet quota failures, 177
      for other illness events, 179-180
  ceilings of, and movement toward other forms
      of activity, 179
  for exercise
      initial treatment and, 171-172
      and performance recording of, 199
  management of failures to meet, 174-179
  in self-control of pain behavior displays, 196
  in shaping rapid walking, 188-189
  variation in, for asymmetrical involvement, 201

R

Recreation and generalization, 217
Reduction of functional imapirment, 109-111
Reduction of pain signals or pain behavior, 105-
      109; *see also* Behavior change; Contigency
      management treatment program
Reinforcement
  for activity and exercise, 173-174
  of activity, and pain behaviors, spouse count of,
      207
  of attention, feedback from performance graphs
      and records in, 197-204
  avoidance learning and, 60-69
  current, 50-60
  delayed (token or point systems), 94-95
  evaluation of, 98-99
  fading and, 93-94
  and feedback from performance graphs and rec-
      ords, 197-204
  function of graphs and, 203-204
  iatrogenic, medication as, 53-57
  interim, 190
  in maintaining operants, 42
  of pain behavior
      childhood experiences and, 46-50
      compensation as, 52-53
      current, 50-60
      direct, 128
          and positive, 45, 46-60
      exercise and activity as, 57-60
      family responses as, 50-53
      iatrogenic, 53-60
      indirect but positive, 45, 46-60, 61-69
  in patient modification of spouse behavior,
      schedule for, 196
  physician-patient relationship as, 190
  schedules of, in behavior change, 89-94
  in self-control of pain behavior displays, 196
  spouse's, of activity and well behaviors, 209-
      210
  of well behavior, failure of, 45

Reinforcer(s), 82-95; *see also* Reinforcement
  attention as, 87-89
  characteristics of, summarized, 85
  identification of, 143
  and maintenance of well behaviors, 118
  natural versus exogenous, 86
  naturally occurring, gaining access to, 97-98
  parents', in childhood, 47
  in patient modification of spouse behavior, 196
  positive, determination of, 82-83
  requirements for, 83-85
  rest or time out as, 86-87
  selection of, 85-86
  in self-control of pain behavior displays, 196
  social responsiveness as, 190
Respondent(s)
  definition of, 37
  and operant, difference between, 41-42
Respondent pain
  behavioral analysis and, 120-121
  behaviors to be changed in, 142-143
  increasing activity in, 153-154
  medication addiction/habituation and, 153-154
  reduction of, 105-108
Response(s) to pain
  anger as, in childhood, 30
  anxiety and, 15, 29-31
  conditioning and, 18-19
  cultural factors in, 15, 23-24
  depression and, 23, 29-31
  discrepant verbal and nonverbal, 12-14
  distractions and, 19
  emotional factors in, 29-32
  expectations and, 20
  social context and, 20-21
  time dimension in, 26-27
Rest
  as pain diminisher, 131
  or time out, as reinforcer, 86-87
Retardation, mental, behavioral concepts applied
    to, 45
Robitussin; *see* Glyceryl guaiacolate

S

Schedules of reinforcement, 89-94; *see also* Rein-
    forcement
  diminishing ratio, 91-93
  fixed interval, 90
  variable interval, 90
Self-control
  in generalization, 96-97
  of pain behavior displays, 195-196
Shaping process, 43-44
  distorted gait as problem of, 184-189
  of rapid walking, procedure for, 188-189
Signal detection theory of pain measurement, 21
  in determining criterion for pain, 24

Sinequan; *see* Doxepin
Social and interpersonal problems of pain patients,
    1-2
Social responsiveness
  attention and, 154-155, 190-210
  procedures for contingent attention and, 192-
    195
  as reinforcer, 190
Specificity theory of pain, 14-15
Spouse(s) of chronic pain patients
  activity modifications of, 135-136
  and attention and social responsiveness, training
    in, 204-210
  behavior of, patient modification of, 196-197
  count of pain behavior and reinforcement of ac-
    tivity by, 207
  direct reinforcement of pain behavior by, 28
  discouraging activity (punishing of well behav-
    ior) by, 128-129
  involvement of, in behavioral analysis, 123-124
  misguided, 144-145
  orientation of, to operant-based treatment ap-
    proach, 150-156
  reinforced, 145
  reinforcement of activity and well behavior by,
    209-210
  responses of, in attention and social responsive-
    ness, 208
Stimulus discrimination between pain and anxi-
    ety, 31-32
Stimulus fading, 44
Supplemental "behavioral" data, 137-140

T

Target behavior(s)
  in behavior change, 105
  identification of, 143-144
  in patient modification of spouse behavior, 196
  in reducing excessive activity, 182
  of spouse and family in attention and social
    responsiveness, 205-206
Techniques of behavioral analysis and behavior
    change, 74-100
Tension and relaxation in behavior change, 132-
    133
Time patterns in pain
  in behavioral analysis, 125-127
  diurnal, 127
  nocturnal, 125
Time-contingent regimen for medications, 159
Token or point systems as delayed reinforcement,
    94-95
Tolerance for exercise, 170
Treatment
  attention and social responsiveness in, 190-210
  of chronic pain, 147-221
    managing pain medications in, 157-167
  of distorted gait, 184-189
  end of, 220-221

Treatment—cont'd
exercise and increase in activity level in, 168-183
generalization and maintenance of performance and, 211-221
goals of, 103-119

V

Variable interval schedules of reinforcement, 90
Verbal and nonverbal pain behaviors, 12-14
Vocational assessment and counseling, 117-118

W

Walking, rapid, procedure for shaping, 188-189
Well behavior(s)
definition of, 117

Well behavior—cont'd
effective, promotion and maintenance of, 117-119
failure of, to receive positive reinforcement, 45
gaps in, 143-144
reduction of, 155
increasing range of, 78
nonreinforcement of, 69-72
positive reinforcement of, 42
punishing of, 128-129
reinforcers and maintenance of, 118
spouse reinforcement of activity and, 209-210
Wheelchair fading and ambulation increase, 187

X

Xylocaine; *see* Lidocaine